BICENTENNIAL
1807
WILEY
2007
BICENTENNIAL

THE WILEY BICENTENNIAL—KNOWLEDGE FOR GENERATIONS

Each generation has its unique needs and aspirations. When Charles Wiley first opened his small printing shop in lower Manhattan in 1807, it was a generation of boundless potential searching for an identity. And we were there, helping to define a new American literary tradition. Over half a century later, in the midst of the Second Industrial Revolution, it was a generation focused on building the future. Once again, we were there, supplying the critical scientific, technical, and engineering knowledge that helped frame the world. Throughout the 20th Century, and into the new millennium, nations began to reach out beyond their own borders and a new international community was born. Wiley was there, expanding its operations around the world to enable a global exchange of ideas, opinions, and know-how.

For 200 years, Wiley has been an integral part of each generation's journey, enabling the flow of information and understanding necessary to meet their needs and fulfill their aspirations. Today, bold new technologies are changing the way we live and learn. Wiley will be there, providing you the must-have knowledge you need to imagine new worlds, new possibilities, and new opportunities.

Generations come and go, but you can always count on Wiley to provide you the knowledge you need, when and where you need it!

WILLIAM J. PESCE
PRESIDENT AND CHIEF EXECUTIVE OFFICER

PETER BOOTH WILEY
CHAIRMAN OF THE BOARD

Health Care Economics

Thomas E. Getzen
Temple University

with Bruce Allen

BICENTENNIAL
1807
WILEY
2007
BICENTENNIAL

Credits

PUBLISHER
Anne Smith

CONTRIBUTING EDITOR
Bruce H. Allen, Ph.D., Professor of Marketing, College of Business Administration, Central Michigan University

CONTRIBUTING WRITER
Jennifer Moore

PROJECT EDITOR
Sarah Wagner

MARKETING MANAGER
Jennifer Slomack

EDITORIAL ASSISTANT
Tiara Kelly

PRODUCTION MANAGER
Kelly Tavares

PRODUCTION ASSISTANT
Courtney Leshko

CREATIVE DIRECTOR
Harry Nolan

COVER DESIGNER
Hope Miller

COVER PHOTO
© VEER. Steve Drake/Photonica/Getty Image, Inc.

This book was set in Times New Roman, printed and bound by R. R. Donnelley.

The cover was printed by R. R. Donnelley Color.

To order books or for customer service, please call 1-800-CALL WILEY (225-5945).

ISBN-13 9780-471-79076-1

ISBN-10 0-471-79076-1

Printed in the United States of America

10 9 8 7 6 5 4 3 2 1

PREFACE

College classrooms bring together learners from many backgrounds, with a variety of aspirations. Although the students are in the same course, they are not necessarily on the same path. This diversity, coupled with the reality that these learners often have jobs, families, and other commitments, requires a flexibility that our nation's higher education system is addressing. Distance learning, shorter course terms, new disciplines, evening courses, and certification programs are some of the approaches that colleges employ to reach as many students as possible and help them clarify and achieve their goals.

Wiley Pathways books, a new line of texts from John Wiley & Sons, Inc., are designed to help you address this diversity and the need for flexibility. These books focus on the fundamentals, identify core competencies and skills, and promote independent learning. Their focus on the fundamentals helps students grasp the subject, bringing them all to the same basic understanding. These books use clear, everyday language and are presented in an uncluttered format, making the reading experience more pleasurable. The core competencies and skills help students succeed in the classroom and beyond, whether in another course or in a professional setting. A variety of built-in learning resources promote independent learning and help instructors and students gauge students' understanding of the content. These resources enable students to think critically about their new knowledge and apply their skills in any situation.

Our goal with *Wiley Pathways* books—with their brief, inviting format, clear language, and core competencies and skills focus—is to celebrate the many students in your courses, respect their needs, and help you guide them on their way.

CASE Learning System

To meet the needs of working college students, *Wiley Pathways Health Care Economics* uses a four-part process called the CASE Learning System:

- ▲ C: Content
- ▲ A: Analysis
- ▲ S: Synthesis
- ▲ E: Evaluation

Based on Bloom's taxonomy of learning, CASE presents key topics in health care economics in easy-to-follow chapters. The text then prompts analysis, synthesis, and evaluation with a variety of learning aids and assessment tools. Students move efficiently from reviewing what they have learned, to acquiring new information and skills, to applying their new knowledge and skills to real-life scenarios.

Using the CASE Learning System, students not only achieve academic mastery of health care economics *topics*, but they master real-world *skills* related to that content. The CASE Learning System also helps students become independent learners, giving them a distinct advantage in the field, whether they are just starting out or seeking to advance in their careers.

Organization, Depth, and Breadth of the Text

▲ **Modular Format.** Research on college students shows that they access information from textbooks in a non-linear way. Instructors also often wish to reorder textbook content to suit the needs of a particular class. Therefore, although *Wiley Pathways Health Care Economics* proceeds logically from the basics to increasingly more challenging material, chapters are further organized into sections that are self-contained for maximum teaching and learning flexibility.

▲ **Numeric System of Headings.** *Wiley Pathways Health Care Economics* uses a numeric system for headings (e.g., 2.3.4 identifies the fourth subsection of Section 3 of Chapter 2). With this system, students and teachers can quickly and easily pinpoint topics in the table of contents and the text, keeping class time and study sessions focused.

▲ **Core Content.** The topics in *Wiley Pathways Health Care Economics* are organized into 14 chapters.

Chapter 1, The Flow of Funds Through the Health Care System, provides an overview of health care economics in society, an explanation of how funds move through the health care system, and a basic understanding of these channels. Important economic principles necessary for the proper study of health care economics are presented, along with six factors that influence the flow of funds. An overview of the major issues in health care financing rounds out the chapter.

Chapter 2, Economic Evaluation of Health Services, discusses the supply and demand of health care. Students learn how to read a demand curve and use marginal revenue to make business decisions.

The supply side of health care, role of price sensitivity in health care economics, and impact of government and insurance regulations on medical pricing are also presented.

Chapter 3, Cost–Benefit and Cost-Effectiveness Analysis, discusses how to make the most of limited funds. Students learn about cost–benefit analysis (CBA) as a means of determining the best use of limited funds and discover the importance of perspective when conducting a CBA. The three major types of medical benefits and the four types of medical costs and how they are valued are also presented, along with information on how economists measure the value people place on life. Students also learn about formulating health policy decisions using CBA, assessing the opportunity costs of policy decisions, and calculating the expected value of uncertain benefits. The chapter concludes with pointers on how to evaluate the potential benefits and costs of policy decisions.

Chapter 4, Health Insurance, reviews the benefits of risk pooling. Answers are provided to important questions, such as: Who takes care of people when they need medical care they can't afford? How does risk pooling make insurance possible? Are people who think they'll become sick more or less likely to obtain insurance? Who pays for losses: insurance companies or the people who buy insurance? Readers learn about the practice of fund pooling to reduce exposure to risks, evaluate the process of adverse selection, argue whether insurance increases or decreases the demand for medical care, and assess whether insurance companies take risks or just put a price on them.

Chapter 5, Insurance Contracts, describes the flow of funds in the insurance industry both within and outside the United States. Information on how patients, providers, and insurance companies benefit from insurance; the difference between traditional indemnity insurance and managed care plans; the types of private and government-funded insurance; and how insurance plans structure incentives are included. The pros and cons of managed care plans are also examined, as are the problems associated with uninsured citizens.

Chapter 6, Physicians, presents the economics of practicing medicine. Students learn how physicians are paid, the cost of running a practice, how doctors act as patients' agents, and the role of licensure in the supply and demand for medical care. The physician payment system is described, and the role that a physician's specialty plays in determining his or her pay is explained. Readers also learn how to calculate the cost of running a physician practice, assess the role of agency and insurance in transferring responsibility from patients, and critique the practice of medical licensure.

Chapter 7, Physician Organization and Business Practice, describes the physician marketplace. Core concepts are discussed, such as the value of a medical education and the role of licensing boards and the federal government in limiting physician supply. The economic benefits of group practices, the role of kickbacks in the flow of funds, and the factors that result in price discrimination are also presented. Students learn how physician supply affects the cost and quality of medical care, analyze physician practice organization and the role of economies of scale, and determine whether more regulations are needed to reduce physician kickbacks.

Chapter 8, Hospitals, focuses on sources and uses of hospital income, major hospital expenses, and hospital financing. Who controls hospitals and the practice of cost shifting are also presented. Students learn about the impact of Medicare and managed care on hospital decision making, why labor makes up the majority of hospital costs, and the effect of an "I'll pay for mine, and you pay for yours" attitude in health care reimbursement. Completing the chapter is a discussion of the role of physicians in hospital management.

Chapter 9, Hospital Costs, describes the factors that contribute to the wide variations in hospital costs, including the size of a hospital, how it manages its budget, and the extent to which it uses economies of scale to run more efficiently. The importance of considering quality and price when assessing hospital care is also included, as is information on how hospitals compete for patients. An overview of government regulation of hospital costs concludes the chapter.

Chapter 10, Managed Care, presents the basics of the HMO revolution, including the reasons for the development of managed care, an explanation of how HMOs reduce costs, the difference between HMOs and less restrictive managed care organizations, and an outline of who wins and who loses in managed care, from the perspectives of patients, hospitals, and physicians. The pros and cons of managed care for various types of patients and the sources and uses of HMO funds are also presented, along with an assessment of the future of HMOs.

Chapter 11, Long Term Care, describes the history and types of nursing homes and other elderly care and how they differ from most other health care. The impact of certificate-of-need legislation on the long term care (LTC) market and Medicaid's role in the LTC boom are also discussed. The chapter presents the controversial topic of whether the government should pay for LTC for middle-class and wealthy Americans and encourages readers to consider the advantages and disadvantages of LTC insurance. Attempts to regulate LTC costs are also discussed, as are estimates of the future costs of LTC.

Chapter 12, Pharmaceuticals, describes the prescription drug marketplace, including the flow of funds through the pharmaceutical industry, the research and development of new drugs, and the major markets for prescription drugs. The role of marketing to physicians and patients, how regulation has changed the industry, and an assessment of why the pharmaceutical industry is so profitable and whether high drug prices are justified are also provided. Predictions regarding the future of the industry, based on current research and development payoffs, conclude the chapter.

Chapter 13, International Comparisons of Health and Health Expenditures, reviews global disparities in health care spending and health throughout the world. Health care spending—and how it is increasing in low-, middle-, and high-income countries—is discussed. Also examined is the relationship between spending, gross domestic product, and a nation's health. International trade in health care, knowledge, and health professionals, along with the concept of health care as a national luxury good, round out the discussion.

Chapter 14, Dynamics of Health Spending, summarizes the present and future of health care economics. It presents the history of cost-control regulations, explains the dynamics of health system changes, describes how economic analysis is used in decision making, and clarifies the difference between individual and national perspectives on health care spending. The role of labor in health care spending, issues involving the allocation of health care resources, and the future of health care are also discussed.

Pre-reading Learning Aids

Each chapter of *Wiley Pathways Health Care Economics* features a number of learning and study aids, described in the following sections, to activate students' prior knowledge of the topics and orient them to the material.

▲ **Pre-test.** This pre-reading assessment tool in multiple-choice format not only introduces chapter material, but it also helps students anticipate the chapter's learning outcomes. By focusing students' attention on what they do not know, the self-test provides students with a benchmark against which they can measure their own progress. The pre-test is available online at www.wiley.com/college/getzen.

▲ **What You'll Learn in This Chapter.** This bulleted list focuses on *subject matter* that will be taught. It tells students what they will be learning in this chapter and why it is significant for their careers. It will also help students understand why the chapter is important and how it relates to other chapters in the text.

▲ **After Studying This Chapter, You'll Be Able To.** This list emphasizes *capabilities and skills* students will learn as a result of reading the chapter. It prepares students to synthesize and evaluate the chapter material and relate it to the real world.

Within-Text Learning Aids

The following learning aids are designed to encourage analysis and synthesis of the material, support the learning process, and ensure success during the evaluation phase:

▲ **Introduction.** This section orients the student by introducing the chapter and explaining its practical value and relevance to the book as a whole. Short summaries of chapter sections preview the topics to follow.

▲ **"For Example" Boxes.** Found within each section, these boxes tie section content to real-world organizations, scenarios, and applications.

▲ **Figures and Tables.** Line art and photos have been carefully chosen to be truly instructional rather than filler. Tables distill and present information in a way that is easy to identify, access, and understand, enhancing the focus of the text on essential ideas.

▲ **Self-Check.** Related to the "What You'll Learn" bullets and found at the end of each section, this battery of short-answer questions emphasizes student understanding of concepts and mastery of section content. Though the questions may be either discussed in class or studied by students outside of class, students should not go on before they can answer all questions correctly.

▲ **Key Terms and Glossary.** To help students develop a professional vocabulary, key terms are bolded when they first appear in the chapter. A complete list of key terms with brief definitions appears at the end of each chapter and again in a glossary at the end of the book. Knowledge of key terms is assessed by all assessment tools (see below).

▲ **Summary.** Each chapter concludes with a summary paragraph that reviews the major concepts in the chapter and links back to the "What You'll Learn" list.

Evaluation and Assessment Tools

The evaluation phase of the CASE Learning System consists of a variety of within-chapter and end-of-chapter assessment tools that test how well students have learned the material. These tools also encourage students to extend their learning into different scenarios and higher levels of understanding and thinking. The following assessment tools appear in every chapter of *Wiley Pathways Health Care Economics*:

▲ **Summary Questions.** These exercises help students summarize the chapter's main points by asking a series of multiple-choice and true/false questions that emphasize student understanding of concepts and mastery of chapter content. Students should be able to answer all of the Summary Questions correctly before moving on.

▲ **Review Questions.** Presented in short-answer format, these questions review the major points in each chapter, prompting analysis while reinforcing and confirming student understanding of concepts and encouraging mastery of chapter content. They are somewhat more difficult than the Self-Check and Summary Questions, and students should be able to answer most of them correctly before moving on.

▲ **Applying This Chapter Questions.** These questions drive home key ideas by asking students to synthesize and apply chapter concepts to new, real-life situations and scenarios.

▲ **You Try It Questions.** Found at the end of each chapter, You Try It Questions are designed to extend students' thinking and are thus ideal for discussion or writing assignments. Using an open-ended format and sometimes based on Web sources, they encourage students to draw conclusions using chapter material applied to real-world situations, which fosters both mastery and independent learning.

▲ **Post-test.** The Post-test should be taken after students have completed the chapter. It includes all of the questions in the pre-test so that students can see how their learning has progressed and improved.

Instructor and Student Package

Wiley Pathways Health Care Economics is available with the following teaching and learning supplements. All supplements are available online at the text's Book Companion Website, located at www.wiley.com/college/getzen.

▲ **Instructor's Resource Guide.** The Instructor's Resource Guide provides the following aids and supplements for teaching an introduction to health care economics course:

- *Sample syllabus:* This syllabus serves as a convenient template that instructors may use for creating their own course syllabi.
- *Teaching suggestions:* For each chapter, these include a chapter summary, learning objectives, definitions of key terms, lecture notes, answers to select text question sets, and at least three suggestions for classroom activities, such as ideas for speakers to invite, videos to show, and other projects.

▲ **PowerPoints.** Key information is summarized in ten to fifteen PowerPoints per chapter. Instructors may use these in class or choose to share them with students for class presentations or to provide additional study support.

▲ **Test Bank.** The test bank features one test per chapter, as well as a mid-term and two finals—one cumulative and one non-cumulative. Each includes true/false, multiple-choice, and open-ended questions. Answers and page references are provided for the true/false and multiple-choice questions, and page references are given for the open-ended questions. Tests are available in Microsoft Word and computerized formats.

ACKNOWLEDGMENTS

Taken together, the content, pedagogy, and assessment elements of *Health Care Economics* offer the career-oriented student exposure to the most important aspects of the field of health care economics, as well as ways to develop the skills and capabilities that current and future employers seek in the individuals they hire and promote. Instructors will appreciate the book's practical focus, conciseness, and real-world emphasis.

Special thanks are extended to contributing editor Dr. Bruce H. Allen, Ph.D., for his assistance in preparing this manuscript. Dr. Allen is a professor of marketing in the College of Business Administration at Central Michigan University. We would also like to thank Jennifer Moore for her invaluable editorial efforts.

We would also like to thank the following reviewers for their feedback and suggestions during the text's development. Their advice on how to shape *Wiley Pathways Health Care Economics* into a solid learning tool that meets both their needs and those of their busy students is deeply appreciated:

- ▲ Gregory O. Ginn, Ph.D., associate professor of health care administration and policy, University of Nevada, Las Vegas
- ▲ Michael A. S. Guth, Ph.D., JD, adjunct professor of financial economics and law, Charter Oak State College and Taft University Law School
- ▲ Craig W. Levin, MBA, accounting manager and instructor, National American University

Finally, we would like to thank Dr. Michael W. Posey, Ph.D., professor and chair of the Health Care Management MBA program at Franklin University, for his invaluable additions to this text.

BRIEF CONTENTS

CONTENTS

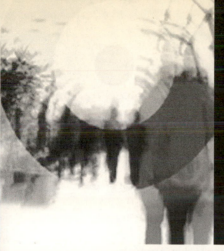

1

THE FLOW OF FUNDS THROUGH THE HEALTH CARE SYSTEM

Applying Economic Principles to Health Care

Starting Point

Go to www.wiley.com/college/getzen to assess your knowledge of the flow of funds through the health care system.
Determine where you need to concentrate your effort.

What You'll Learn in This Chapter

▲ The role of health care economics in society
▲ The value of following money through the health care system
▲ What factors influence the flow of funds
▲ Important economic principles that are necessary for the study of health care economics
▲ Important health principles that influence people's health care decisions

After Studying This Chapter, You'll Be Able To

▲ Assess the economic issues that are exclusive to the health care industry
▲ Prepare a list of factors that influence the flow of funds through the health care system
▲ Analyze major issues in health care financing
▲ Analyze medical decisions, using basic economic principles
▲ Evaluate the field of health care, using basic health principles

INTRODUCTION

Who gets a heart transplant? Why does surgery cost so much? Will insurance pay for AIDS treatment? How many children get immunized? Is Senator Smith's health plan worth voting for? People grapple with these sorts of questions every day in hospitals, in doctors' offices, in the halls of Congress, and in their own homes. These questions are the subject of health economics, along with the more ordinary decisions that together have an even greater impact on an individual's personal health: how much exercise to get, the value of reducing cholesterol in the diet, whether to study until 3 a.m. or get a good night's sleep, and so on.

In this book we discuss hospitals, nurses, ambulances, drugs, sex, extortion, kickbacks, government, family ties, love, international trade, sports injuries, and the next generation—the makings of several box office hits. We look at all these topics from the perspective of an economist, seeing them in terms of economic concepts, such as opportunity cost, budget constraints, monopoly, and marginal productivity. Some people claim that this takes all the fun out of drugs, sex, and business intrigue. Not so. Economic principles provide the motivations that shape this story, giving it character development and structure rather than just one scene after another, as in some forgettable action movie.

At its most basic level, health care is a handful of economic transactions, in which patients purchase insurance, physicians and hospitals provide services, pharmacies provide medications, and insurance companies pay for those goods and services. So to understand health economics, you must follow the money. In this book, we look carefully at how people engage in financial transactions with physicians, with hospitals, and with each other to improve their health. Following the trail of money, or what economics call the *flow of funds*, through the health care system makes it possible to apply economic principles to situations involving life and death, not-for-profit organizations, professional licensure, addiction, and other issues. We will look at how medical transactions are like and yet unlike most of the rest of the economy.

When someone says *economics* or *economic behavior,* the sorts of things that probably come to mind—interest rates, unemployment, stock markets—seem far removed from the hospital emergency room. If I asked about your most recent contribution to the health sector of the economy, you might not even think of the little line on your paycheck stub labeled "HI" or "FICA:M" or "Medicare." Yes, that's 1.45 percent of your gross income that's taken out for Medicare. No, it's not your health insurance because you don't become eligible for Medicare until you reach age 65 or become permanently disabled. Health care doesn't always easily fit the standard models economists use to analyze buying and selling wheat, or renting property, or the price of gold. However, money drives the health care system just as it does many other activities in society.

The flow-of-funds approach to health care economics allows us to follow the trail of money through the health care system to study the financial transactions that take place between patients, doctors, hospitals, and third parties, such as private insurers and the government. Who pays for what has changed dramatically in the past 60 years. Whereas in the past, the majority of individuals paid their medical bills with private funds, today insurance companies and other third parties cover the majority of payments, with individuals paying only a small fraction of the total flow of funds with private money. Just as the source of funds has changed, so has the use of those funds. Increasing intensity in the quality of medical services has resulted in increases in medical spending that surpass increases in inflation, wages, and even the use of health care services.

Several factors affect the size and direction of the flow of funds, including the value we place on our health, the quality of medical care we seek, and medical innovations. When any of these factors take on greater or lesser importance, they affect how much money flows through the system and to whom it flows.

Economists readily acknowledge that health involves more than money, but a few health principles fall within the economic realm. For instance, it's true that health is priceless, but how much money we have often plays a large role in determining our health. The final section of this chapter touches on these and other health principles related to the field of economics.

1.1 What Is Economics?

The essence of economics is trade, or "making a buck." Economists focus on the **market,** which is the point at which buyers and sellers exchange dollars for goods and services. Without buyers and sellers, there would be no economy— no wealthy surgeons, no insurance companies, no hospital billing departments. The following sections offer a brief overview of important economic principles and concepts.

1.1.1 The Fundamental Theorem of Exchange

For a surgeon to be a seller, the patient must be a buyer. They must agree on a price so that an exchange can occur. The surgeon would probably prefer that the price be higher, and the patient would probably prefer that it be lower, but both must be satisfied in order for a trade to take place. Economists observe that because a transaction takes place, there must have been mutual agreement that made both the buyer and the seller better off. If the surgeon would rather have watched television than perform another operation, she would have turned down the case. If the patient would rather have saved the money or gone to a different surgeon, he could have done so. The insight that both parties must be benefiting if they freely agreed to make a trade is central to an economic vision of the world and is known as the **fundamental theorem of exchange.**

1.1.2 Trade

The **terms of trade** specify what the buyer is to give to the seller and what the seller is to give to the buyer in return. When you buy a common item in a store, such as aspirin, a price of $2.29 per bottle of 50 may tell you everything you need to know about the transaction. For services, and for medical care in particular, the transaction is apt to be much more complex. For example, consider the transaction for an operation to implant an artificial intraocular lens (IOL) in a patient's eye to replace a natural lens that has become clouded by cataracts. The patient is to pay a $200 deposit up front and $800 more within 30 days after the surgery is completed and all sutures are removed. Reduced to its simplest level, the terms of trade in this exchange can be expressed as a monetary price of $1,000 for the IOL implant. Yet much more than the $1,000 is being agreed to in this transaction. The physician agrees to provide not just any artificial lens but to choose the correct one, continuously monitor the quality of the operation, and control adverse reactions to postoperative medications. The patient agrees to make payment in two parts, with a time limit, and may assume that the operation will be redone without further charges if the first attempt isn't satisfactory. Many of the agreed-upon conditions (that the physician is licensed, will use only qualified assistants, will not try to boost the bill needlessly to increase her fees, and will keep the patient informed of any possible adverse consequences, and that the patient will wear bandages as long as necessary and not go skydiving) will never be specified explicitly unless some disagreement and subsequent legal action force the doctor and patient into court.

The simplest form of trade is a **two-party transaction,** as shown in Figure 1-1, in which consumers buy from businesses, exchanging money for goods and services:

▲ Consumers make up the **demand side** of this simple market.
▲ Sellers (often referred to as *firms*) make up the **supply side.**

When you purchase a bottle of aspirin from Walgreens, you are engaging in a two-party transaction. Similarly, when Walgreens purchases the aspirin from a wholesaler or directly from the aspirin manufacturer, it is involved in a two-party transaction.

Figure 1-1

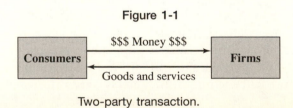

Two-party transaction.

Figure 1-2

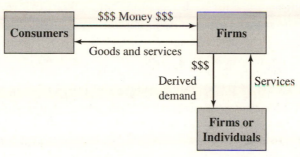

Derived demand between firms.

To get the labor, land, and other supplies needed for production, the firm (the seller) in Figure 1-1 must also be a buyer, as shown in Figure 1-2. These secondary two-party transactions are examples of **derived demand,** purchases made as a step in the production process rather than for final consumption. Continuing with our aspirin example, the aspirin manufacturer must buy the ingredients to make the aspirin, as well as the bottles to hold the tablets and labels to identify them. It must also hire employees to run the equipment that produces the aspirin. These exchanges are all examples of derived demand.

Firms are owned by individuals (or other firms) who provide the capital (money), labor, and organizational effort necessary to get them started and keep them running. Thus, every dollar that a consumer gives to a firm, whether used for wages, profits, or purchase of goods and services from another firm, ultimately ends up in the hands of someone who wants to spend it. When workers or owners spend money, they become consumers and therefore complete the **circular flow of funds** through the economy, as shown in Figure 1-3.

Figure 1-3

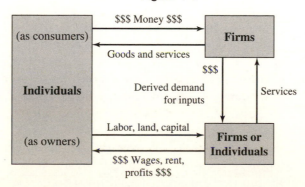

Circular flow of funds.

In a very basic model of marketplace behavior, price is the only thing that matters in a transaction, and both the buyer and seller are "price takers." That is, there are so many buyers that whether one person buys or not has little influence on the price in the market; therefore, buyers must "take" the price as given. Similarly, there are so many firms selling the same product that no single firm can affect prices; hence, all firms must take the price as given.

This uncomplicated model of the marketplace comes close to capturing what happens when you buy a bottle of aspirin. The model works reasonably well for most of the purchases made by consumers, so it can be used to understand the economy as a whole. Yet most medical decisions are far more complicated than buying a bottle of aspirin, and this simple model fails to capture many of the essentials when life-and-death decisions are being made. Organizations adapt creatively to the special demands of health care. Studying such adaptations reveals the potential of economics as a discipline in a way that the analysis of more standard markets cannot.

1.1.3 Contracts

A **contract** is an agreement to trade. In most daily transactions, the contract is often so simple that it's never written down and can be stated in only a few words (e.g., "Will you take $5 for that lamp?"). Buying a new car is more complicated. There's almost always a sales agreement, the terms of which must be agreed to by a manager, and the real seller isn't the salesperson but a corporation. Taxes must be paid. The buyer has a warranty against defects and malfunction, and in some states has a legal right to return the car without penalty within the next three days. Buying a house entails an even more intricate set of contracts, with obligations involving many firms and the government.

The shape and responsiveness of an economy—its information structure— is determined by the contracts that link parties. It is made up of all the contractual entities: people, partnerships, corporations, government agencies, courts, constitutional conventions, legislatures, and so on.

Medical care is part of, and contractually connected to, the larger economy as a whole.[1] Medicine is more special than most other types of economic activity, however, because of extreme information requirements and risks entailed in treating disease. No one needs a prescription to rent a DVD. You don't have to have insurance or sign a consent form to have your car's fuel pump worked on, and almost anyone can cut your hair without a license. The degree of trust in a surgeon, and the reliance on professionals to enforce standards and maintain quality within the operating room, is quite special. To meet such special needs, society has introduced a wide variety of contractual structures, including professional licensure, hospital staff bylaws, and regulatory review.

FOR EXAMPLE

Where Economists Get Their Data

To analyze U.S. health care, economists must have access to information on health care spending. One reliable source of information is the National Health Expenditure Accounts series, which is the most comprehensive source of health care expenditure data in the United States. Published by the U.S. Department of Health and Human Services, it aims to "identify all goods and services that can be characterized as relating to health care in the nation and [to] determine the amount of money used for the purchase of these goods and services." The series is available online at www.cms.gov/statistics/nhe.

SELF-CHECK

- Explain the role that **contracts** play in the **market**.
- Give an example of **derived demand** and the **circular flow of funds**.
- Describe a **two-party transaction** and identify the **supply side** and the **demand side** of the transaction.
- State the **fundamental theorem of exchange**.
- Explain how health care economics differs from most other marketplace behavior.

1.2 The Flow of Health Care Funds

To follow the flow of funds through the health care system, we must not only understand *how* transactions take place between buyers and sellers but also *how much* money flows through the system, the sources of those funds, and how those funds are used (see Figure 1-4).

1.2.1 Health Care Spending in the United States

Medical care in the United States is a trillion-dollar business, with an estimated average of $7,556 spent per person in 2007.[2] The 307 million citizens of the United States received services from more than 4,000 hospitals, 30,000 nursing homes, 750,000 physicians, 2.2 million registered nurses, and 8 million other health care workers. The major sources and uses of health care funding in 2007 are indicated in Table 1-1. Individuals paid $262 billion, or 11 percent of total funding; private (mostly employer-based) health insurance paid 35 percent; and the government, the largest payer, paid 47 percent (19 percent Medicare, 15 percent Medicaid,

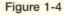

Figure 1-4

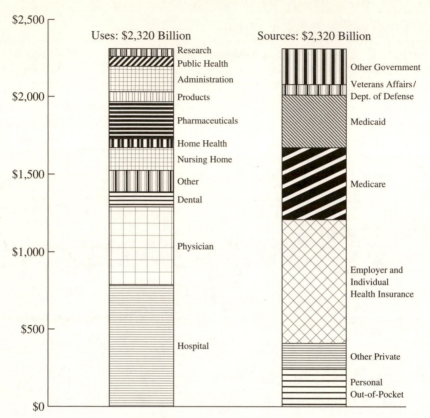

Sources and uses of health care funds, 2007.

13 percent other government programs). The remaining 7 percent of total health care funding came from a variety of other private sources (i.e., philanthropy, industrial clinics, interest and rental income of providers). The largest use of funds was the $709 billion spent on hospital care, which accounted for 31 percent of the total.

Every dollar spent by a patient, an insurance company, or a government is recorded as a cost but is also recorded as income to a physician, a hospital, an agency, an administrator, or another health employee. The flow of money is circular. Money itself is only a way of keeping track of all the obligations within the economy. Every dollar spent by one person is, of necessity, a dollar of income for someone else. Tracing the flow of funds through this complex system provides some sense of the forces that shape the economy.

1.2.2 Sources of Funds

Health care spending has grown enormously. In 2007, it was 16.8 percent of the U.S. gross domestic product (GDP). That growth is due in part to the shift from

Table 1-1: U.S. Health Care Spending, 2007

$2,320 billion total; average of $7,556 per person

Uses of Funds	Percentage of Total	Amount per Person	Sources of Funds	Percentage of Total	Amount per Person
Hospital	34%	$2,585	Medicare	19%	$1,442
Physician	22%	$1,652	Paycheck deduction		$ 937
Dental	4%	$ 330	Medicaid	15%	$1,131
Other	6%	$ 429	VA & DOD	3%	$ 214
Nursing home	6%	$ 474	Workers comp.	2%	$ 135
Home health	2%	$ 187	Other govt.	8%	$ 604
Drugs	10%	$ 771	**Total government**	**47%**	**$3,526**
Products	3%	$ 199	Employer insurance	35%	$2,626
Admin. costs	7%	$ 535	Self-paid	11%	$ 853
Public health	3%	$ 235	Charity, etc.	7%	$ 550
Research	2%	$ 159			

Based on a projected U.S. population of 307 million.

Source: U.S. Office of the Actuary, National Health Projections, http://www.cms.gov/NationalHealthExpendData/

individual payments to third-party financing, such as private insurance companies and government. In 1929, 81 percent of medical expenditures came directly from individual "out-of-pocket" payments and only 19 percent from government and other third-party organizations (see Table 1-2). This ratio has long-since been reversed, with individuals in 2007 paying only 11 percent directly and the remaining 89 percent of funds flowing through third-party transactions involving government, not-for-profit organizations, and insurance.

All the important features of health care (physicians, hospitals, insurance, and so on) in 2007 were present in some form 100 years ago, but their relative importance to the flow of funds has changed so much that the transactions look entirely different today.[3] Physicians, who in 1900 were tradespeople sometimes making do with partial payment in eggs or flour, have become highly paid and technologically sophisticated professionals who rarely talk to their patients about paying the bills. Hospitals, once minor supports for a few disabled and disadvantaged individuals, are now technological palaces of intensive treatment and the largest users of U.S. health care funds. Whereas in 1900 hospitals were financed by a few donors and some patient fees, they are now financed almost entirely by third parties: either by government insurance such as Medicare and

Table 1-2: Sources of Payment in 1929, 1970, and 2007

	1929	1970	2007
Total health spending (millions)	$ 3,656	$ 75,111	$2,319,640
Adjusted for inflation (2002 dollars)	35,900	320,756	2,319,640
Per capita (adjusted)	295	1,525	7,556
As a % of GDP	3.5%	7.2%	16.8%
Percentage paid by			
Self (out-of-pocket)	81%	33%	11%
Third parties	19%	67%	89%
Government	13%	38%	47%
Private insurance	<1%	21%	35%
Philanthropy, other	6%	8%	7%

Medicaid or by private insurance provided through employment or purchased directly by consumers (see Figures 1-5 and 1-6). For every $100 spent in the hospital, less than 2 percent comes from charitable donations. And much of the 3 percent paid for by patients out-of-pocket consists of copayments, deductibles, and other fees related to third-party insurance payments.

Figure 1-5

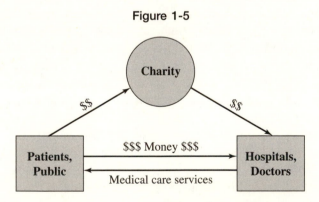

Health care flow of funds, circa 1900.

Health care spending has grown rapidly for a number of reasons, including the following:

▲ As people become wealthier, they are willing to spend more money on all goods and services. After people's basic necessities, such as food and housing, are taken care of, they are willing to spend extra on health care.

Figure 1-6

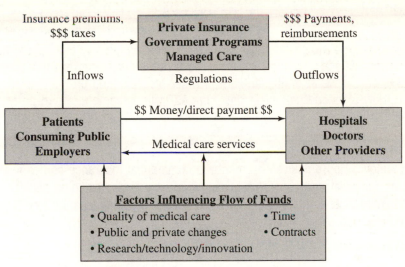

Health care flow of funds, circa 2007.

The picture isn't altogether rosy, however, as it's also the case that record numbers of people are unable to pay their medical bills.

▲ Technological advances make modern medicine more desirable. For instance, arthroscopic knee surgery makes it possible for surgeons to make a small incision and insert a tube-like instrument into the knee to diagnose and repair tissues. The shorter recovery period of this less-invasive procedure makes it more appealing than traditional knee surgery requiring large incisions.

▲ An aging population favors health care over other goods. An 80-year-old woman suffering from arthritis is likely to spend her limited income on pain medicine and other treatments rather than on a plane ticket to Bermuda.

FOR EXAMPLE

Going Broke for Health Care

According to a study by researchers at Harvard University, the average out-of-pocket medical debt for those who filed for bankruptcy was $11,854. Surprisingly, 68 percent of those who filed for bankruptcy had health insurance. In addition, the study found that 50 percent of all bankruptcy filings were partly the result of medical expenses. The average debtor was a 41-year-old woman with children and at least some college education. Most debtors owned their homes and were predominantly middle or working class.[4]

INSURANCE: A WRENCH IN THE TWO-PARTY TRANSACTION

Insurance shifts the burden of paying for health care from the individual to a third party. Because of this "cost-shifting" in the payment system, almost no one knows who is paying for what.[5] Billed charges bear little resemblance to what is paid or what the health care provider receives, and provider revenues are usually identified not as "income" but as "reimbursement." Third-party payments are made with the following funds:

✔ Taxes paid to government agencies
✔ Employer and employee payments to commercial insurance companies and for-profit and not-for-profit managed care firms, including health maintenance organizations (HMOs), preferred provider organizations (PPOs), and other organizations
✔ Philanthropic contributions to charities

These major categories of third-party payments all have a similar purpose: pooling funds from many people to pay the bills of the few patients who need care. Who gets care and what kind of care are decisions made according to the rules of the group and the opinions of the professionals who run the health care system. In each case, indirect third-party payment weakens the monetary linkage between buyer and seller that characterizes the direct two-party transactions typical in most other sectors of the economy. For most medical transactions, there is no exchange of money between the recipient of services and the provider. The patients (or their families) pay insurance premiums and taxes, and the doctors and hospitals are paid by the government and insurance companies. In the absence of a direct link between the amount paid and the resources used in treatment, "prices" become more ambiguous and less important to the transaction than ongoing relationships of trust and professional behavior. One of the purposes of this textbook is to explain how economic forces continue to operate when prices don't function in a normal way and how other organizing principles (e.g., professionalism, licensure, regulation) serve as replacements.

▲ Insurance now covers more of the cost. Shifting the financial burden from individuals to third parties through insurance not only changed the way funds flowed but made more funds available so that the health care system could grow rapidly and absorb an ever-larger share of total economic output.

1.2.3 Health Care Providers: The Uses of Funds

Payments by patients, government, and insurance companies have increased 200-fold over the past 60 years; thus, payments received by doctors, hospitals, and other care providers have increased by the same amount (see Table 1-3). In general, both the public, as users of the system, and providers, as suppliers of care, have been happy with this large increase in spending. The public has gotten a health care system that is technologically advanced and responsive to their needs. Providers have gained glory in the fight against disease and substantial gains in income, making them eager to continue the struggle.

After adjusting for changes in inflation, health care wages, and use of services, spending has still increased dramatically over the past 30 years—more than 250 percent. How can spending increase so much more rapidly than the increase in the number of services or in the wages of those who provide them? The intensity and quality of services have increased. More tests are done for a patient in a modern intensive care unit during a single day than were done for a patient

Table 1-3: Changes in the Use of Health Care Funds Over Time

	1929	1970	2007
Spending per person (in 2002 dollars)	$295	$1,525	$7,558
Percent usage			
Hospital	23%	44%	34%
Physician	36	20	22
Dental	12	6	4
Drugs	18	7	10
Other	1	3	6
Nursing home	N/A	5	6
Home health	N/A	N/A	3
Products	3	6	3
Admin. and insurance costs	3	4	7
Public health	3	2	3
Research	1	3	2
Total	*100%*	*100%*	*100%*
Hospital days per person	0.9	1.2	0.6
Hospital employees per patient	<0.5	3.1	8.3
Physician visits per person	2.6	5.0	3.9

over the course of a month in his or her wooden bed in 1929. Many of those tests (e.g., MRIs, blood glucose tests, heart monitoring tests) weren't available back then. The physician who drove to the patient's house and worked alone out of a black bag has been replaced by a team of therapists, technicians, and support staff assisting a group of physicians, many of whom are specialists using a wide variety of sophisticated medical equipment.

Another factor that explains some of the growth in spending is that, as some common, acute (short-term) diseases have become curable or preventable, medical care is increasingly applied in cases of chronic diseases that were once considered hopeless. The shift from simple caring to technologically sophisticated curing is reflected by shifts in the categories of expenditure; more is going to institutional care in hospitals and nursing homes, while the share devoted to personal services by doctors has declined. The fraction of the health care dollar spent for manufactured goods such as drugs has also fallen, while the cost of labor-intensive services has risen.

SELF-CHECK

- How much do experts estimate will be spent on medical care per person in the United States in 2007?
- List four reasons why health care spending has increased in the United States.
- Explain why health care spending has increased so much more rapidly than the number of services or the wages of those who provide them.

1.3 Major Issues in Health Care Financing

When tracing the flow of funds through the health care system, it's important to be aware that the money trail is constantly shifting, changing direction (e.g., who makes the payments and who receives them) and size (e.g., how much money flows through the system). The following sections identify several of the factors that influence the flow of funds.

1.3.1 The Value of Health

Why does health care cost so much? Because we place great value on our health. Health is so precious to us that its value exceeds that of the things we possess. After all, what benefit do I get from spending my money on books or art or cars or clothes if I am dead? Sick and in pain, confronted with the possibility of death, people would be willing to spend almost any amount of money to get their health back. Health care costs so much because people are willing to pay for it. The many years a surgeon spends in training, the billions of dollars government spends on public health, and the comprehensive health insurance plans provided by employers are consequences of the value we as a society place on health care. They're effects rather than causes. We're willing to spend so much on physician training, public health, and health insurance because what they produce is valuable to us.

1.3.2 Time: A Scarce Resource

Time is more limited than money. You have just 24 hours each day. To use your money as a consumer, you must have time. Given time, you can get money. Or you can spend your time meditating, hunting for berries in the woods, or writing poems in the sand. At least you're alive. If you have money but no time, the money is worthless. Death is the ultimate budget constraint. When your time is up, there are no second chances, no credit advances, and no more decisions to make. While all economists acknowledge that a lifetime is a scarce resource, health economists are acutely aware of this fact because the business of medical care centers on life-and-death decisions.

It is difficult to improve your health after it has deteriorated. Spending money on medicine when you are seriously ill is a little like spending money on your car after the engine has begun to burn oil: Regular maintenance is a lot cheaper. How healthy you are when you get old depends not so much on the medical care you get then as on what you have done to and for your body over the years. Taking some of your time each week to exercise and giving up some tasty junk food (e.g., donuts, fries, ice cream sundaes) can help you live longer and feel better in the future. Some people would call such behavior health consciousness or following a healthy lifestyle. As economists, we call it savings and investment. If I reduce consumption now (less ice cream), I can consume more (have greater enjoyment) in future years. I invest in my body by exercising, just as a firm invests in a manufacturing plant by doing maintenance and construction. Most readers of this textbook are studying now for a future reward: knowledge, grades, a degree, career advancement. You are investing, giving up time (and money) now to obtain more value in the future.

Medical school is a form of investment, usually a very good one. Similarly, the research done by pharmaceutical companies is an investment: forgo current profits to discover a new drug that will begin to sell 15 years from now. In a society, the money used for medical schools and research, the loss of life due to trials of experimental drugs, and the difficult learning curve of surgeons in training (somebody has to be the first patient) are investments in the future of medical care. Losses are real, and staggeringly large, but the rewards exceed the losses. Imagine how many of your parents or your classmates would be dead if we decided as a society to stop the losses and practiced the best nineteenth century medicine for the next 100 years.

1.3.3 How Quality Factors In

Medicine often involves life-and-death decisions. In these situations, quality is crucial, and quantity doesn't matter. It doesn't help if a mediocre surgeon offers to give you a second operation at half price. A patient usually consumes one and only one "unit" of care—an operation, in this case—for each illness. The only trade-off made is in the quality, not the quantity, of the procedure. Having budget decisions made over quality rather than quantity tends to make the economist's job more difficult. While it's reasonable to assume for most other goods that price per unit remains constant as the quantity increases or decreases, any change in quality must change the price. Quality cannot simply be added up or multiplied to arrive at a total spending limit the way quantity can.

The quality of medical care has increased over the past 30 years. But has it increased as much as, or more than, the cost? While measures such as the consumer price index (CPI) attempt to deal with these issues, there is no consensus on how accurate they are, or even on what these measures should be. Can quality be measured by the number of lives saved, the number of lives saved per dollar spent, the number of tests or services provided, the level of physician knowledge (and should this count if the patient dies?), or patient satisfaction? Historically, most emphasis on quality was at the level of the individual: a procedure, a patient, or a physician. Was the surgery done properly? Did the patient heal well and was he satisfied with the care he received? Was the doctor adequately trained for the procedure, with a certified supporting staff? Recently, economists have shifted the focus from the individual to the group. The tools of population health allow economists to ask the following kinds of questions: What percentage of patients suffer infections as a result of surgery? What percentage of patients require a second operation? How do these rates compare with those of surgeons and hospitals in other states or countries?

Even though quality of care can mean the difference between life and death, it's important to remember that medical care can't permanently save a life because we will all die eventually. What medical care can do is prolong a life and make it more productive. The extension of life isn't, however, unambiguously good. Increasingly, we are asked to make decisions about end-of-life care, release from suffering, and quality of life not in terms of morbidity and mortality but in terms of relationships, social connections, and spiritual concerns.

1.3.4 Public vs. Private Goods

For some goods, there is only one unit, which we consume collectively. The atmosphere is an example. It doesn't make sense to talk about quantities of atmosphere. Having "more" by breathing deeply, turning on a fan, or opening a window doesn't add value if the problem is pollution. *Quality* is the only thing that matters. When discussing goods, it is important to distinguish between those goods shared by the public collectively and those owned by people individually.

▲ Air quality, the legal system, national defense, cancer research, transportation, and other goods that are similarly universal in consumption are known as **public goods**.

▲ Unlike public goods, **private goods** can be owned and consumed individually.

Just because public goods are universally consumed doesn't mean that they can't become scarce. Scarcity of air quality (i.e., pollution) can be addressed through various improvements, each of which has a cost. Public funds, although much greater than those of any individual, are still subject to budget constraints. The price of better air must be paid by giving up some other public goods or by all of us giving up some of our private goods by paying higher taxes.

"Private" and "public" are polar concepts. Few goods are so purely private that they're entirely unregulated regarding safety, ingredients, and disposal, and few goods are so public that there are no differences among individuals regarding use or quality.[6] Medical care clusters more services toward the public end than is immediately apparent. Even though each of us goes individually to the hospital emergency room, in a small city, we must all go to the same emergency room, and we therefore get pretty much the same quality of care. In a large city with many hospitals, there is somewhat more variation, but patients are rarely able to choose their surgeon, nursing staff, or room. Contrast that with the purchase of a coat, a birthday cake, or even a wheelchair, in which case there are many more choices and there is much more individual control over quality.

Payment systems also tend to make medical care a public good. All employees in a firm often have the same insurance plan. Therefore, the mail clerk and the executive vice president are equally valued customers of the hospital. In Chapters 4 and 5 we examine how the pooling of funds through insurance can make medical care into a form of public good even though services are provided and consumed in private transactions between doctors and patients.

1.3.5 Research, Technology, and Innovation

Technology has been the driving force in the health care system—saving babies, lengthening lives, creating hospitals, linking medical records worldwide, and raising the American public's willingness to spend more than $2 trillion a year. One can easily imagine that spending would be doubled again without complaint if the research laboratories could come up with a vaccine for AIDS, a cure for cancer, and a reversal of Alzheimer's disease. Medical discoveries have often been unexpected outgrowths of other activities (e.g., Pasteur's discovery of bacteria grew out of an investigation into the causes of spoiled wine and beer) or the refinement of insights from patient care. Historically, what little direct funding there was for research came mostly from philanthropists. Today, taxpayers are the largest source of pure research funding, through support of the National Institutes of Health and similar government-funded programs. However, a much larger portion

FOR EXAMPLE

National Institutes of Health

The National Institutes of Health (NIH) is the primary federal agency for conducting and supporting medical research. It is composed of 27 institutes and centers, including the National Cancer Institute, the National Eye Institute, and the National Institute on Aging. The NIH received $28.6 billion in federal funding in 2006. What do U.S. taxpayers get for their money? NIH scientists investigate ways to prevent disease as well as the causes, treatments, and even cures for common and rare diseases. Eighty percent of NIH funding is distributed as research grants to all 50 states and several foreign countries. Based in Bethesda, Maryland, the NIH employs 18,627 people.

of research funding is hidden in the cost of patient care, as the work of physicians to develop and refine new technologies is covered through reimbursement. Similarly, most of the research and development (R&D) at pharmaceutical companies is buried as an overhead cost in the production of drugs.

The cost of continually innovating and changing medical treatments and delivery systems is staggeringly high, yet the cost of *not* innovating is much greater. What athlete injured today would wish to forgo arthroscopic knee surgery and accept a hot mustard plaster? Senior citizens may say they want to turn back the clock to the good old days, but any politician who threatens to take away Medicare, or even to cut benefits slightly, gets defeated at the polls. The American public demands a modern, constantly updated health care system. Research into new therapies and new forms of organization is the force that has made it worth spending $2.3 trillion today versus $4 billion 100 years ago. Yet the flow of funds into research is hard to trace, and the connection between spending and benefits is difficult to make.

SELF-CHECK

- How does the value we place on our health influence the cost of health care?
- Distinguish between **public goods** and **private goods**.
- In life-and-death situations, which is more important—quality or quantity?
- What is the largest source of funding for pure research? List two other sources of funding.

1.4 Economic Principles as Conceptual Tools

The question of whether the side effects of a course of highly toxic chemotherapy are worth the possibility of living another eight months is highly personal, yet the principles involved are common to most economic problems: balancing costs and values within a set of constraints imposed by the situation. It can be analyzed like other decisions, such as whether to apply to graduate school, how many risks to take while skydiving, and the choice between buying health insurance and taking a vacation. A list of principles that are useful as "conceptual tools" for analyzing decisions is provided in the following sections.

1.4.1 Trade: Benefiting from Exchange

People engage in trade—exchanging things, time, favors, money, and information—because it makes them better off. Both sides must benefit, or they wouldn't agree to trade. This is the fundamental theorem of exchange and perhaps the most basic principle of economic reasoning.

1.4.2 Choice: Are Benefits Greater Than Costs?

Every decision involves a trade-off, giving something up in order to get something else, choosing the option that means more to the individual. This is obvious when you engage in trade with someone else. It's true whenever you make a choice, even though you "trade" only with yourself (e.g., giving up a workout at the gym in order to study, passing up a new CD in order to buy dinner at a restaurant, giving up some of your savings in order to take a trip to Cancun). Economists assume that people tend to make choices that make them better off in a way they value (not necessarily financially). This is known as the **benefit–cost principle.**

1.4.3 Opportunity Cost: What Do I Have to Give Up?

The best measure of what something costs is what one has to give up to get it, which is what economists call the **opportunity cost.** The opportunity cost of a trip to Cancun might be $750 in savings; the opportunity cost of an extra weekend date might be an A as your grade falls to a B+ because you gave up study time. Conversely, you might say that the decision to study to get an A cost you a date. The decision you make, not the price tag or money, determines the opportunity cost of something. The primary cost of attending this class is the time it takes (the fun you could have had and/or the money you could have earned), not the amount spent on tuition and books.

FOR EXAMPLE

A Scarcity of Nurses

Registered nurses (RNs) make up the largest group of health care providers in the United States. In 2000, 59 percent of RNs were employed in hospital settings, with a smaller percentage of RNs working in health care settings such as ambulatory care, home health care, and nursing homes.[7] Authorities have warned that the United States could fall 275,000 nurses short by 2010. The predicted shortage will be due in part to increasing health care demands from a growing elderly population and in part from dissatisfaction among RNs, who often complain of understaffing and low pay and benefits. In the face of these shortages, many hospitals and other health care institutions are recruiting foreign nurses from less developed countries, such as Mexico, the Philippines, and India.[8]

1.4.4 Scarcity: Working Within the Limits

Why does a decision always involve giving something up? Because reality imposes limits, or constraints, on what you can do. The most basic limit is time. You have only 24 hours per day, and when your days are gone (due to death) you have no more life to use in production or consumption. Your income and your bank balance, the place you live, the things and friends you have, and even your credit rating all put limits on what you can do to make yourself better off. Economists call them budget constraints. This term applies not only to money but also to time, things, relationships, and any other kind of constraint.

SELF-CHECK

- Explain the **benefit–cost principle.**
- Indicate what defines the **opportunity cost** of any action.
- List three typical budget restraints.

1.5 Health Principles

Medicine isn't entirely, or even mostly, about money. Science, caring, professionalism, and even religious concerns regarding birth and death can be more important than dollars. Economics gives one important and clear perspective, but it's a limited view—similar to the kind of limited view that an x-ray provides of a person. Economics has expanded to examine social relationships, politics, and the financing of technological advances. Yet no matter how powerful economics is for analyzing decisions, it still remains just one piece of a larger picture. Most of medicine and health lies outside the scope of this textbook, but five simplified health principles within the expanding realm of economics are noted here.

1.5.1 Health Is Priceless

In a crisis, people pay almost anything for medical care. The opportunity cost is too great to bargain over "how much" when your mother's or daughter's life is at stake. People don't want to make difficult decisions regarding trading off dollars for health. This is why virtually every modern economy offers emergency medical care on demand and extensive programs of health insurance.

1.5.2 Money Still Determines Health

Although demographic factors such as age, sex, and race are important in determining health, money plays a big role. Everywhere we look, the rich are typically healthier than the poor. In unsophisticated rural villages and modern cosmopolitan cities, with health insurance or without, the rich tend to do better in terms of both mortality (i.e., death rates) and morbidity (i.e., illness rates). A particular rich person may be in worse health than a poor person, but in general, money has a strong positive impact on physical condition.

1.5.3 Health Risks Are More Public Than Private

Your income depends more on the economy into which you were born than on your individual skills and effort. So, too, does the state of your health. Compared with starting your life in Switzerland, being born in a rural village in the Sudan severely limits both your earning power and your life expectancy.

1.5.4 Individual Choices: Lifestyle Is More Than Medicine

People's lifestyle plays a large role in their health care choices. The United States has a high-quality and highly regulated health care system, and so our choices regarding "better" care usually have a lot more to do with personal satisfaction than they do with whether we live or die. Branch Creek Hospital versus University Hospital? Generic naproxen sodium versus Aleve? Doctor at the local health department clinic versus specialist in private practice? Our choices don't tend to have a major impact on death rates, although they may have a lot to do with personal satisfaction and the quality of the experience. Flying first class on a major carrier is more comfortable than flying cut rate in economy class, but the safety (i.e., the likelihood of dying in a crash) is about the same.

FOR EXAMPLE

Medical Bargains or Boondoggles?

Prices for medical procedures are often far lower abroad than in the United States, but there's no guarantee that the quality elsewhere will be on par with procedures here. Would you be willing to have a coronary bypass done in South Africa to save $63,000? Here are a few price comparisons to consider:

Procedure	Cost in the United States	Cost Elsewhere
Coronary angiogram	$25,600	$ 2,450 (Singapore)
Coronary bypass	$86,000	$23,000 (South Africa)
Knee replacement	$36,300	$ 2,100 (Mexico)
Hip replacement	$40,800	$ 7,200 (Singapore)
Facelift	$ 6,800	$ 3,000 (India)
Lasik (per eye)	$ 2,000	$ 750 (Thailand)
In vitro fertilization	$12,000	$ 7,800 (Canada)[9]

1.5.5 Measurable Differences in Quality over Time or Regions Are Greater Than Most Differences in Choices Faced by Patients

Heart surgery in 2007 will be so much better than the kind practiced in 1962 that no one would choose the latter. Rich patients may fly from Guatemala to the United States for superior medical care, but few U.S. tourists would decide to have knee replacement surgery done in Guatemala while on vacation to save a few dollars. Individual market choices for quality are important and persistent for goods such as clothing and housing, but medical care is more like the market for computers and video equipment: Most people pay for what is newest.

SELF-CHECK

- List and explain five health principles.
- Briefly explain how a person's lifestyle influences his or her health care decisions.

SUMMARY

For people to get what they want from the health care system, patients and health care providers must engage in trade. Health economics is the study of how those transactions are made and of the bottom-line results.

The terms of trade are the specifics of a transaction. Only in a very simple exchange are all the terms of trade captured in the money price. The fundamental theorem of exchange states that for a trade to take place, both the buyer and the seller must believe that the trade makes them better off.

Goods and services are only worth as much as people are willing to pay for them. Health care costs so much because people place so much value on their health. As a wealthy country, the United States will spend more than $2 trillion on health care in 2007, supporting a dynamic and technologically sophisticated health care system. Health care costs have consistently risen 3 to 5 percent more rapidly than incomes and now account for 16.8 percent of GDP. Government is the largest provider of health care funds (47 percent), and hospitals are the largest users (34 percent). Research into new drugs and treatments is very expensive, but the forgone opportunity cost of not innovating would be much greater.

Economists must tackle two major complexities when studying the economics of health. First, most people make health care choices based on quality rather than price or quantity. Second, the effects of medical care on health are uncertain.

KEY TERMS

Benefit–cost principle	The principle that people tend to make choices that make them better off in a way they value.
Circular flow of funds	A system in which every dollar that a consumer spends ultimately ends up in the hands of someone else who wants to spend it.
Contract	An agreement to trade.
Demand side	The consumer.
Derived demand	Demand for a good due to its use rather than for itself (e.g., the demand for x-ray film is derived from the demand for medical diagnoses, which in turn are derived from a consumer's demand for health).
Fundamental theorem of exchange	A theorem stating that any voluntary exchange between persons must make both of them better off because they willingly agreed to trade.
Market	The point at which buyers and sellers exchange dollars for goods and services.

Opportunity cost	Something that must be given up in order to do or obtain something; the highest valued alternative which must be foregone. For example, the opportunity cost of taking a final exam may be missing out on a trip to Bermuda.
Private goods	Goods that are consumed or financed individually.
Public goods	Goods that are consumed or financed collectively (e.g., clean air, national defense, discovery of penicillin) either because it's impossible to include/exclude any consumer who doesn't pay or because once the goods are produced, there's no additional cost for additional consumers.
Supply side	The seller.
Terms of trade	Terms that specify what the buyer is to give the seller and what the seller is to give the buyer in return.
Two-party transaction	An exchange between a buyer and seller, usually trading money for goods or services.

ASSESS YOUR UNDERSTANDING

Go to www.wiley.com/college/getzen to evaluate your knowledge of the flow of funds through the health care system.
Measure your learning by comparing pre-test and post-test results.

Summary Questions

1. A contract is the point at which buyers and sellers exchange dollars for goods and services. True or False?

2. Most medical decisions can be captured by a simplified model of market-place behavior in which price is the only thing that matters. True or False?

3. The fundamental theorem of exchange states that
   (a) every dollar that a consumer spends ultimately ends up in the hands of someone else who spends it.
   (b) the essence of economics is trade.
   (c) both parties in a transaction must be benefiting if they freely agreed to make a trade.
   (d) to understand health economics, you must follow the money.

4. In a two-party transaction, consumers make up the supply side and sellers make up the demand side. True or False?

5. The largest single share of total personal health expenditures in the United States comes from
   (a) out-of-pocket spending by consumers.
   (b) private insurance.
   (c) Medicare.
   (d) Medicaid.

6. The largest single share of expenditures for health services in the United States is for
   (a) physicians.
   (b) hospitals.
   (c) drugs.
   (d) long term care.

7. The primary cause for the high price of health care is
   (a) the many years a surgeon spends in training.
   (b) the billions of dollars government spends on public health.
   (c) the comprehensive health insurance plans provided.
   (d) the value we place on our health.

8. You go to a free beach, put on suntan lotion, and play music on your radio. Which of the items in this scenario are public goods and which are private goods?

   (a) Public goods: lotion, beach; private goods: music

   (b) Public goods: lotion; private goods: beach, music

   (c) Public goods: beach; private goods: music, lotion

   (d) Public goods: beach, music; private goods: lotion

9. The best measure of what something costs is what one has to give up to get it. This is what economists call

   (a) the cost–benefit principle.

   (b) opportunity cost.

   (c) a budget constraint.

   (d) the fundamental theorem of exchange.

10. People tend to make choices that make them better off in a way they value. True or False?

11. Because health is priceless, economic factors such as wealth don't have any influence on people's well-being. True or False?

Review Questions

1. List some contractual structures society has introduced to handle the complexity of health care transactions.

2. Have health care costs increased or decreased in the past 100 years? List explanations for the change.

3. Explain how insurance weakens the monetary linkage between buyer and seller that characterizes the direct two-party transactions typical in most other sectors of the economy.

4. The text speaks of a "derived demand" for inputs. Is the demand for health services a derived demand? Why or why not?

5. If good health is priceless, why are there prices for doctor visits, hospital stays, and drugs?

6. In 1929, 81% of health spending was out-of-pocket, which means it didn't involve the huge administrative costs associated with insurance or government payment programs. What caused us to move to an apparently less efficient system in which less than 20% of health spending is out-of-pocket?

7. List an example of quality of care in the delivery of medical care and discuss why a patient might be willing to pay more for it.

Applying This Chapter

1. Compare the terms of trade when purchasing a pair of reading glasses for $7.99 from a drug store versus buying a pair of prescription glasses for $159.99 from an optician.

2. Approximately how much was spent on health care costs for you in the past year? What percentage did you pay out-of-pocket? What percentage did private insurers pay? What percentage did the government pay? How does the total amount compare to the national average for 2007?

3. What is the opportunity cost of going to a doctor to be examined for skin cancer?

4. What is the primary budget constraint facing an 84-year-old billionaire?

5. Would eliminating research reduce or increase the cost of U.S. health care? Why?

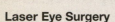

Laser Eye Surgery

Laser eye surgery to correct poor eyesight is an elective operation that often costs from $1,500 to $5,000 and is rarely covered by medical or vision insurance. When such surgery is successful, however, patients are no longer required to buy and wear glasses or contacts—and the surgery has a high success rate, although there is some healing time, and the procedure itself is daunting for many people. What are the costs (financial and opportunity costs) of choosing to undergo laser eye surgery over wearing glasses or contacts? Conversely, what are the costs and benefits of sticking with glasses or contacts?

Health Care as a Drain on the Economy

Automaker General Motors employs approximately 150,000 people. In 2005, the company spent $5.4 billion in health care costs. Those expenses account for about $1,500 of the cost of each vehicle produced in the United States. Such expenses are often characterized as a "drain on the resources" of General Motors and of consumers who buy cars. For instance, if General Motors didn't have such high health care costs, it could price vehicles more competitively and thus work to regain market share lost to foreign automakers. Similarly, the $1,500 of consumer money that goes to GM's health care costs could instead be used to pay for college tuition or to purchase other goods and services to help fuel the economy. In a brief essay, consider how such health care expenses might be recharacterized as contributing to, rather than draining from, the economy.

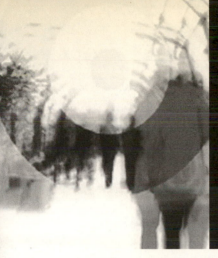

2

ECONOMIC EVALUATION OF HEALTH SERVICES
The Supply and Demand of Health Care

Starting Point

Go to www.wiley.com/college/getzen to assess your knowledge of how economists evaluate health care.
Determine where you need to concentrate your effort.

What You'll Learn in This Chapter

▲ The difference between need and demand
▲ How to read a demand curve
▲ How to use marginal revenue to make business decisions
▲ The role of price sensitivity in health care economics
▲ The supply side of health care

After Studying This Chapter, You'll Be Able To

▲ Predict how the quantity of services used varies as price changes, using the concept of demand
▲ Estimate marginal revenue and marginal cost
▲ Appraise the price sensitivity of a product or service
▲ Analyze the impact that government and insurance regulations have on medical pricing

INTRODUCTION

Health economists use the concept of demand to ask how the quantity of services used varies as price changes. The concept of a demand curve yields two fundamental insights: (1) Providing more medical treatment means giving up something else, and (2) as more and more care is provided, the benefit of each additional unit becomes smaller and smaller. Health economists focus on trade-offs, choices that must be made, scarcity of resources, and allocating resources among competing needs, not on defining one specific need.

2.1 Need vs. Demand

When considering medical care, economists and doctors ask different questions. Doctors ask, "If money is no problem, what should I do for *this patient*?" Economists, even health economists, aren't trained to answer such a question. They try to answer a different question: "Given that there isn't enough for everyone to have all that they need, who should get treated? How should resources used for medical care vary across groups?" These two questions demonstrate the difference between *need* and *demand*:

▲ **Need** is as a professional determination of the quantity that should be supplied. Doctors tend to consider medical decisions in terms of need.
▲ **Demand** is the relationship between price and quantity. Economists consider medical decisions in terms of demand.

When doctors consider a patient's needs, they are determining the level of care necessary to heal the patient's illness. Doctors don't consider the cost of the treatment, patients' ability to pay for the treatment, or anything else having to do with the price of the care. Their job is to do whatever they can within their power to heal their patients. Because physicians are supposed to act in a patient's best interest, they try to behave as if they have no financial stake in the treatment and as if the patient can pay for whatever treatment is recommended.

For decisions regarding individual patients, a need-based medical perspective is appropriate. If we look beyond the individual patient to the health care system as a whole, however, this need-based perspective is no longer adequate. Although we don't ask doctors to determine what is best for taxpayers or employers or insurance companies, someone must tackle these issues. That job is left to health economists.

Economists consider systemwide medical decisions in terms of demand. Economists think about how choosing one set of insurance regulations means more children will get immunized, but fewer elderly people will receive home care, while another plan might protect accident victims, reduce taxes, or provide more incentives to work. The trade-offs between medical care and other goods, among different groups of patients and different types of care, are the issues that health economics is designed to address.

Need and demand are different, yet complementary, perspectives on the complex set of human, financial, and scientific exchanges that constitute medicine. It could be said that, to some extent, doctors ignore economics, while economists ignore medicine. Health economists try to bring the two disciplines together by applying economic models to the science of medicine.

2.1.1 The Demand Curve

When economists talk about "demand," what they are really talking about is a **demand curve.** A demand curve is a graph that shows the total quantity of a good that buyers wish to buy at each price. For example, a demand curve for artificial hearts tells us the total quantity of artificial hearts that buyers wish to buy at various prices (see Figure 2-1).

Demand curves always slope downward. Demand curves are downward sloping because the quantity demanded always falls as prices rise (assuming that all other conditions remain constant), a generalization known as the **law of demand.** For example, if each artificial heart cost $1 million, they would only be used in matters of life and death. If further development reduced the cost of artificial hearts to $100,000 each, more people would get them. The artificial hearts would still be used only for people with serious illnesses, but they might be implanted long before a person's natural heart gave out. If the cost of artificial hearts dropped to $100, a new heart would be readily available to anyone who needed it. Consider what would happen if the cost of artificial hearts dropped to $10 and they could be easily implanted during a 15-minute visit to the doctor. Some people who had never been ill but were just worried, or who thought that they were weak and wanted a supercharger to help them run faster, might have new hearts implanted.

Figure 2-1

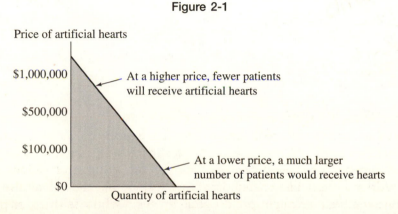

The demand curve for artificial hearts.

MARGINAL BENEFITS

People engage in trade to make themselves better off. What principle determines when to stop? When the benefits from the next step are outweighed by the costs. Each decision increment (e.g., read one more page, eat one more slice of pizza, play one more game) adds a little value, which economists refer to as a **marginal benefit.** Each step also takes a little more time or money, called a **marginal cost.** The real issue isn't whether something (e.g., grades, food, playing time) is good but whether you would be better off with more or less of it. As more and more is done, a point at which the benefits of each additional step become smaller and smaller (diminishing marginal returns) is usually reached, and the costs of an additional unit become greater. *Maximum net benefits are obtained by pushing to the point at which rising marginal costs equal falling marginal benefits.*

The demand curve is a marginal benefit curve that traces how much each additional unit of service is worth. At a price of $1 million, the artificial heart would be implanted only in people who believed they would receive more than $1 million in benefits. At a price of $100,000, the artificial heart would be implanted in people whose perceived benefit ranged from $1 million to $100,000. At $50,000, the artificial heart would be implanted in a few more people, whose marginal benefit would fall to between $100,000 and $50,000, who would be willing to pay for the operation, and so on. Note that the demand curve implies that the value of an artificial heart depends on its scarcity and on how many are already in use. If only a few hearts were sold, their value would be fantastically high; they would cost millions and millions of dollars each. After many artificial hearts were sold, their marginal value— the value of each additional sale—would be quite low. Another way to look at marginal benefit is to look at an example involving aspirin: If you feel well, you'll derive no real benefit from the aspirin, so you wouldn't pay very much for it. But if you were up late drinking the night before, that aspirin would be quite valuable to you.

2.1.2 Derived Demand

People want health, not medicine. You get medical care only if you need it, if you think that it will improve your health. No one buys heart surgery, chemotherapy, or x-rays just because these are fun things to have or because the hospital is having a sale. Economists would say that the demand for medical care is derived demand and depends on the usefulness of the treatment in providing health. As noted in Chapter 1, economists define derived demand as demand for a good due to its use, rather than for itself. The demand for x-ray film is derived from the demand for medical diagnoses, which in turn are derived from a consumer's demand for health. This is the case with most goods. A cast-iron skillet is bought not for the metal but as a utensil for cooking food. Skis are bought for skiing, not to take up space in the closet. The business of health, the actual transactions observed—doctor visits, surgery, prescriptions—are in the derived realm of medical care; they are not direct trades for health itself. If we could simply buy health—adding to life expectancy the way one picks up a three-year guarantee on a new computer—then much of what makes health economics special would simply fade away.

When medical care is viewed as derived demand, other health-determining factors—genetics, nutrition, lifestyle, environment—are seen as substitutes for that care. That is, instead of going to the doctor, we could try to eat right, exercise, and start life with better parents. The cumulative impact of these other factors is much greater than any differences in the amount or quality of care received in the current U.S. health care system. Why then is so much money spent and attention focused on medical care, an input that makes such a relatively limited contribution to health?

At the moment of need, medical care is perhaps the only thing we can buy to make us better. The other factors that determine health (e.g., genetics, lifestyle, accumulated exposure to pollutants, luck, nutritional history) cannot be purchased on demand. None of us can buy new parents. In the United States, however, most of us can buy the surgical care needed to mend and straighten a broken nose.

FOR EXAMPLE

Your Insurance Company Wants You to Go on a Diet

Insurance companies are acutely aware that medical care is often a substitute, or derived demand, for good health and that healthy choices such as eating right and exercising can often achieve the same goal at a far lower cost. If more of their policyholders ate low-fat, high-fiber diets and ran three miles a day, fewer of them would have high cholesterol, have high blood pressure, or suffer from coronary artery disease. This would mean fewer expensive prescriptions and medical procedures. Recognizing the financial benefits of a healthy lifestyle, many large insurance companies, such as BlueCross and BlueShield and Kaiser Permanente, actively promote healthy lifestyles through outreach and education programs. One such program is the BlueCross BlueShield Association's Walking Works program, which touts the benefits of incorporating a daily walking routine and offers advice for getting started.

2.1.3 Individual, Firm, and Market Demand

So far, we have been rather casual about the distinction between the demand of an individual and the demand of a group. Let's be more precise. The definition of *demand* depends on the decision being made. To determine how many times Alice Anderson will visit the doctor, we look only at Alice's behavior. This is an example of **individual demand.**

To estimate the use of ambulance services in Lockport, Maine, we look only at people in the town and the surrounding area, not the entire state. To project how a change in the hospital deductible for Medicare will affect spending, it's necessary to look at the entire elderly population of the United States. The **market demand** is the sum of all individuals in that market. It's the decision being analyzed that defines the market. It may correspond to a geographic area, a group of friends, or all the people who visit a particular Web site.

If there were only one pharmacy in Lockport, it would be a monopolist (sole seller), and the demand of the market as a whole would be the same as the demand for the firm. **Firm demand** is the demand for each firm in a market. Suppose instead that there are four pharmacies in Lockport. What demand curve is relevant to them? The pharmacies are concerned with more than individual demand because each of them has many customers. Yet none of them fills all the prescriptions in Lockport; therefore, a pharmacy's own business isn't the same as market demand. Rather, each pharmacy can sell a greater or lesser fraction of all the drugs sold in town by changing prices. Economists say that the pharmacy "faces a firm demand curve" of potential customers (which is some fraction of the entire market). If one pharmacy's prices are much lower than those of the others, it will get the bulk of business. Conversely, even a pharmacy that charges high prices will get some business from customers who live nearby or if it's the only one open in the middle of the night.

SELF-CHECK

- Distinguish between **need** and **demand.**
- Explain what a **demand curve** is.
- State the **law of demand.**
- Explain the relationship between **marginal benefits** and **marginal costs** with regard to obtaining maximum net benefits.
- Give an example of each of the following kinds of demand: **individual demand, market demand,** and **firm demand.**

2.2 Marginal Revenue

A firm's profits depend not on how many units are sold but on the amount of money it brings in (revenue). In deciding whether to sell more, not only does price matter, but how much prices must be lowered to increase sales also matters. If a pharmacy sells two bandages at $10 each, its total revenue is $20 (2 × $10). To sell three bandages under the same circumstances, the pharmacy would have to lower the price to $8. At the lower price, the pharmacy's total revenue will rise to $24 (3 × $8). The gain in total sales is just $4 ($24 – $20). This gain in total sales is the marginal revenue of the third unit of sale.

▲ **Marginal revenue** is the change in a firm's total revenue that results from a one-unit change in sales.

One way of looking at marginal revenue is that to increase sales, the $8 received from the additional unit sold is partially offset by the $2 price reduction (from $10 to $8) of the other two units, so that the net gain is just $4.

The way to maximize profits (*total revenues – total costs*) is to sell additional units, as long as the marginal revenue is greater than the marginal cost.

▲ **Marginal cost** is the increase in total costs caused by the production of one more unit.

When marginal revenue is less than marginal cost, the sale is a loser, even if the price is still above cost.

The concept of marginal revenue takes a while to grasp but is essential for understanding business decisions. The relevant decision is about a bit more or a bit less and how total revenue will change as a result: a decision at the margin.

2.2.1 Price Sensitivity

When economists consider demand, they care more about change than about any particular quantity or price. To study change, economists need to measure how price increases or decreases affect people's buying decisions; in other words, they need a tool to measure price sensitivity. Economists use the concept of elasticity to measure price sensitivity.

▲ A demand curve indicating that the quantity demanded will change a lot for any small change in price is said to be **price elastic**.
▲ If the quantity demanded barely budges when the price rises, demand is said to be **price inelastic**.

More precisely, price elasticity is measured by the percentage change in quantity demanded for each 1 percent change in price, as shown in the following equation:

$$\text{Price elasticity} = \frac{\%\ \text{change in quantity}}{\%\ \text{change in price}}$$

If the percentage change in price is equal to the percentage change in quantity, demand is said to be **unit elastic.**

Elasticity can be used to study the similarities and differences in demand. If Alice's demand for Flonase is likely to decline by 25 percent if the price increases by 10 percent, then her elasticity is –2.5. If Alice's response is pretty much average, then even though we may be talking about thousands of prescriptions, the effect on the market as a whole will still be a 25 percent decline for a 10 percent price increase.

What about the firm demand for Eastside Pharmacy in Lockport? Chances are, it will be more price sensitive than the individual or market demands. If Eastside Pharmacy raised prices, many customers would start buying from Central Pharmacy instead. Only if all four pharmacies in Lockport raised prices by 10 percent would it be likely that all four would experience a 25 percent decline in demand. Why is firm demand so much more price sensitive than the other types? Because the other firms in the market are good substitutes. The more substitutes available, the more price sensitive demand is.

To see how substitution affects price sensitivity, consider what would happen if there were 10 percent increases not just in the price of Flonase but also in the prices of all allergy medications. Alice wouldn't be so quick to cut her purchases of Flonase because all her alternatives would have also increased in price. Considering the range of substitution provides more insight into why so much medical care is price inelastic. If I think that a particular medication or treatment is best for me, or that my doctor is the only one who can understand my headaches—that there are no good substitutes for the care she provides—I'm not likely to be very sensitive to price. On the other hand, if I consider all doctors and allergy medications to be pretty much the same, or if I'm willing to seek alternative therapies such as homeopathic treatments, I'll be happy to switch to save a few dollars.

The change in demand due to a change in price also depends on the amount of time available to find a substitute. Acute need (e.g., heart attack, stroke) makes it impossible to shop around for the best price in medical care. However, you

FOR EXAMPLE

Substitutes—Generics vs. Brand-Name Drugs

Newly introduced drugs enjoy U.S. patent protection and market exclusivity. After their patent expires, however, manufacturers can begin selling generic equivalents of the brand-name drugs. These generic equivalents serve as good substitutes for their brand-name counterparts, often at much lower prices. The availability of substitutes forces manufacturers to lower prices of their brand-name products to stay competitive. For instance, the introduction of a generic version of the cholesterol-lowering drug Zocor (generic name simvastatin), which totaled $4.4 billion in sales the year prior to the patent expiration, lowered the price of Zocor by as much as 80 percent.

might have a long time to look for a surgeon to operate on your sore knee or to find a nursing home for your grandfather. With more time available, demand is more sensitive to price.

2.2.2 Price Elasticity and Marginal Revenue

Firms facing inelastic demand find that total revenue goes down when they sell more units. Firms facing elastic demand find that revenues increase when prices are reduced to sell more units. Firms facing unit elasticity find that total revenues remain unchanged.

Most medical care is relatively inelastic. Pain, critical needs, fear of uncertainty, and insurance tend to reduce the role of price in patient decision making. Note what happens to a firm that sells more of an inelastic good: Because increasing the quantity sold by 2 percent requires a large decline in price, perhaps 10 percent, the firm actually loses money.

Most hospitals face very inelastic demand, especially for emergency services, yet they charge less than profit-maximizing prices. Why don't they charge more if doing so would increase profits? The reasons are many, ranging from desire to help the poor to administrative controls over allowable changes. Also, the sensitivity to price change today is significantly less than the ultimate response to a price change in the long run (e.g., after people organize protests, build another hospital, or shift their business across town).

Some medical goods—especially those for which consumers have several choices and good information in advance of purchase, such as allergy medications—are price elastic. For these goods, total revenues would decline if prices were increased. Thus, it's more likely that a medical provider facing elastic demand is behaving more like a standard profit-maximizing firm. However, price controls, informal norms about overcharging, and other deviations from perfect competition may still be significant, even in the more price-sensitive medical markets.

2.2.3 Price Discrimination

A firm doesn't necessarily face the same price elasticity in each market it operates in. Where should it try to raise prices? In the market that's least price sensitive. Consider a young radiologist, Dr. Almon, who is starting a practice in Los Angeles. He works at a posh Beverly Hills clinic on Tuesday and Thursday, seeing a few patients. On Monday, Wednesday, and Friday, he works in a crowded clinic in east L.A., seeing dozens of patients. Initially, he charges $25 to read a routine x-ray in both places. He finds that raising prices to $35 makes little difference in Beverly Hills, but he loses half his clients in east L.A. when he does this. He can increase the profits of his overall practice by raising prices in Beverly Hills to $45 and lowering prices to $20 in east L.A. He's just as busy as he was before, but he's making more money.

Charging different prices in different markets is a standard strategy that both business and nonprofit organizations use to increase revenues. The practice is known as **price discrimination.** Hot dogs cost more in baseball parks, clothes cost less if you work in the store (e.g., being there gives you great information and increases price sensitivity, and you may get an employee discount), and scholarships reduce the price of a college education for students who have the most choices (i.e., athletes and scholars). Price discrimination is socially accepted and widespread in medicine. The most common form—charging patients with higher incomes and/or better insurance more than others—has the advantage of appearing socially beneficial and fair. Even the federal government practices price discrimination, making higher-income states pay a higher proportion of Medicaid expenditures.

It seems right to charge less to those who can afford less, but is it? Stores don't sell milk and bread at a discount to people with less money, so why should radiologists or physical therapists discount their services? One major reason is that any attempt to sell bread and milk cheaper would be undercut by people shopping for the best deal: rich people would drive to east L.A. for low-priced groceries.

Why wouldn't people drive from Beverly Hills to east L.A. for the cheaper services at Dr. Almon's east L.A. clinic? Some patients will switch clinics to obtain a lower price, but only a few. Service markets are much easier to separate for purposes of price discrimination than goods markets because the patient actually has to show up at the office to receive services. The patient must find out that the price difference exists and then be willing to go through the hassle of getting to the more distant location.

Dr. Almon can charge more in Beverly Hills than in east L.A. because his patients are less price sensitive there, not because they have higher incomes, can afford more, or deserve to pay more (even though these reasons may count for something as well). He can choose to set prices in each market relative to the price elasticity demand among consumers there. He can raise prices where demand is inelastic and reduce prices where demand is elastic.

Just as firms can use price discrimination based on location, they can also do so based on time. Movies are cheaper in the afternoon than in the evening because customers are more price sensitive then—and they can't transfer the picture to view it later in the evening. Dining out is often less expensive during the week than on Saturday night for the same reason. Some forms of time-based price discrimination are discouraged. For instance, it would be considered highly unethical for a doctor to charge a patient more during an emergency than for similar services on a routine visit, even though it's clear that patients are very price inelastic during a medical emergency.

The frequency with which price discrimination is practiced in medicine was one of the factors that first convinced economists that physicians had a substantial monopoly power, even though there are many physicians competing for patients in every city. (See Chapter 6 for more on physician monopolies.) The evidence that physicians use monopoly power to increase their incomes is well established but tells only a small part of the story because there is even more persuasive evidence that physicians don't behave as profit-maximizing monopolists. Charging lower prices in poor neighborhoods may help increase total revenues, but providing care for free (which many physicians routinely do) is altruistic behavior inconsistent with profit maximization. As noted earlier, physicians also tend not to exploit patients' willingness to pay more during medical emergencies. Even more interesting to many economists is the evidence that for much of the medical care provided in hospitals and doctors' offices every day, demand is inelastic, but prices don't rise. A profit-maximizing firm would keep raising prices in the face of inelastic demand until it reached an elastic portion higher up the demand curve. It is evident that, while demand and supply analysis can tell us a lot about the economics of medicine, it doesn't account for many of the features that make medicine a notable profession with a special place in human society rather than just another way to make money.

2.2.4 Is Price All That Matters?

What does it mean to pay for something? To a politician, it may mean losing some votes or giving up a pet project. To a student going out partying on Sunday night, it may mean a headache and a lower grade on Monday's exam. To someone who wants a driver's license, it may mean hours of anxiety. In each case, something has to be given up to get something else. Economists often use the term *price* to refer to anything one has to give up to get some desirable good in trade. For medical care, it is common to talk about time, pain, and risk of death as prices of treatment.

Services can be allocated to patients through time, pain, and risk just as they can through money. In Canada, where patients don't pay directly for most doctors' services, waiting times have increased. By discouraging those who aren't willing to spend time waiting for care, the number of patients treated is limited just as effectively as it is when price is used to discourage those who aren't willing to pay money for care. An example of allocation by pain is provided by pain clinics that insist on screening patients with an uncomfortable diagnostic procedure known as an electromyelogram (EMG). Patients who aren't willing to undergo an EMG can't obtain clinic services.

An important difference between a money price and a time price or a "pain price" is that the money price is paid to the other party in the transaction. If an arm brace costs $10, the store receives $10. In contrast, if a patient has to wait six extra hours in the waiting room, no one receives those six hours. If an EMG is painful, a patient's willingness to undergo it may convince the therapist that the patient needs services, but the pain doesn't yield pleasure to the therapist. The patient's time and pain is a personal cost that doesn't directly benefit the provider. Economists tend to favor money prices as a way to allocate goods and services because they entail fewer such "deadweight" costs.

SELF-CHECK

- Explain the difference between **marginal revenue** and **marginal cost.**
- Describe the characteristics of a demand curve that is **price elastic,** a demand curve that is **price inelastic,** and a demand curve that is **unit elastic.**
- Explain the concept of **price discrimination.**

2.3 Supply, Demand, and Market Prices

Competitive markets use prices to allocate goods and services to consumers who want them the most (in monetary terms) and to pay suppliers for producing those goods and services. Most real markets, and virtually all medical markets, depart to some degree from the model of perfect competition. Nevertheless, it's a useful starting point for analyzing the economic forces that shape human transactions, even when time, pain, uncertainty, and tradition cause substantial deviations from the simple model.

The demand curve has been discussed at length. But what about supply? Again, it's vital to note that the economic concept of supply is always a supply curve. A **supply curve** is a graph (or schedule) that shows the total quantity of a good that sellers wish to sell at each price. This curve emphasizes change, allowing us to focus on a range of responses indicating how firms will vary the amount supplied as the price increases or decreases. Just as the demand curve is a marginal benefit curve, showing how people in the market are willing to pay for one more unit of a good, under perfect competition, the supply curve is a marginal cost curve, showing how much must be paid to induce firms in the market to supply one more unit.

In most competitive markets with which you are familiar, firms set whatever price they choose, and consumers decide how much to buy. Firms experiment with different prices to maximize profits, just as consumers experiment with different patterns of consumption to maximize the benefits they can obtain within their budgets. Price is the point at which all the stresses are met and balanced. The decision for a profit-maximizing firm is quite simple: Sell more (lower your price) if the marginal revenue (MR) obtained is greater than the marginal cost (MC) of providing the goods. The firm will continue to lower price until the gains from additional sales are offset by the costs—that is, where MR = MC.

In medical care, hospitals and doctors are often not allowed to set their own prices but must accept prices that are set administratively by government or insurance companies. Patients buy what is needed (i.e., what sellers think patients should buy) and don't pay any price directly; rather, they pay some amount indirectly through taxes and premiums. The transactions are highly regulated, and some of the funding comes from grants and philanthropy rather than sales.

FOR EXAMPLE

Medicare Limits What Physicians Can Charge

The 1989 Omnibus Budget Reconciliation Act (OBRA 89) included physician payment reform, part of which put limits on how much physicians can charge Medicare patients for services covered by Medicare. Physicians are permitted to charge only 15 percent more than the Medicare-approved amount. In northeastern Michigan, the Medicare-approved amount of a lowest-level office visit (sometimes called a nurse visit) is $20.63. The limit a physician can charge a Medicare patient for this service is $23.72. In comparison, a physician practicing in northeast Michigan would typically charge $29 for this service.

SELF-CHECK

- Briefly explain the role of prices in competitive markets.
- What is the purpose of a **supply curve**?

SUMMARY

The concept of need—a professional assessment of the quantity of services required, regardless of price or other trade-offs—is appropriate for individual decision making when price, cost, budget constraints, and other monetary factors have already been decided. The concept of demand is more useful for decisions that balance the need for medical care with other goods or allocating care among groups of people.

The demand curve is a marginal benefit curve that traces how much each additional unit of service is worth. Much of the total value of health care may lie in only a few units of service, targeted to those most in need, with many subsequent services provided to a large number of people for little additional benefit. Some things that are essential to health (e.g., nutrition, exercise, preventive care) are plentiful and trade at a very low price in the market, while some services that make only a marginal contribution but are scarce (e.g., neurosurgery for someone who is already seriously ill) command a high price.

Marginal revenue, the additional revenue that can be obtained by selling one more unit, is always less than average revenue (price) because a firm must reduce the price of goods to sell more. A firm facing elastic demand that raises prices will see total revenues fall because the quantity demanded will fall by a larger percentage than the increase in price. A firm facing inelastic demand can raise prices and increase revenues because there will be only a small decrease in quantity sold.

For manufactured goods, supply and demand are clearly separated, with interaction occurring only through market forces. For health care, several factors make such a separation difficult: a strong physician–patient relationship of trust, the difficulty of making choices and obtaining information about life-and-death matters, and pervasive uncertainty. The tools of supply and demand analysis must be used with care and sometimes must be modified to conform to the realities of the health care market.

KEY TERMS

Demand	The relationship between price and quantity.
Demand curve	A graph that shows the total quantity of a good that buyers wish to buy at each price.
Firm demand	The demand for each firm in a particular market.
Individual demand	The demand by each individual in a particular market.
Law of demand	A concept stating that the quantity demanded will always fall as prices rise (assuming that all other conditions remain constant).
Marginal benefit	The increase in total benefit that results from adding one additional unit.
Marginal cost	The increase in total cost caused by the production of one more unit.
Market demand	The sum of all individuals in a market.
Marginal revenue	The change in a firm's total revenue that results from a one-unit change in sales.
Need	A professional determination of the quantity that should be supplied.
Price discrimination	The practice of charging different prices in different markets to increase revenues.
Price elastic	Demand in which the quantity demanded changes a lot for any small change in price.
Price inelastic	Demand in which the quantity demanded barely budges when the price rises.
Supply curve	A graph showing the total quantity of a good that sellers which to sell at each price.
Unit elastic	Demand in which the percentage change in price is equal to the percentage change in quantity.

ASSESS YOUR UNDERSTANDING

Go to www.wiley.com/college/getzen to assess your knowledge of how economists evaluate health care.
Measure your learning by comparing pre-test and post-test results.

Summary Questions

1. Demand is the relationship between price and quantity. True or False?
2. Doctors are more concerned with demand; economists more are concerned with need. True or False?
3. The demand curve:
   (a) always slopes downward.
   (b) shows the total quantity of a good that buyers wish to buy at each price.
   (c) is a marginal benefit curve.
   (d) always slopes downward, shows the total quantity of a good that buyers wish to buy at each price, and is a marginal benefit curve.
4. Health can be seen as derived demand for medical care. True or False?
5. Firm demand is:
   (a) the sum of all individuals in a market.
   (b) demand by one firm in a market.
   (c) the sum of all firms in a market.
   (d) an individual in a market.
6. Marginal revenue is the change in a firm's total revenue that results from a one-unit change in sales. True or False?
7. Once marginal revenue is more than marginal cost, the sale is a loser, even if the price is still above cost. True or False?
8. A demand curve indicating that the quantity demanded will change a lot for any small change in price is said to be:
   (a) price elastic.
   (b) price inelastic.
   (c) unit elastic.
   (d) price inelastic and unit elastic.
9. Firms facing _____ find that total revenue goes down when they sell more units.
   (a) elastic demand
   (b) inelastic demand
   (c) unit elastic demand
   (d) elasticity

10. It is illegal for physicians to engage in price discrimination. True or False?

11. Medical services can be allocated to patients through:
    (a) time.
    (b) pain.
    (b) pain and money.
    (d) time, pain, and money.

12. Medical markets are perfectly competitive marketplaces, in which prices are used to allocate goods and services to consumers who want them the most (in monetary terms) and to pay suppliers for producing those goods and services. True or False?

Review Questions

1. What is the difference between a patient's demand for physical therapy and his or her need for physical therapy?

2. In the year 2007, in Anytown, suppose that one person is willing to pay $1,000 for relief from hay fever; another two are willing to pay $350; about five more are willing to pay $50; one is willing to pay $40; one is willing to pay $35; one each is willing to pay $34, $32, $30, and $28; about a dozen are willing to pay $10; four are willing to pay $5; and half of the rest of the town (another 75 people) are willing to pay $1.
   (a) Draw the demand curve for hay fever relief in Anytown.
   (b) What is the potential total benefit from relief of hay fever if the medication is provided to everyone who asks? To everyone willing to pay $35 or more?
   (c) If the price of hay fever medication is $20, what is the quantity demanded? What is the quantity demanded if the price is $50? If it is $5?

3. In what units is Prozac purchased? What are the units in which psychotherapy is purchased?

4. If the price of a postoperative follow-up visit is reduced from $40 to $30, the number of patients returning for follow-up increases from 18 to 25.
   (a) What is the marginal revenue (MR)?
   (b) What is the price elasticity?
   (c) What would your estimate of MR and price elasticity be if the quantity demanded moved from 18 to 20 (instead of 25)?

5. Which are more elastic, dental visits or visits for the treatment of diabetes? Physician visits or hospital days? Psychiatry visits or orthopedics visits? Why?

6. If the price of office visits increases from $20 to $22, and the number of visits per family per year declines from 12 to 10, what is the price elasticity of demand?

7. Dr. Old requires that all services be paid for at the time of treatment, in cash. If he decides to allow patients to pay with credit cards, will this increase or decrease demand? Will it increase or decrease price elasticity?

8. Which is more price elastic, the demand for Cesarean sections or the demand for vaginal deliveries? Why?

Applying This Chapter

1. Ask four people what they have paid for (a) a drug, (b) minor care (e.g., an office visit, a physical therapy session), and (c) major care (e.g., hospitalization, a surgical procedure). Find out how price sensitive they think they were for each. Do they think that everyone else receiving similar care paid the same amount as they did?

2. Our Lady of Dollars Hospital needs to increase total revenue to build a new chapel. The hospital wants to keep the total number of patients in each service area (e.g., emergency room, obstetrics ward, operating room, laboratory, cardiac ward) the same. How can the hospital use price discrimination to achieve this objective?

3. If people are healthier, will their demand for medical care increase or decrease? (Be careful; this is a tricky question. Consider some analogies: If people become more coordinated, will their demand for athletic equipment rise or fall? If they become more knowledgeable, what happens to their demand for books?)

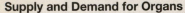

YOU TRY IT

Supply and Demand for Organs

Each year, thousands of people die while on the waiting list for donor organs. Aside from the high cost of organ transplants, the most pressing constraint is the number of donors. Because organ donation arrangements can easily be made when getting a driver's license, write a brief paper discussing why you think such an organ shortage exists. If people had a financial incentive, such as a reduction in the cost of their driver's license, do you think more people would agree to donate their organs? Why or why not?

What's It Worth to You?

People sometimes criticize British and Canadian health care because patients must often wait for tests that are available quickly in the United States. What those critics often fail to mention is that health care costs in Britain and Canada are much lower than those in the United States. Is the delay worth $1,000 in savings each year? $10,000? Prepare a brief report comparing the U.S. health care system to that of Canada. What are the pros and cons of each system?

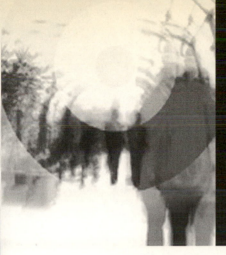

3

COST–BENEFIT AND COST-EFFECTIVENESS ANALYSIS
Making the Most of Limited Funds

Starting Point

Go to www.wiley.com/college/getzen to assess your knowledge of cost–benefit analysis and cost-effectiveness analysis.
Determine where you need to concentrate your effort.

What You'll Learn in This Chapter

▲ How to use cost–benefit analysis (CBA) as a means of determining the best use of limited funds
▲ What the three major types of medical benefits are and how they are valued
▲ What the four major types of medical costs are and how they are valued
▲ How economists measure the value people place on life
▲ The importance of perspective when conducting a CBA

After Studying This Chapter, You'll Be Able To

▲ Formulate health policy decisions, using CBA
▲ Assess the opportunity costs of policy decisions
▲ Calculate the expected value of uncertain benefits
▲ Evaluate potential benefits of a policy decision
▲ Evaluate potential costs of a policy decision

INTRODUCTION

Health economist Bengt Jönssen said that the purpose of health economics is to save lives. He was referring specifically to the use of economic evaluation tools to determine the most appropriate allocation of resources to health and among competing health applications. The tools of the health economist for this purpose are primarily cost–benefit analysis (CBA) and cost-effectiveness analysis (CEA). CBA comes closest to replicating the logic of the market, by considering a potential use of resources and asking, "Is this worth what it costs?" Unless the decision is necessarily "all or nothing," CBA is also used to answer "How much is enough?"

To undertake a CBA, you must first know the value of costs and the benefits. The economic concepts of opportunity cost and marginal analysis come into play. The appropriate measure of economic cost is opportunity cost, determined by the highest-valued alternative given up when a decision is made. Marginal analysis is used to determine the value of one more unit of service. The estimate of what's likely to happen is called the expected value.

Health care has three primary benefits to people, the most obvious of which is our health. But how do you put a value on health? On a life? Everything we do, every decision we make, is a judgment about value. When people act, they show by that act that they think the gains are worth more than the costs. Economists look at decisions patients and physicians have made in the past to estimate the value they place on health outcomes.

3.1 Cost–Benefit Analysis

> It is best to think of the cost–benefit approach as a way of organizing thought rather than as a substitute for it.
>
> —Michael Drummond[1]

Every choice involves a trade-off, giving up something to get something else. People make these sorts of decisions every day. **Cost–benefit analysis (CBA)** is a set of techniques for assisting in the making of decisions that translates all relevant concerns into market (dollar) terms. It's a way of formalizing the decision-making process—the balancing of pros and cons, of advantages and disadvantages. Insurance companies and governments use CBA all the time to determine how to spend their limited funds on the wide variety of health care goods and services on the market. CBA is also used for public decision making to protect the interests of children, homeless people, people with mental illness, and other individuals who aren't able to make decisions in their own best interests.

Every decision—whether in the market, the public sector, or the family—involves a form of CBA. Usually, the consideration of costs and benefits is informal and internal, so we aren't even aware we're doing it. When this happens, we can only observe the behavior that results from this internal weighing of costs and benefits.

Cost-effectiveness analysis (CEA) is a form of CBA that analyzes the cost side of the decision but doesn't translate the benefits (e.g., lives saved, illnesses prevented, a patient's additional days of activity, the extent to which a patient's sight is restored) into dollars. CEA is used in decision making to determine which alternatives are cheaper yet effective. A study evaluating whether hypertension screening, nutrition counseling, medication, or cardiac bypass surgery would provide the most additional years of life expectancy for each dollar spent is a cost-effectiveness study. A study evaluating whether cardiac bypass surgery adds a sufficient number of years to life expectancy to justify its cost is a cost–benefit study.

3.1.1 An Everyday Example: Knee Injury

Life, and the health care system in particular, confronts us with difficult choices every day. Is it worth taking three hours, and possibly paying $400, to go to the emergency room (ER) so that a doctor can examine the throbbing knee you injured playing soccer? Because pain makes it difficult to think, it can be helpful to make a list of the pros and cons of each alternative, as follows:

Pros (Go to ER)	Cons (Don't Go to ER)
It might stop the pain.	It might cost up to $400.
It could prevent long-term injury.	It will take at least 2 and maybe 4 hours.
I will feel stupid if something was wrong and I didn't go.	Even if the injury is serious, surgery could make it worse.
I can't get any work done anyway, while I sit here worrying.	My friends on the team will think I'm a wimp.

If you believe that the benefits of going to the ER outweigh the costs, you'll go to the ER. Even if you don't write down the pros and cons, a similar sort of balancing takes place inside your head. CBA is the explicit and formal presentation of that mental balance sheet.

Economics doesn't provide answers or make it easier to take bitter medicine, but it does clarify how to ask the questions to make decisions more rational and more consistent. First, you must identify the benefits and costs. Then, you must quantify each benefit and cost as accurately as possible, given what's known about the situation. For example, it's impossible to determine exactly how long an ER visit will take, but you might think a range of two to four hours is likely. You must then place a value on each benefit and cost. A balance sheet can be added up only if every line is expressed in the same terms, usually dollars. It doesn't make much sense to compare a benefit of $50 with a cost of ¥910 (yen), and there's no rule for determining how many hours of pain are worth avoiding a permanent limp; however, it's clear that a cost of $500 is less than a benefit of $1,000.

Let's use this example of a knee injury to better understand CBA:

▲ You expect that the direct dollar cost of the ER visit (after insurance) is about $80, and you expect to wait for three hours. Because you could have been at a job where you were making $7 per hour, we can add $21 for the *opportunity cost* of the waiting time. (We consider the fact that surgery could make you worse instead of better in Section 3.1.2.)

▲ Feeling that you aren't as tough as other members of the team seems silly, but it's worth something. How much? Suppose you were willing to pay $40 for crutches you really didn't need, just to keep your friends from making fun of you. This $40 reveals your dollar value of avoiding a "wimp" label.

▲ Adding all the items, your estimated total cost for going to the ER is $80 (charges) + $21 (time) + $40 (fear of being called "wimp") = $141. (See Table 3-1.)

Table 3-1: Knee Injury as an Example of CBA

Scenario: I injured my knee playing soccer this afternoon. I called and got an appointment to go to the orthopedics/sports medicine clinic in ten days, next Thursday. However, my knee has now begun to hurt a lot and I wonder if I should go to the emergency room (ER) right away.

CONS (don't go)		
The ER visit will cost $50, $100, or more. (Direct personal cost; ignores cost to insurance)	Average =	$80
I will have to wait for at least 2 and maybe up to 4 hours. (Opportunity cost)	3 hours × $7 =	$21
My buddies on the team will think I am a wimp. (Willingness to pay $40 for crutches just to look good)	Willingness to pay =	$40
Even if the injury is serious, surgery could make it worse. (The issue is treatment today vs. Thursday, rather than treatment vs. no treatment, so only incremental costs count.)	Sunk cost =	$0
	Total cost =	$141

Table 3-1: *(continued)*

PROS (go to ER now)		
It might stop the pain. (Pills stop pain with certainty; going to the ER gives just a 1-in-3 chance)	$150 \times 1/3 =$	$50
It could prevent long-term injury. (WTP $50,000 for knee surgery, 1/200 chance, discount 7 years @ 5%)	$50,000 \times 1/200 \times .71 =$	$178
I will feel stupid if something was wrong and I did not go. ("Worried well" WTP for regular office visit)	Willingness to pay =	$20
I can't get any work done anyway while I sit here worrying about it. (Time has same $ value for benefits and costs)	6 hours $\times$ $7 =	$42
	Total benefits =	**$290**

Observed behavior just gives us a lower bound that benefits exceed costs (>$141). Another observation, that I did not go when the wait was 5 hours and ER charges were $250, could provide an upper bound as well (<$325).

What's it worth to stop the pain? Suppose that instead of going to the ER, you call the clinic and ask that someone phone in a prescription to the pharmacy. How much would you be willing to pay (WTP) to get the prescription rather than endure the pain? It's difficult to study, and it may be impossible to work, when you are in pain. It's also difficult to sleep or even enjoy watching television. You might be willing to pay as much as $150 for relief from pain. This WTP is the correct measure of the value of benefit received.

You may not realize it, but every decision you make can be quantified by using a CBA. Your action (in this case, going to the ER) reveals that your estimate of total benefits outweighs your estimate of total costs. You don't find yourself being wheeled into the ER, saying "I'm happy because I've got a projected consumer surplus from coming here." You just do it, or you don't. An economist considers your choice the true indicator of your personal and largely unconscious CBA.

3.1.2 Opportunity Cost: Looking at Alternatives

Growing old is a pretty lousy thing to have happen to you, until you consider the alternative.

—George Burns

> ### FOR EXAMPLE
>
> #### How CEA Has Had an Impact on Heart Attack Treatment
>
> CBA and CEA can play a large role in the development and adoption of medical innovations. They can help determine whether new therapies offer good value for the money. Consider the application of CEA to two different drug therapies for heart attack patients: low-tech bacterial enzyme streptokinase, which costs about $300 per treatment, and high-tech genetically engineered recombinant t-PA (tissue plasminogen activator), costing about $2,200. A large patient trial showed that patients given t-PA had a 1 percent better chance of still being alive within 30 days of receiving the drug than patients who were administered streptokinase. CEA based on the results of this study and the cost of the drugs showed that t-PA provided an extra life year at an estimated cost of $33,000, so t-PA was judged to be an economically attractive therapy. Prior to the trial, t-PA had had a 55 percent U.S. market share, with streptokinase having the remaining share. After the trial, recombinant t-PA and similar drugs increased their market share to 96 percent, leaving streptokinase with just 4 percent. It is estimated that this decision adds about $627 million annually to the national health budget.[2]

Costs and benefits don't have value in and of themselves; instead, their value depends on the alternatives. When a patient is diagnosed with pancreatic cancer or human immunodeficiency virus (HIV) infection, all the alternatives are pretty bad, but four years of life might be a lot better than two years of life, and the ability to play tennis a lot better than continuous nausea. On the other hand, all the alternatives facing a student graduating with a master's degree in medical information systems may look good, yet living in San Francisco might be more appealing than living in San Antonio, and the possibility of moving up into corporate systems management within a national health care chain might be more appealing than remaining the director of records in a small community hospital.

To make a decision, the relevant question isn't how good or how bad the situation is, but rather: What are the options? The appropriate measure of economic cost is **opportunity cost,** which is defined as what must be given up in order to do or obtain something; in other words, an opportunity cost is the highest-valued alternative given up when a decision is made. In choosing a $45,000 job in San Francisco, the graduating student who gives up a $50,000 job in San Antonio is "paying" an opportunity cost of $5,000. The cost of not taking an experimental drug to treat HIV is the forgone chance of living an extra two years or feeling better.

3.1.3 Expected Value: What's Likely to Happen

The goal of using CBA is to make a decision in which benefits (B) are greater than costs (C), or B > C. But suppose benefits or costs are uncertain. For example, 20 milligrams of methotrexate might cure you, but it might also leave you in the same condition. Surgery may cause you to miss one or five weeks of work. You must make a choice, based on the best possible information or the best guess, long before you know the outcome of the treatment. The estimate of what's likely to happen is called the **expected value.** If the analysis concerns many people, the expected value is just the average.[3] For a single person facing an event that either will or will not happen, the expected value is the value of that event (benefit or cost) multiplied by the probability that the event will occur:

$$\text{Expected Value of Z} = (\text{Probability Z will occur}) \times (\text{Value of Z})$$

A patient receiving chemotherapy who has a 70 percent chance of death may live, while a patient receiving surgery who has a 20 percent chance of death may die. Yet the treatment decision must be made in advance and should maximize expected outcomes in the face of this uncertainty. Of course, after the fact, the patient's family may wish that they had done something differently. To say that the optimal choice sometimes turns out worse is simply to recognize that life is full of risks. CBA is based on the best available estimate of what's likely to happen. It may be a guess or, preferably, based on well-designed studies. "I don't know" and "I need more information" are not valid responses because a decision is going to be made, regardless of how much is known. The job of the analyst is to get the best estimate and to explain the alternatives. An option is chosen if:

$$(\text{Probability of Gain}) \times (\text{Benefit}) > (\text{Probability of Loss}) \times (\text{Cost})$$

Notice how this formula separates the uncertainties (probability of gain/loss) and the values (benefit/cost) that are involved in the decision-making process. Judgmental advice, such as "it's better to get the operation and risk dying than not get the operation and remain impaired," jumbles probabilities and values together, hiding information and increasing the difficulty of communication. Such jumbled statements don't make the patient think about how much it's worth to live impaired compared with dying or to consider specifically the percentage probability of partial recovery or death. Clearly identifying the benefits, costs, and risks provides a better ground for shared decision making between the physician and patient.

3.1.4 Maximization: Finding the Optimum

More medical care usually makes people healthier. Physicians, rightly, concentrate on benefits as opposed to costs and often try to do as much as possible. However, people who use more resources to obtain medical care have fewer resources available for food, entertainment, housing, and other goods they want. Economics is concerned with trade-offs. What's the appropriate balance between medical care and other goods? How many doctors, nurses, and hospitals should there be? Economists insist that both costs and benefits be considered in making a decision. Economists also approach the decision differently from most physicians, asking not what's right or wrong but whether a little more or a little less would make things better or worse. An economist studies the changes in costs and benefits to optimize, moving toward a maximum net benefit in small steps.

To estimate the maximum net benefit of a decision, economists must ignore some of the complexity of medical conditions and frame the issues in terms of dollars. Prices, costs, taxes, bids, contracts, and so on are the language used by economists to communicate human desires and limitations. The task of CBA is to make that language clear and applicable to the situation at hand and to present the essential facts and trade-offs in a way that is easily understood by physicians, the public, and politicians.

Defining the Margin: What's the Decision?

The term **margin,** much favored by economists, means "the change in *xxxx*." The decision being made determines the margin. Sometimes, the margin is how many patients should be admitted for treatment. Economists use the following rule to simplify decision making: *The decision between alternatives depends only on factors that change.* Therefore, it's not necessary to examine the full range of possibilities but only to look at doing a little more or a little less (i.e., to consider changes at the margin) to determine whether a decision is optimal. If the marginal benefits of a therapy are greater than the marginal costs, more should be done. If marginal costs are greater than marginal benefits, less should be done.

Declining Marginal Benefits

The **marginal benefit** is the value to consumers of one more unit of service. People are less willing to pay for additional care as more and more is provided; therefore, the curve slopes downward. It looks like the demand curve; in fact, the marginal benefit curve and the demand curve are the same. To understand why, remember that the demand curve is a graph showing what quantity a consumer will buy at different prices. As long as the marginal benefit exceeds the price, consumers will continue to buy. The quantity at which they have had enough and stop buying is the quantity at which the marginal benefit has fallen to the point where it's just equal to price. The quantity bought at a price, $P, is the same as the quantity at which the marginal benefit is $P; the marginal benefit (stated in dollars) of one more unit for a consumer who already has quantity Q is the same as the price the consumer is willing to pay for one more unit.

Even though society benefits from having more medical care, the additional increment of benefit from each additional hospital day or doctor visit tends to become smaller and smaller as more services are provided. There are two reasons for declining marginal benefits:

▲ As more treatments are provided, they are given to less and less severely ill people, who are less likely to benefit. In ERs and Army field hospitals, the process of giving treatment first to those in most dire need of medical help is known as triage, and although it doesn't use all the mathematics or technical terminology, triage operates on the same principles as economic maximization.

▲ For any single person, the benefit from having one more medical service tends to decline as more and more services are used, just as the benefit from consuming additional pizzas or sodas or pretzels per day tends to decline as the second, third, and fourth are consumed.

In Figure 3-1, the fact that more medical care will improve health is shown by the rise in the total benefit curve. The fact that marginal benefits become smaller as more and more services are used shows up as a lower rate of increase, reducing the slope to make it flatter.

Maximizing Costs vs. Benefits

Costs are the other side of the decision from benefits. Every additional unit of treatment adds to total costs. After startup, the marginal cost of producing another unit of medical treatment is usually constant or rising as the total number of treatments increases. Each additional hospital bed tends to cost as much as or more than the last one, and each additional nurse who is hired expects to get paid as much as or more than the last one hired. At some point, the additional costs of extra treatments will outweigh the additional benefits. An **optimum** is where the net gain (i.e., benefits − costs) is largest.

If the additional (marginal) benefit from providing one more treatment is larger than the additional (marginal) cost, providing more treatments will make society better off. If the additional benefit from providing one more treatment is smaller than the additional cost, providing more treatments will make society worse off. At the optimum, the additional benefit will just offset the marginal cost; therefore, there is no change in net gains (i.e., marginal gain = 0).

3.1.5 Average, Total, and Marginal Costs for Society

A society that uses average benefits and average costs to make medical decisions usually ends up providing far too much medical care. To see why, consider the following example. Suppose that a new operating suite for cardiac surgery is built. The first operation will be performed on the patient who needs it the most, one who gets a major reduction in mortality (i.e., risk of dying from cardiac disease), perhaps 50 percent. The next patient selected will not need the operation as much and will obtain a significant, although smaller, reduction in mortality, perhaps 40 percent. The third and fourth patients will obtain mortality reductions of 30 percent and 20 percent, respectively. At this point, the operating suite is full. How much benefit would be obtained by increasing capacity so that a fifth patient could be treated? If expansion allowed a fifth patient, whose mortality will be reduced

Figure 3-1

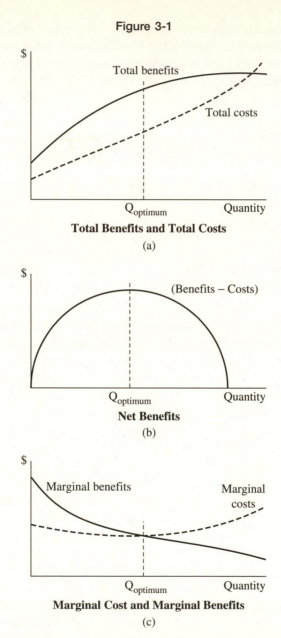

Total Benefits and Total Costs

(a)

Net Benefits

(b)

Marginal Cost and Marginal Benefits

(c)

Total, net, and marginal benefits and costs.

by 10 percent, to be treated, the marginal benefit is 10 percent. However, the average mortality reduction is much greater (50% + 40% + 30% + 20% + 10% ÷ 5 = 30%), making the expansion appear much more worthwhile than it really is. Whether that extra patient is scheduled to come in first or last does not matter. The relevant issue is that the more limited operating room space would be given to the patients who need the operation most; therefore, the marginal benefit of adding one more patient (10 percent gain) is less than the average benefit (30 percent gain). In other words, the overall average gain per patient treated is a poor indicator of the marginal benefit to be gained by treating one more patient.

SELF-CHECK

- Explain the difference between **CBA** and **CEA** and give an example of each.
- Explain the role of **expected value** in CBA.
- Describe where the **optimum** is located on a graph.

3.2 Measuring Benefits

In any CBA, you must identify and quantify both the benefits and the costs. For most medical programs, there are three major types of benefits:

▲ Health
▲ Productivity
▲ Reductions in future medical costs

3.2.1 Health

Better health is the most direct and important gain from medical care. Yet it's often difficult to determine how much change in health status actually results from medical care and how much results from waiting for things to heal, random variation, nutrition, and other factors. If a cancer patient lives eight months, is that six months longer than the patient would have lived without treatment, or is it four months fewer because chemotherapy is so toxic? Such obstacles to valid measurement of the effects of treatment usually limit CBA to studies of large groups of patients where statistics can be used to estimate average effects. After the effect of therapy is measured, the problem of placing a dollar value on the improvement in health must be faced. If faster treatment can give the average heart-attack victim four more months of life, is that worth $1,000? $100,000? $1,000,000? Or perhaps $19.95?

Most people would agree that gaining an extra year of life is worth more than $1,000 and less than $1,000,000. Deciding exactly where, within that range, the appropriate value lies is crucial in determining whether it's worth spending $50 million to upgrade the 911 emergency telephone system in order to treat people more quickly. Some innovative techniques for measuring the value of life are explored in Section 3.4, but it's important to recognize now how difficult and ambiguous the measurement process is. Most health care provides more subtle gains (e.g., physical therapy improves mobility, medication lessens the pain from a headache), which are even more difficult to measure in dollar terms.

A significant number of all visits to the doctor, perhaps as many as half, don't make a difference in health status. Either the symptoms that led people to seek care weren't caused by anything serious or the condition was such that medical care couldn't change the course of the disease. These visits still provide a benefit in the form of subjective feelings of care, reassurance, and social support, but they don't provide a cure. The benefits of caring are often left uncounted because they are small relative to the gains from a dramatic cure. However, when you consider how many more people obtain the benefits of caring from medical professionals than obtain large health gains from cures, the importance of the subjective feelings of care, reassurance, and social support look quite large.

3.2.2 Productivity

The earliest economists weren't as interested in the value of health itself as they were in how much a healthier workforce could contribute to the economy. When modern economists turned their attention to evaluating health programs in the 1950s and 1960s, the difficulty of directly measuring and valuing health improvements led them to consider increases in earnings due to greater life expectancy and reduced sick days as substitute measures. Such gains can be measured with precision and are easy to obtain from existing labor statistics. These advantages made earnings the primary measure of benefits in CBA for the next 20 years, but now earnings are considered an inadequate measure. Are women's lives worth less than men's because women's earnings are lower on average? Are elderly people worthless when they stop working? Contributions to society through the labor market are a clear benefit of health care but by themselves form an incomplete and biased measure.

3.2.3 Reductions in Future Medical Costs

Many diseases are less costly to treat if care is given early and if treatment is done correctly the first time. Vaccination now can prevent hospitalization in the future. Better infection control allows patients to be discharged from the hospital sooner. Yet good medical care isn't always, or even usually, cheaper. The least expensive way to treat heart attacks is never to attempt resuscitation. A transplant may mean 10 more years of life, but it will certainly mean hundreds of thousands of dollars in additional care. Reductions in cost, while not insignificant, can hardly constitute the primary justification for medical care.

FOR EXAMPLE

Health Care Value

Researchers at Harvard University and the University of Michigan measured the cost of medical care that extends the average person's life by one year. They calculated that Americans of all ages spent an average of $19,900 on medical care for each extra year of life expectancy gained from 1960 to 2000.[4] The nearly $20,000 spent for each extra year of life—when averaged over 40 years—would be widely considered a reasonable value. Many public and private insurers routinely pay for treatments that cost up to roughly $100,000 for each additional year of life.

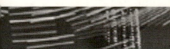

SELF-CHECK

- List three primary benefits of medical care.
- Identify one of the shortcomings of using productivity to define the benefit of medical care.
- Identify one of the shortcomings of using reductions in cost to define the benefit of medical care.

3.3 Measuring Costs

When determining the costs involved in any CBA, economists typically consider the following types of medical costs:

▲ Medical care and administration
▲ Follow-up and treatment
▲ Time and pain of the patient and his or her family
▲ Provider time and inconvenience

3.3.1 Medical Care and Administration: Charges vs. Costs

Unlike prices for other goods, most medical prices are overstated to cover related expenses for education, research, community outreach, and care for patients who can't pay. Health economists use three methods to determine the direct costs of medical care[5]:

▲ **Adjusted charges:** Adjusted charges for U.S. hospital care are usually estimated by multiplying billed charges by the Medicare cost-to-charge ratio (see Section 8.1). The actual cost of hospital services is, on average, only about 60 percent of billed charges. The cost of some services, such as laboratory work and drugs, may be as little as 15 percent of charges, while for ER and obstetric services, actual costs may be as much as 125 percent of billed charges. Per-unit costs are always estimates and are subject to interpretation.

▲ **Cost accounting:** Cost accounting for CBA uses the same principles as job costing in other industries. Resources (e.g., nursing hours, technician time, space, supplies) are estimated from direct observation, and their costs are estimated using prevailing wages, prices, and so on. An overhead charge is then applied for administration, utilities, and other central services.

▲ **Extrapolation from comparable services:** Extrapolation from comparable services is used when charges aren't available and cost accounting is too time-consuming. For example, the cost of keeping patients in the hospital when they need only custodial care could be extrapolated from the cost of a day in a nursing home.

3.3.2 Follow-up and Treatment

While direct costs are almost always counted when determining the price of medical care, most medical care creates secondary treatment costs, which aren't always counted. In screening for colon cancer, for example, the largest cost might not be the screening test itself but the additional laboratory work done on those who never had the disease but whose initial tests indicated a false positive. Similarly, the surgical cost of a knee operation for a 70-year-old widower may be much less than the cost of postoperative admission to a nursing home for weeks of recovery because he can't climb the stairs of his apartment. With surgery, it's usually necessary to include as a cost the possibility of serious complications and death, which are worse than the condition being treated. The point is that most medical care (and other human attempts to do good) involves many secondary or unintended effects that must be included to ensure that the cost accounting is comprehensive.

3.3.3 Time and Pain of Patient and Family

The time patients lose and the pain they suffer often outweigh direct medical costs. It's common to value patient time at the average wage rate for all employed workers. Pain, suffering, anxiety, and death are most appropriately valued according to a person's willingness to pay. An economist doing a CBA might not consider a particular patient's point of view and his or her specific pain and time costs, which could explain why people don't take advantage of many beneficial treatments.

3.3.4 Provider Time and Inconvenience

Some medical activities aren't undertaken because providers aren't compensated for their time and inconvenience. For example, while there is a tremendous need for organ donations, the physicians who must obtain the families' consent are the ER doctors, neurosurgeons, and internists present at death who find it burdensome to speak with the families and try to get them to agree to donate their loved ones' organs. Taking time to explain the issues, dealing with emotional distress, and facing frequent refusals are costs for which they obtain no direct benefits. Such "hassle costs" are a disincentive that greatly reduces the number of organs made available for transplant. Similarly, the requirement that every hospital admission or referral to a specialist be documented imposes a hassle cost on the primary physician and leads, predictably, to a lower number of hospital days and specialist referrals. This reduction in services may make it look as if managed care plans ration the number of services to reduce costs and make profits. However, it's important to remember that the services forgone are those that the patient's physician was unwilling to write a letter or make a phone call to support and, therefore, are unlikely to have been considered critically important.

FOR EXAMPLE

The 80-20 Rule in Health Care

For years, management consultants have called attention to the 80-20 rule of business: that 20 percent of something will lead to 80 percent of something else. For example, 20 percent of customer complaints will consume 80 percent of your time in resolving complains, or 20 percent of your clients will generate 80 percent of your income. With health care costs, the same model holds true, but it is closer to a 90-10 rule: Fewer than a dozen disease categories consume 80 to 89 percent of all health-related costs. These diseases include heart disease and atherosclerosis (i.e., hardening of the arteries), cancer, stroke, pneumonia and influenza, chronic obstructive lung disease, accidents, diabetes, septicemia (blood poisoning), and kidney disease.

3.4 The Value of Life

> *A man who knows the price of everything and the value of nothing.*
> —Oscar Wilde, definition of a cynic

Isn't health priceless? Some patients and physicians protest that it's impossible to measure the priceless benefits of medical care with the crude yardstick of money. Regardless of whether people think it's right or proper, their actions place a dollar value on human life when they make a decision to provide or deny treatment. If an 87-year-old patient in heart failure is transferred from a nursing home to a cardiac care unit for 10 days, the physician affirms through his or her actions that living another 6 months in a nursing home is worth more than $15,000. Immediately discharging this patient with instructions to take four aspirin every 6 hours affirms the physician's belief that it's not. Our actions place a dollar value on life, even if we choose not to recognize this fact. We live in a world of scarce resources and must make decisions within these limitations. We use money to place a value on (and a limit on the value of) health, whether we wish to or not. Perhaps the most important role of economists in the CBA of health care is pointing out this reality.

The task of putting a value on human life is difficult, to say the least. It's relatively easy to tie specific dollar amounts to goods and services that are traded in the market, such as medical care, work time, drugs, and transportation. The process isn't so clear-cut when it comes to putting a dollar value on life and death or pain and suffering. Because there's no organized market like the New York Stock Exchange for postoperative pain and mortality, economists must find a way to reflect the value that people place on these events. By choosing to buy a car that is less expensive but less safe than another, a person is making an implicit trade between money and the risk of dying. People also make this trade when buying smoke detectors, choosing to accept a more dangerous job assignment for higher pay, refusing to fill a prescription because it costs too much, and flying to a distant facility to get the best possible treatment for a rare disease. In other words, people buy and sell health all the time, but they don't do so in an organized market like the New York Stock Exchange. Economists don't put a value on life or illness;

FOR EXAMPLE

Putting a Price Tag on Life

One attempt to put a dollar value on life arose from the observation that people would run across a highway (at a small but noticeable risk of dying) rather than spend the time going around to a pedestrian overpass. Through observations and questionnaires, it was established that people were willing to accept a risk of .000002 of death to save seven minutes (0.117 hours) of walking. Valuing the people's time by an average wage rate of $20 per hour, the value of life was calculated to be $1,170,000. Other studies have estimated values of life from $800,000 to $6 million.[6]

they measure the value that consumers put on life and illness, as shown by their behavior.

We all must die sometime; therefore, no medical treatment can truly save a life. The real task of medicine is to reduce suffering and anxiety while extending the expected length of life by a few months or years. Economists use the decisions made by state legislatures, families, and patients to show that they value the length and quality of life, which can be changed by medical care, rather than the fact of mortality, which can't.

SELF-CHECK

- Briefly describe the process by which economists measure the value that people put on life.
- List some things you do everyday that can be used to determine how much value you place on your life.

3.5 CBA Perspectives: Patient, Payer, Government, Provider, and Society

How much has to be paid for treatment and how much the treatment is worth depend on whose perspective the cost–benefit analyst is taking. From the patient's point of view, treatment that makes an infectious disease less communicable is of no direct benefit, and medical costs may be relatively unimportant if the person has insurance. From a group perspective, reducing communicability to neighbors is a major benefit of treatment, and hospital charges are important because total insurance premiums for the group as a whole will rise. The narrowest perspective is that of the individual. The broadest perspective is that of society as a whole, including future generations.

Many of the conflicts over health policy arise from the difference in perspectives of different groups. For gay men in San Francisco, many of whom are infected with HIV, research and prevention of AIDS is the most important health issue of our time, while finding drugs to assist in stroke rehabilitation is not.[7] For residents of the Christian Acres Retirement Community in a small Midwestern town, these priorities may be reversed.

3.5.1 Distribution: Whose Costs and Whose Benefits?

In the real world, people may think that they should consider benefits to society as a whole, but they act according to a more immediate calculus of benefits and costs to themselves as individuals and to the groups (e.g., teenagers, steelworkers, residents of Lancaster, Hispanics, senior citizens) to which they belong.

A major barrier to actually implementing a project is raised by the question: What about the losers? Laser surgery for cancer may help thousands of people who wouldn't have survived with the chemotherapy previously used, but it will kill some people who would have lived. Development of a new home health system means that the hospital down the street will find even more of its beds empty and will have to lay off some employees. It is almost impossible to make a major change that hurts no one.

3.5.2 CBA: A Limited Perspective

While CBA is a powerful tool, it can be quite limited. It's impossible to do an economic analysis unless the medical facts are well known. How many people have the disease, what is the cure rate from therapy, and what levels of disability are likely to result? These clinical questions must be answered before any assessment of costs and benefits is attempted. The strength of CBA as a tool lies in its ability to interpret medical issues as choices in a market. Yet to do so, it must force health and human caring into such a rigid economic model that it tends to overemphasize efficiency and may entirely fail to recognize the most important ethical and social values that underlie medical practice. Medicine as a profession rests on the dignity and sanctity of life, a philosophy and practice that resists overt commercialization.

3.5.3 CBA and Public Policy Decision Making

CBA is a way of looking at past behavior, at decisions actually made, so that future decisions can become more clear, rational, and consistent. A decision being made by a single person was used in the knee injury example in Section 3.1.1. In practice, CBA is almost never done for a single case because it takes too long, costs too much, and depends on statistical assumptions that are more valid for large groups. When a single person is involved, that person knows his or her personal costs and willingness to pay better than any analyst. Formal analyses are apt to be most useful under the following circumstances:

▲ Large amounts of resources (e.g., millions or billions of dollars) are involved.

▲ Responsibility for decisions is fragmented (e.g., government agencies, large corporations).

▲ The goals and objectives of different groups are at odds or unclear.

▲ Alternative courses of action are radically different.

▲ The technology and risks underlying each alternative are well understood.

▲ A long time frame is involved.

Is screening blood donors for HIV and hepatitis worthwhile? How often should they be screened, and with what tests? Is inpatient alcohol treatment better than outpatient and, if so, is it enough to justify the increase in costs? The treatment of millions of people costing billions of dollars over many years is involved in these issues, each of which has been given full formal CBA. The test of what's important ultimately lies in the judgment of those who are most affected by the decision. Health CBA almost always counts two factors—death and money—because they are routinely recorded. A good analysis is able to capture other factors that are significant and yet keep the presentation simple enough that the costs and benefits of alternative courses of action are clearly seen.

FOR EXAMPLE

The Cost-Effectiveness of HIV Screening

A study published in *The New England Journal of Medicine* examined the costs, benefits, and cost-effectiveness of screening for HIV in health care settings now that highly active antiretroviral therapies are available to treat patients. The study found that screening cost approximately $15,000 per increased additional year of life. The researchers concluded that the cost-effectiveness of routine screening in health care settings is similar to that of other commonly accepted screening procedures and should be expanded.[8]

SELF-CHECK

- Indicate the narrowest and broadest perspectives a CBA can take.
- List two medical facts that must be known before a CBA can take place.
- Give an example of a medical issue to which CBA has been applied to help decide policy.

SUMMARY

Cost–benefit analysis (CBA) organizes the facts provided by clinicians and the public's values to present data in a way that is useful for making policy decisions. The appropriate measure of costs is the opportunity cost (i.e., what's given up). The appropriate measure of benefits is the willingness to pay— what the patient or society is willing to give up to attain an improvement in health. In choosing between alternatives, it's the change in benefits (i.e., marginal benefits) and the change in costs (i.e., marginal costs) that matter, not the average or per-person value. However, benefits are rarely certain. The expected value of a medical treatment is the product of the likelihood of success multiplied by the magnitude of the health gain that will occur if treatment is successful.

The primary benefits to be accounted for in health care projects are health, productivity, and reductions in future medical costs. The major categories of costs are medical care and administration, side effects, patient and family time and pain, and provider time and inconvenience.

KEY TERMS

Cost–benefit analysis (CBA)	A set of techniques for assisting in the making of decisions that translates all relevant concerns into market (dollar) terms.
Cost-effectiveness analysis (CEA)	A form of CBA that analyzes the cost side of a decision but doesn't translate the benefits (e.g., lives saved, illnesses prevented, a patient's additional days of activity, the extent to which a patient's sight is restored) into dollars. CEA is used in decision making to determine which alternatives are less expensive yet effective.

Expected value	An estimate of what is likely to happen.
Margin	The change in *xxxx*. A one-unit increase.
Marginal benefit	The value to consumers of one more unit of service.
Opportunity cost	What must be given up in order to do or obtain something; the highest-valued alternative that must be forgone.
Optimum	The point at which the net gain (benefits– costs) is largest.

ASSESS YOUR UNDERSTANDING

Go to www.wiley.com/college/getzen to evaluate your knowledge of cost–benefit analysis and cost-effectiveness analysis.
Measure your learning by comparing pre-test and post-test results.

Summary Questions

1. Cost–benefit analysis (CBA) is a set of techniques for assisting in the making of decisions that translates all relevant concerns into market (dollar) terms. True or False?

2. Cost-effectiveness analysis (CEA) is a form of CBA that analyzes the _____ side of the decision but doesn't translate the _____ into dollars.
   (a) cost; benefits
   (b) benefit; costs
   (c) government; individual decisions
   (d) individual; government decisions

3. A society that uses average benefits and average costs to make medical decisions usually ends up providing far too little medical care. True or False?

4. An opportunity cost of attending medical school is
   (a) the forgone earnings from another career.
   (b) the forgone time spent with family and friends.
   (c) the forgone money spent on medical school tuition.
   (d) all of the above.

5. An estimate of what is likely to happen is called the
   (a) opportunity cost.
   (b) expected value.
   (c) marginal cost.
   (d) marginal benefit.

6. Marginalism is used to determine whether a decision is good or bad. True or False?

7. For most medical programs, the major types of benefits are
   (a) health, productivity, and reductions in future medical costs.
   (b) productivity and reductions in future medical costs.
   (c) reductions in future medical costs.
   (d) health and productivity.

8. When determining the costs involved in any cost–benefit analysis, economists typically consider all types of medical costs except
   (a) medical care and administration.
   (b) time and pain of patient and family.

(c) provider time and inconvenience.

(d) health and productivity.

9. It is impossible to place an economic value on human life. True or _False_?

10. The determination of costs or benefits is always based on point of view. True or False?

Review Questions

1. What are some economic concepts that economists use in a CBA to capture human desires and limitations?

2. "A society that uses average benefits and costs as a guide to decisions will usually end up providing far too much medical care." Why?

3. What is the cheapest way to treat someone who is having a severe heart attack? Is this treatment also the most medically desirable option?

4. When considering the cost of surgery, what kinds of costs must be taken into account?

5. If it's true that no medical treatment can truly save a life, what is the purpose of medical care?

6. Are cost–benefit analyses effective at the individual level? Why or why not?

Applying This Chapter

1. Successful rehabilitation of a shoulder injury avoids the need for reconstructive surgery costing $6,000. However, rehabilitation is successful only 70 percent of the time. What is the expected value of rehabilitation?

2. A course of chemotherapy costs $8,000. If given to patient A, it will increase life expectancy by two months; for patient B, by six months; for patient C, by one month; for patient D, by five months; and for patient E, by four months.

   (a) If all five patients are treated, what is the average cost per year of life gained?

   (b) If only one patient can be treated, which one should it be?

   (c) If only two patients are treated, which ones should they be?

   (d) What is the marginal cost per additional year of life for the patient who is most likely to benefit?

   (e) What is the marginal cost per additional year of life for the patient who is least likely to benefit?

   (f) Draw the total and marginal benefit curves (label the y axis "Years of life gained" and the x axis "Number of patients treated").

   (g) If all five patients are treated, what is the average cost per year of life gained? What is the marginal cost?

(h) If patients are treated in alphabetical order, which one determines the marginal cost per year of life gained—patient A, patient E, or some other patient?

3. Government programs that send doctors to reduce infant mortality direct most of the doctors to poorer neighborhoods. Pediatricians setting up new practices are more likely to locate in wealthier neighborhoods. Explain why both doctors can be said to be obeying the "law of downward-sloping demand," even though they move toward opposite ends of the income distribution.

4. A school district determines that fewer than 70 percent of first-grade students have completed all recommended immunizations. A task force suggests two ways to reach the goal of 95 percent immunization: (1) Hire 20 visiting nurses to do outreach in the community or (2) pass a law mandating that children won't be allowed to attend school unless they bring documentation showing evidence of complete immunization. Which plan is more cost-effective? How is the distribution of costs and benefits different under the two plans?

5. The World Health Organization (WHO) is considering sending a team of experts to deal with an outbreak of schistosomiasis in a distant country. Sending a larger team will allow WHO to prevent more fatalities, and WHO estimates the following effectiveness:

# of Team Members	# of Deaths
0 (i.e., no action)	1,200
5	500
10	200
15	100
20	60
25	40
30	30
35	25
40	22
45	20
50	20

(a) It costs $5,000 for each team member sent. Calculate the total, average, and marginal costs of life saving through this effort and display them on a graph. If saving a life is valued at $100,000, what is the optimal number of people WHO should send to combat the epidemic? If saving a life is valued at $10,000, what is the optimal number? What team size gives the most "bang for the buck" (i.e., the largest number of lives saved per dollar spent)?

(b) Each person sent must be taken away from a disease-fighting team at work elsewhere in the world. What is the appropriate opportunity cost measure of sending people to fight the new epidemic—the transportation cost of $5,000 or the reduction of life-saving efforts from the job they are pulled away from?

6. Treatment for endocarditis is risky. The patient will either die in the hospital, partially recover, or fully recover. With full recovery, the patient can expect to live for another 20 years, but only 25 percent of patients fully recover. With partial recovery, the patient can expect to live 10 more years. However, 20 percent of patients die in the hospital. Assuming that patients usually live just 1 year without treatment, what is the expected value of the treatment, expressed as additional years of life?

7. Many experts recommend that people get at least 30 minutes of vigorous exercise three to five times a week; however, actual participation in exercise is less than the amount (a) needed or (b) demanded. Why do most college students get more exercise in summer than in winter? Does need, demand, or a difference in the opportunity cost of time account for the fact that most actors get more exercise than most accountants?

YOU TRY IT

Identifying the Important Costs

Suppose the state legislature is considering a measure that would effectively set a minimum size for nursing homes (presumably in order to gain economies of scale). Write a brief report indicating what sorts of costs would be important to consider in a cost–benefit analysis of the proposal. Be sure to explain your choices.

Economic Evaluations of Childhood Immunization

Suppose your state were to establish something called the Health Effectiveness Analysis Program (HEAP), whose purpose would be to look for areas of intervention that would promote health and save money for the state and its people. You have been asked to write a brief background paper for state government. Using the example of childhood immunizations, identify and briefly discuss three or more issues or questions that are likely to arise in making economic evaluations (e.g., cost–benefit or cost-effectiveness analyses) of health interventions.

Comparing Different Economic Evaluations

Every economic evaluation of a health program, medical procedure, drug, device, and so on must confront certain issues. Select and review three articles of your own choosing that present economic evaluations.

1. Explain the following problems in economic evaluation and compare, contrast, and evaluate how your articles deal with them:
   a. Identification of costs and benefits/outcomes
   b. Measurement of costs and benefits/outcomes

2. What unique or additional issues or problems are raised by the articles you have chosen, and how successfully do you believe they are handled?

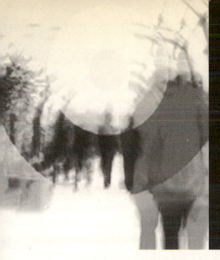

4

HEALTH INSURANCE
The Benefits of Risk Pooling

Starting Point

Go to www.wiley.com/college/getzen to assess your knowledge of the health insurance industry.
Determine where you need to concentrate your effort.

What You'll Learn in This Chapter

▲ Who takes care of people when they need medical care they can't afford
▲ How risk pooling makes insurance possible
▲ Whether people who think they'll become sick are more or less likely to obtain insurance
▲ Who pays for losses: insurance companies or the people who buy insurance

After Studying This Chapter, You'll Be Able To

▲ Defend the practice of pooling of funds to reduce exposure to risks
▲ Evaluate the process of adverse selection
▲ Argue whether insurance increases or decreases the demand for medical care
▲ Assess whether insurance companies take risks or just put a price on risks

INTRODUCTION

Breaking a leg, developing pneumonia, having a heart attack—when these bad things happen, most people rely on insurance to cover the financial obligation. From an individual perspective, insurance generates net benefits by allowing trade between two possible states of the world: A little money in the usual state (i.e., when a person is healthy) is given up to get a lot of money in the unusual and more difficult state (i.e., when a person is sick). From society's point of view, insurance is a method of pooling risk so that one person's loss is shared across many people rather than being borne by that person alone. The entire cost of medical care, including the costs of administration and use of financial capital, is paid through premiums, taxes, or patient coinsurance (e.g., deductibles, copayments) collected for services rendered.

People prefer having an income that is certain rather than the same average income subject to random fluctuations. As a consequence, consumers are willing to pay more than the expected value of a loss to obtain insurance coverage. All participants gain peace of mind, knowing that they can obtain necessary medical care with limited financial risk.

4.1 Protection Against Risk

What would you do if you broke your leg or came down with a serious illness and had to take an unpaid leave of absence from your job while you recovered? If you needed someone to help take care of you, how would you pay that person? How would pay your food, housing, and other bills, including your medical bills, which, even just for a broken leg, are likely to be large?

The chance that you might become injured or sick is a *risk,* as is the chance that you might have significant expenses when you have no income. In most cases, injuries and illnesses are accidents, so it's difficult to protect yourself against them, except through the general strategy of being careful. There are, however, various methods of protecting yourself against unanticipated expenses. In this section, we briefly discuss four possible sources of funds to cover unanticipated medical expenses: savings, family and friends, charity, and insurance.

4.1.1 Savings

People save so they'll have money to pay for goods and services in the future, either to cover a planned expense (e.g., retirement, a vacation) or to protect themselves against a risk (e.g., getting fired, suffering an injury or illness). In terms of risk protection, however, saving has two serious disadvantages:

▲ Payments still come entirely out of your own pocket. The only difference from paying out of current income is that, with savings, in effect, you pay before you incur the expense.

▲ Expenses can easily exceed your savings—especially medical expenses associated with a serious illness or injury.

Certainly, savings can provide some buffer against unexpected expenses so that you can still, for example, pay the rent if you incur a $600 bill for emergency dental work. But for most people, savings won't come close to covering the enormous costs of modern medical care—doctors, tests, hospitals, drugs, and so on. Just the $20,000 or so required to treat a broken leg would be beyond what most people could save and then afford to use, and the expenses associated with a serious illness would exceed the financial capabilities of all but the wealthiest individuals.

4.1.2 Family and Friends

Often, people who haven't been able to save money on their own ask family or friends for financial help to cover unexpected costs. Such help may be freely and generously given, but as a method of risk protection, it has many of the same disadvantages as using your own savings. After all, if you haven't been in a position to save much, how likely is it that your family or your friends will be in such different positions as to let them cover very large expenses for you without serious negative consequences for themselves? Also, help of this kind creates obligations—if not the obligation to pay back what you've been given, then the obligation to offer similar help when family or friends need it in the future.[1]

Of course, a person in need can ask for help from more than one family member or friend at a time and in this way spread the expense across multiple parties. But this doesn't change the basic issue in terms of protection against the risk of large medical expenses: Such expenses are often so large that even spreading them among several individuals doesn't make them manageable. (Note, however, that this notion of spreading expenses across multiple parties is central to the idea of insurance, as we'll discuss later in this chapter and throughout this text.)

4.1.3 Charity

Charity for individuals in need can be private (i.e., given by people who have resources to spare) or institutionalized (i.e., given by organizations that have raised funds for that purpose); of course, the funds raised by charitable institutions also, ultimately, come from individual people. In either case, the people supplying the funds feel an obligation to help others that extends beyond friends and family, to people they've never met and who can do nothing for them in return. This sort of caring for others is part of what makes a group of people a society rather than just a collection of individuals.[2] (And again, note that charitable giving also generally spreads expenses across multiple people;

rarely does a single individual directly provide all the aid needed by another single individual.)

From the perspective of meeting people's medical needs, it's interesting to note that the first hospitals were charitable institutions, substitute homes for people who didn't have homes and for people who were ill or disabled and whose families couldn't take care of them. This type of charity predates health insurance by thousands of years, but it's clearly not an adequate solution to today's medical needs; even the enormous funds commanded by charitable individuals and institutions would fail by a large margin to cover everyone's medical expenses.

4.1.4 Insurance

In modern society, the most common method of protection against the risk of large medical costs is insurance, which comes in two forms: social insurance and private insurance.

Social insurance extends and formalizes the informal obligations of citizens to society expressed in charitable giving.[3] The main U.S. social insurance programs that cover medical expenses are Medicare, Medicaid, and Social Security:

▲ Medicare covers medical expenses for elderly people.
▲ Medicaid covers medical expenses for poor people.
▲ Social Security, along with the related Supplemental Security Income (SSI) program, covers medical expenses for disabled people.

Contributions to these programs are not voluntary but mandatory through the tax system: Virtually everyone who earns an income must contribute some amount. Who contributes (and how much) and who receives benefits (and how much) are determined by legislation and court decisions.

Private health insurance is based on a contract between an individual and an insurance company. In traditional private insurance plans, also known as indemnity plans, the contract simply called for the insurance company to pay for all (or a defined part) of the medical bills a person incurred. Such plans have become rare because people today want their health insurance company to do more—for example, to bargain for lower prices with hospitals and physicians, to evaluate whether a new drug is really worth twice as much as the old one, and to process all the paperwork. Managed care plans, which were developed in response to these needs, provide a package of such services at a reasonable cost. (See Chapter 10 for more discussion of managed care plans.) In the United States, most people who have private health insurance have it through an employer, in which case the contract is between the employer and the insurance company, but the employee, too, must agree to be bound by the contract.

The U.S. health care system is based on a blend of social and private insurance. Far more people are covered by private insurance than by social insurance, but unlike social insurance programs, private insurance does nothing for people who can't afford to buy insurance or for people excluded from purchasing insurance (e.g., many people with disabilities). Private insurance doesn't pay for medical research or for educational programs to promote healthy lifestyles, nor does it provide outreach to teenage mothers or to people who have mental illness. In short, private insurance does nothing to strengthen the social bonds among the nation's people or the sense that we can look to each other for support. Private health insurance does benefit the people who purchase it and the companies that provide it, but the idea that the health of individuals is a matter of public concern is so strong that even when insurance is privately paid for and is managed by profit-making firms, government regulations mandate who must be offered coverage, what coverages must be offered, and how prices must be set. In this way, even private insurance is forced to at least partly conform with the principles of social insurance.

Neither private insurance nor social insurance programs are perfect. As the number of people covered increases, social insurance tends to become less connected to personal empathy, becoming just one more government service provided through the political process. As taxpayers, we tend to be willing to provide some medical care for everyone—but not necessarily the best quality of care. And some taxpayers are hostile to social insurance in any form, asking, for example, why society should spend huge amounts of money caring for irresponsible people with unhealthy lifestyles. Truly comprehensive and effective social insurance would require what may seem impossible—that society reach a consensus on who deserves what level of medical care and on how that care should be delivered.

FOR EXAMPLE

Why Do Police Officers and Firefighters Have Such Comprehensive Insurance?

Medical coverage for those who put their lives on the line for the good of the community remains comprehensive even at a time when many employers and government agencies are cutting back on benefits. There is a symbolic importance to this insurance that goes beyond financial considerations: If the community isn't willing to do everything possible to protect the health of these public servants, why should these servants continue to risk their lives to save the lives of others? Similar considerations lie behind the $20 billion system to care for disabled veterans, given the willingness of military troops to go to great lengths to recover a wounded or dead comrade when such efforts don't seem to be worthwhile from a cost–benefit perspective.

SELF-CHECK

- List four possible sources of funds to cover unanticipated medical expenses. Identify the pros and cons of each.
- List two types of insurance in the United States and explain each.
- List three types of **social insurance** programs in the United States.

4.2 The Economics of Private Health Insurance

Consider 100 middle-aged senior executives at Xumma Corporation. They are aware of certain health statistics for people like them. For example, they know it's likely that several of them will get sick during the next year, some with minor illnesses and a smaller number with more serious illnesses. They also know there's a good chance that at least one of them will have a heart attack, in which case a coronary artery bypass graft (CABG) could save the person's life. These executives are well paid and are therefore willing to take the risk of having to pay the medical expenses associated with getting sick, but a CABG plus the necessary continuing care would cost about $50,000, and they aren't willing to take the risk of having to pay that. How can they protect themselves against that risk? One of the executives has an idea: "Let's form a club," she says. "Each of us will put in $500, and if one of us has a heart attack, we can use the money to pay for the surgery."

4.2.1 Risk Pooling

The executive's idea—forming a group so that individual risk can be shared among many people—is known as **risk pooling** and is an essential feature of all insurance. In insurance terms, each person in the insured group (i.e., each policyholder) pays money (i.e., premiums), which the insurance company uses to cover the costs of everyone in the group actually affected by the risk (i.e., each person with medical expenses is reimbursed, or receives benefits).

In the real world, an insurance company with only 100 policyholders (like the Xumma executives' club with 100 members) couldn't survive economically because with a small group, the chance would be too great that actual costs would exceed the expected (average) costs indicated by statistics. In terms of our example, if, by chance, 3 or more of the executives needed a CABG in the first year of the club's existence, there wouldn't be enough money to pay for all the operations, and the club would go broke. But if the number of policyholders is large enough, the chance that actual costs will significantly exceed expected costs is quite low.

4.2.2 Premiums

Insurance companies not only like to sell insurance to large groups of people with predictable (average) medical costs, but they also try to do the best job possible of predicting those costs so they can price premiums to cover all the costs and ensure some profit. The specialty responsible for predicting medical costs is actuarial science, which uses information on previous costs for groups of people with known characteristics to predict future costs for similar groups.

In our example of the club formed by Xumma executives, the predicted medical cost is $50,000 because that is the cost of one CABG, and information on previous costs for groups like this indicates that one CABG will be needed. This lets us determine the **actuarially fair premium:** the predicted cost divided by the number of people in the group, or $50,000/100 = $500.

However, insurance premiums must be greater than the actuarially fair premium, not only to cover the costs associated with the risk being insured against but also to provide profit to the owners or shareowners of the insurance company, to cover the company's administrative expenses, and to provide a cushion against unpredicted expenses. The difference between the actual premium and the actuarially fair premium is known as the **loading factor.** In the case of the Xumma executives' club, they might be wise to establish a premium of $1,000 rather than $500 (i.e., a premium with a loading factor of $500, or 100 percent), to guard against the possibility that more than one CABG would be needed.

4.2.3 Variation in Medical Expenses

Health insurance became more of a necessity as medical care became more expensive, with the potential cost of illness gradually increasing from burdensome to overwhelming. In 1929, for example, $200 was an unusually large medical bill, but even after adjusting for inflation, there's no comparison between then and now; in today's high-tech medical arena, costs of $100,000 or more are common. Few people can afford to pay for modern treatment of serious (or even not-so-serious) illness, but few are willing to forgo treatment if they become ill. Only insurance, by spreading the cost of care across the entire employed population, can make it possible for most people to obtain good medical care when they need it.

Of course, insurance wouldn't be necessary (at least not insurance as we know it) if everyone's medical expenses were near the average of about $7,556 per person per year. In reality, however, there's a great deal of variation—much more than the variation for food, housing, clothing, transportation, and other major expenses—as shown by the following projected U.S. statistics for 2007 (see Figure 4-1 for a graphical depiction of the individual variation in medical expenses):

▲ 15 percent of people had less than $300 in total medical expenses for the year.

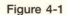

Figure 4-1

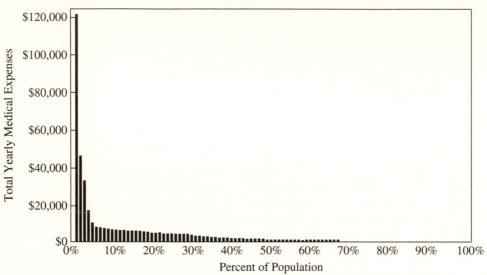

Note: The 1 percent of individuals with highest cost consume approximately
30 percent of total services, and the top 5 percent consume about 50 percent.

Distribution of individual medical care expenditures.

▲ 75 percent of people averaged almost $3,000 in total medical expenses
  for the year.
▲ 9 percent of people had more than $35,000 in medical expenses for the
  year, accounting for 40 percent of all medical expenses.
▲ 1 percent of people accounted for nearly 30 percent of all medical
  expenses.[4]

Most of us can afford to pay for at least some of the cost of the care we
expect to receive if we get sick. And most of us—even those who are healthy
and have minimal medical expenses—accept the idea that we should contribute
something toward the total medical expenses of all the people in our country.
But how much can we afford? A $150,000 medical bill would be staggeringly
difficult for most of us to pay. And many people would have trouble paying even
the $7,556 average annual cost of medical care per person. But whether we like
it or not, that average amount per person is extracted through taxes, bills paid
by individuals, insurance premiums paid by employers or individuals, or some
other means, such as charitable giving.

4.2.4 How Risk Pooling Reduces the Effects of Variation

The chance that an insured group will have extraordinarily high or low losses
declines sharply as the number of people in the group increases. This is illustrated

Figure 4-2

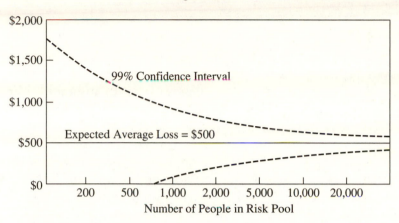

Variability declines as the size of the risk sharing pool increases.

in Figure 4-2, which is based on the assumption that each person in an insured group (i.e., the risk pool) has a 1 in 100 chance of incurring $50,000 in medical expenses in a given year. Thus, the expected (average) annual medical costs per person is $500, regardless of the number of people in the group, as indicated by the solid horizontal line in Figure 4-2. The dotted lines in the figure are called 99 percent confidence intervals: They show how the size of the risk pool reduces the effects of variation in medical expenses. That is, for any given number of people in the risk pool, we can be 99 percent confident that average annual medical expenses per person will be some amount between the dotted lines (or between $0 and the upper dotted line because it doesn't make sense to talk about negative medical expenses). For example, as the figure shows:

▲ With just 20 people in the risk pool, all we can be 99 percent confident of is that average annual medical expenses per person will be somewhere between $0 and about $1,700.

▲ With 200 people in the risk pool, we can be 99 percent confident that average expenses will be between $0 and about $1,500.

▲ With 2,000 people in the group, we can be 99 percent confident that average expenses will be between about $200 and $750.

▲ With 20,000 people in the risk pool, we can be 99 percent confident that average expenses will be between about $370 and $630.

This dramatic decline in variation as the size of the pool increases is shown in the figure by the way in which the dotted lines narrow toward the $500 expected average.

FOR EXAMPLE

Everyone Pays

Employers pay about $2 an hour (or about 8 percent of compensation) per employee for health benefits, reducing the amount that can be paid out as wages.[5] Even if an employer doesn't provide health insurance, money is deducted each week as taxes, often labeled "H.I." or "FICA:M" on a paycheck. This is hospital insurance—not for the employee, but for the elderly and people with disabilities on Medicare. Even when senior citizens pay thousands of dollars out of pocket, more than 90 percent of hospital bills, half of nursing home bills, and almost one-third of the costs of their drugs are being borne by other people, mostly younger working people.

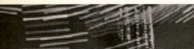

SELF-CHECK

- Indicate how an **actuarially fair premium** is determined.
- Define **loading factor.**
- Briefly explain how **risk pooling** reduces the effects of variation in medical costs.

4.3 Risk Aversion

To the extent that people can easily pay for routine losses (e.g., with personal savings or regular income), they are not willing to pay insurance premiums that include a loading factor, as all real premiums do. It's as if the person were saying, "I know I'm likely to incur X amount (i.e., the expected [average] amount) in routine losses, but I can afford to pay that amount, and the likelihood of a really large loss of this type is very small. So why should I pay premiums that total greater than X?" Thus, most people choose not to buy insurance against routine losses (e.g., losing a textbook that costs $100 to replace). Instead, most people choose to insure themselves against potentially catastrophic losses only, such as the losses they would suffer if their house burned down, their car were wrecked, or they came down with a serious illness. This reflects **risk aversion,** the willingness to incur a relatively small but certain expense (the premium) to avoid the risk of a catastrophic loss.

Some people are very averse to risk and will go to great lengths to avoid it. But even people who can accept some risk (and that includes most people) choose not to take financial chances unless they have to or think they have a decent chance of being well paid for doing so. For example, a person might invest money in a company's stock (a risky investment compared, say, to buying government bonds) if it seems likely that the price of the stock will rise or that the investment will pay significant dividends. People's degree of risk aversion also depends to some extent on their income and savings. For example, a person with an annual income of $200,000 (and savings to match) might be willing to risk losing a $100,000 investment in a promising new company, whereas a person with an annual income of $20,000 (and savings to match) would probably be very unwilling to put $10,000 into a similarly risky investment.

Given that most people are risk averse to some degree, how can we explain the fact that almost everyone who has the opportunity to buy affordable health insurance does so? First of all, as noted earlier, risk aversion actually motivates people to insure themselves against the catastrophic losses associated with serious medical conditions. With insurance, people can obtain worthwhile medical care they otherwise couldn't afford. What does "worthwhile" mean? Suppose that you have a serious liver disease, that you value your life at $100,000 per year (see Chapter 3 for a discussion of what it means to set a monetary value on one's life), and that a $350,000 liver transplant could extend your life expectancy by 10 years. The expected benefit of the transplant ($100,000 × 10 = $1,000,000) is greater than the cost, so the transplant is clearly worthwhile. That is, if you had $350,000, you would willingly spend it on the transplant, and if you have the right kind of health insurance, you can have the transplant even if, like most people, you don't have $350,000. Insurance gives you the peace of mind that comes from knowing you'll be properly cared for if you become seriously ill.

We can see another reason for the prevalence of health insurance by comparing it to property and casualty insurance. With most property and casualty insurance, people are insuring themselves against expenses that are large, infrequent, and unpredictable (e.g., the expenses arising from a house fire or an auto accident). Many of the medical expenses that we insure ourselves against fit this description, but some don't. For example, expenses for visits to your family doctor (or primary care physician) for colds and the flu are usually small, not infrequent, and fairly predictable. There are three main reasons health insurance is so extensive, covering minor and routine services as well as catastrophic events:

▲ There is a widespread belief that everyone has a right to medical care.
▲ Medical providers (e.g., doctors, hospitals) promote insurance because it benefits them—for example, it guarantees payment and it avoids sullying the doctor–patient relationship with the taint of commercial trade and haggling over price.
▲ It is nearly impossible for people to be informed consumers and smart shoppers when it comes to medical services. What medical care do I really need? Is treatment A, which costs $1,500 less than treatment B,

FOR EXAMPLE

Are You Risk Averse?

Here's an easy test: Imagine your boss offering to flip a coin to determine whether to double your monthly paycheck or take it away. If the prospect of losing your paycheck is much more unpleasant than the chance of doubling it, you, like most people, are risk averse and a good candidate for insurance. Yet, even if you're risk averse, you probably "gamble" by investing a portion of your retirement savings in stocks because you're compensated by getting, on average, higher returns that you could with less risky investments.

really just as good? Will having an operation now save money in the long run, without jeopardizing my health? For most of us, answering questions like these is just too difficult, so we turn to intermediaries— doctors and insurance plans—to answer them for us.

SELF-CHECK

- Explain what it means to be risk averse.
- List three reasons health insurance is so extensive.

4.4 Adverse Selection

What if you knew that you were much more likely than the average person to have a heart attack or some other serious illness? (And some people do, effectively, "know" this because of their family history and other risk factors.) In this case, you would make sure that you got health insurance, even if you had to pay a very high premium. In contrast, if you were quite sure that your health was going to remain excellent, you might not be willing to pay even a low premium for insurance. This illustrates what common sense tells us: When people have a choice about whether to pay for health insurance, those at high risk for medical problems are more likely to buy insurance than those at low risk.

This type of situation is called **adverse selection** because the characteristics of the group that selects the option to buy insurance are disproportionately adverse from the point of view of the insurance company. That is, the average medical expenses for the insured group are likely to be greater than the average medical expenses for the entire group that had the option to buy insurance (and thus the insurance company is likely to suffer greater-than-average losses). For this reason, insurance companies that provide group insurance for businesses typically require that at least a majority of the employees, if not all employees, be insured. If young, healthy workers could decide not to participate, premiums would have to increase to cover the higher-than-average losses. At the extreme, the insured group might include only those who were certain to collect benefits because they were already ill or sure to become ill—in which case, premiums would have to increase to the point where having insurance would be as expensive as not having insurance.

In many situations, adverse selection isn't a problem, as long as both the insurance company and the higher-risk individuals are aware of and acknowledge the reasons for higher risk. In that case, premiums can be adjusted to account for varying risk categories. For example, pricing by age is common because older people tend to incur higher medical expenses than younger people; thus, the monthly premium might be $300 for people 35 and younger, $500 for people 35 to 50, $650 for people 51 to 60, and $850 for people 61 and older. Adverse selection creates difficulties in two main situations:

▲ When the people buying insurance know about risk factors that the insurance company doesn't know about (e.g., the insurance company may not know your chest hurts every time you go walking or that your diet consists almost entirely of fried foods).

▲ When both parties know about the risk factors but raising premiums enough to compensate for these factors is considered unfair (e.g., charging males significantly more than females of the same age, doubling the premium when a person reaches age 61, charging unmarried men more than married men because unmarried men are at higher risk for contracting HIV/AIDS).

Adverse selection also comes into play when an employer offers two kinds of plans, a basic plan and a more comprehensive plan for which employees pay extra. In this case, adverse selection is involved because the following scenario is likely to develop:

1. A disproportionate number of high-risk individuals (for example, those who are older or overweight) tend to buy the comprehensive plan.

2. As more high-risk people sign up for the comprehensive plan, their medical expenses exceed the expected value, and even the "high" premium isn't sufficient to pay the bills. Thus, the extra premium for comprehensive insurance has to be raised still higher.

3. As the premium goes up, fewer and fewer low-risk people are willing to pay for the better coverage. Eventually, only those who know they are certain to incur large medical expenses sign up for the comprehensive plan. This defeats the principle of risk pooling, on which insurance depends, and leads to the termination of the more comprehensive plan.

FOR EXAMPLE

How Do They Know?

Actuaries have found that people who buy life insurance are more likely than average to die prematurely, due to the nature of adverse selection.[6] For example, people who know that their heart palpitates or know they have had a lack of physical activity since they turned 50 are more apt to buy life insurance when it's offered. Conversely, those who buy annuities (policies that pay insured individuals a certain amount per year as long as they live) show positive selection and are less likely than average to die prematurely. In this way, individuals may have private knowledge that they can use to select coverage that is most favorable to them but more costly to the insurer.

SELF-CHECK

- Define **adverse selection**.
- Describe two situations in which adverse selection causes difficulties.

SUMMARY

From an individual perspective, insurance is a form of trade between time periods or between different possible states (i.e., healthy or sick) in the future. From a societal perspective, insurance is a method of pooling risks so that the burden of financial loss is distributed over many people. Private insurance contracts spread risk through organized markets. Social insurance uses taxation to spread risk over all citizens.

Because of risk aversion, consumers are willing to pay more than the expected value of a loss to obtain insurance coverage. People who know that they are likely to sustain a loss are more likely to purchase insurance, resulting in adverse selection.

KEY TERMS

Actuarially fair premium	The predicted cost divided by the number of people in the group.
Adverse selection	A situation in which those at high risk for medical problems are more likely to buy insurance than those at low risk.

Loading factor	The difference between the actual premium and the actuarially fair premium.
Private health insurance	Insurance that is based on a contract between an individual and an insurance company.
Risk aversion	The willingness to incur a relatively small but certain expense (the premium) to avoid the risk of a catastrophic loss.
Risk pooling	Forming a group so that individual risk can be shared among many people.
Social insurance	Insurance that extends and formalizes the informal obligations of citizens to society expressed in charitable giving.

ASSESS YOUR UNDERSTANDING

Go to www.wiley.com/college/getzen to evaluate your knowledge of the health insurance industry.
Measure your learning by comparing pre-test and post-test results.

Summary Questions

1. The U.S. health care system is based entirely on social insurance programs. True or False?

2. Medicare and Medicaid are social insurance programs. True or False?

3. Adverse selection in insurance means:

   (a) the choice by consumers of an insurance plan that is insufficient to meet their needs.

   (b) the choice by insurance plans not to cover medical conditions that exist at the time a person begins coverage with the insurance plan.

   (c) the systematic choice of a particular insurance plan by persons with higher-than-average risks.

   (d) the choice by insurance plans to require certain persons to have their premiums determined on an individual basis.

4. Which of the following would be part of the loading portion of the premium for insurance?

   (a) The expected loss from occurrence of the insured hazard

   (b) The transaction costs of the insurance business

   (c) Profit for the insurance company

   (d) The transaction costs of the insurance business and profit for the insurance company

5. To be financially feasible, insurance premiums must be greater than the actuarially fair premium. True or False?

6. The willingness of consumers to pay more than the expected loss in order to obtain insurance coverage is an example of:

   (a) irrational evaluation of risk.

   (b) the market power of insurance companies.

   (c) adverse selection.

   (d) risk aversion.

7. The actuarially fair premium is:

   (a) one in which the loading includes only the actual administrative costs, not profit for the insurer.

   (b) the premium that minimizes the chance for welfare loss due to insurance.

(c) equal to the underwriting gains of the insurer.

(d) equal to the expected loss from the risk being insured.

8. Pricing an insurance policy based on age is an example of:

(a) adverse selection.

(b) risk aversion.

(c) unfair age discrimination.

(d) risk pooling.

Review Questions

1. What systems—formal and informal—are in place to take care of people when they need medical treatments?

2. The private insurance contract is only one way of dealing with uncertainty and risk. Identify two other mechanisms and discuss their relative strengths and weaknesses compared to the insurance contract.

3. Are people who think they will become sick more or less likely to buy insurance? Is this an example of adverse selection?

4. Who ultimately pays when an insurance company suffers a loss due to an unusual number of heart attacks requiring surgery: the insurance company or the people/companies who are buying the insurance?

5. If such insurance were available, rational consumers would gladly purchase insurance covering 100% of their health care expenditures. True or False? Why?

6. The more likely you are to suffer a loss, the more likely you are to need compensation, and therefore the more you are willing to pay for insurance protection. True or False? Why?

7. If almost all persons are risk averse, why aren't all risks insured? Identify three examples (that are significantly different from each other) of risks that are typically uninsured and discuss why this is so.

8. Which situation would post the largest problem regarding adverse selection at a small company: inclusion of maternity coverage in the standard benefits package or an optional rider providing maternity coverage for an additional premium?

9. How might the widespread belief that everyone has a right to medical care contribute to increased insurance costs?

Applying This Chapter

1. Suppose an insurance company last year had claims costing $660,000 for a company with 100 employees and expects costs to rise 4% in the coming year. The company intends to charge $72 per person per month. What is the load above the actuarially fair premium?

2. A company with 1,204 employees had the following experience this year:

	Cost Each
29 hospitalizations	$5,980.00
1 transplant	$287,000.00
52 physical therapy sessions	$320.00
21 births	$2,100.00
4.1 physician visits per employee	$52.35
2.7 prescriptions filled per employee	$27.80

Assuming that the cost of medical care rises 8 percent over the next year, what would the actuarially fair premium per employee be for the next year?

3. If the insurance company in Question 1 charges $76.42 per person per month, what is the loading factor?

4. Explain why paying $1,000 per year to insure a $200,000 house—a common occurrence in the United States—is actually an example of risk aversion.

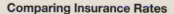

YOU TRY IT

Comparing Insurance Rates

Visit the website of ehealthinsurance.com (www.ehealthinsurance.com) and click the "Get Quotes" button. Plug in the appropriate data to get insurance rate quotes for two different individuals living in your ZIP code:

(a) A 55-year-old man who has used tobacco products within the past 12 months

(b) A 22-year-old woman who hasn't used tobacco and who is a full-time college student

Prepare a report detailing the types of plans available for each individual. In your report, indicate whether there is a significant rate difference for the man and the woman. If so, explain why that might be the case.

The Massachusetts Universal Health Insurance Law

In 2006, Massachusetts became the first state in the nation to require all residents to buy health insurance or face legal penalties. The law calls for all uninsured adults in the state to buy some kind of insurance policy by July 1, 2007, or pay a fine. Choices include a range of new and inexpensive plans from private insurers, subsidized by the state. Write a paper considering the pros and cons of such a plan.

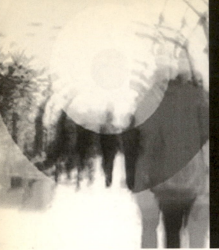

5

INSURANCE CONTRACTS
The Flow of Funds in the Insurance Industry

Starting Point

Go to www.wiley.com/college/getzen to assess your knowledge of insurance contracts and the flow of funds in the insurance industry.
Determine where you need to concentrate your effort.

What You'll Learn in This Chapter

▲ How patients, providers, and insurance companies benefit from insurance
▲ The difference between traditional indemnity insurance and managed care plans
▲ Types of private and government-funded insurance
▲ How insurance plans structure incentives

After Studying This Chapter, You'll Be Able To

▲ Assess health care in the United States compared to that of other industrialized countries
▲ Analyze the pros and cons of managed care plans
▲ Evaluate the problems associated with having so many uninsured individuals in the United States
▲ Evaluate insurance policies based on their incentive structures

INTRODUCTION

In a standard market, consumers determine demand and sellers determine supply, and money flows between the two groups. Insurance changes the standard market model by redirecting the flow of money and introducing inefficiencies in the health care system. Insurance changes who negotiates prices, who bears responsibility for mistakes, and who has the right to profit from directing business to one hospital instead of another. In the medical world, patients receive care but don't directly pay for it; insurance companies neither supply nor consume, but they pool risk and profit from handling funds; and providers are reimbursed by a third party—insurance—on behalf of a group of patients rather than being paid directly.

Recognizing the inefficiencies of traditional indemnity insurance, insurance companies introduced managed care organizations (MCOs), which take an increased role in scrutinizing medical care and services and limiting the types of payments made. The government also has a significant effect on the ordinary operation of the market. By offering tax incentives to employers to provide health coverage for their employees, the government essentially subsidizes the price of insurance. Finally, insurance contracts don't just pool risks, they also change the incentive structure—and sometimes these changes are quite deliberate and favor one party over another.

5.1 How Insurance Benefits Everyone Involved

When insurance companies are involved in health care, the flow of funds changes, as illustrated in Figure 5-1.

What does each of the three parties—patients, providers, and insurance companies—involved in an insurance contracting network gain?

▲ Patients gain by pooling risks to eliminate financial uncertainty and make expensive treatments affordable (see Chapter 4).

Figure 5-1

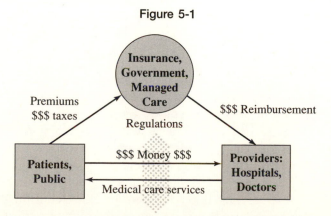

How insurance redirects the flow of funds.

▲ Insurance companies benefit from profits. Even when the underwriting gains (i.e., the difference between premiums paid in and benefits paid out plus administrative costs) are negative, an apparent loss, companies may still make money because they will hold the premiums for 6 to 24 months before paying out benefits. In addition, insurance companies usually get higher returns on investments than individuals because insurers are so large, with better opportunities and specialized investment staffs.

▲ Providers gain from an increase in demand and regularity of payment. When patients are covered by insurance, they are more apt to come in for care and less likely to argue about price. Traditionally, patients expected doctors and hospitals to be more lenient than landlords and bankers about late payment, and many medical bills went unpaid or were paid only in part.

5.1.1 The Role of Government

Many governments provide medical care directly, as is done by the National Health Service in the United Kingdom and by the Swedish health system. Some countries have chosen to build on employee health insurance plans to create universal coverage for all citizens, such as the German Krankenkassen or the Japanese employment societies.

The United States is somewhat unique in that insurance is encouraged but not universally required. The U.S. government, through Medicare, directly provides insurance for all people 65 and older and, through Medicaid, provides insurance for many people who are poor or disabled. The U.S. government also provides tax incentives for many others to be insured through the private sector. The primary tax incentive is that health benefits are nontaxable compensation for employees but still allowed as deductible expenses for the employer. This tax break for employer-paid health insurance is a substantial and important part of the voluntary system of health care that Americans have come to depend on. Without the tax incentive, most working people wouldn't have health insurance as an employee benefit.

5.1.2 Who Pays? How Much?

People often mistakenly believe that when insurance pays for something, it's free. Even if you don't pay cash out of your pocket for your medical care, every dollar spent on medical care is paid by you, or by me, or by someone just like us. Insurance companies and the government never really "pay" for anything. For the most part, individuals pay for medical care by paying higher taxes and/or taking home lower wages. Even the tax advantage for employee benefits doesn't mean that we get something for nothing. (There are no free lunches!) The government still has to pay its bills. If fewer dollars are collected through wage taxes, more dollars must be collected through gasoline taxes, property taxes, income taxes, Social Security taxes, or other taxes to make up the difference. When a

> ## FOR EXAMPLE
>
> ### Japan vs. the U.S.: Comparing Health Insurance Coverage
>
> Life expectancy in Japan is the highest in the world: 78 years for men and 85 years for women. However, the level of health care spending is only half that of the United States, about $2,080 per person, accounting for 6.7 percent of gross domestic product. The technology used in the Japanese health care system is similar to that used in the United States, but the organization and flow of funds and, hence, the quantity and intensity of use, are considerably different. In Japan, all citizens are covered by some form of insurance and are able to choose any physician or hospital they wish, with no bills other than modest copayments per visit or per day. Japan's universal health insurance system functions as more than just a financing mechanism; it also functions as the means of health policy implementation. By using a uniform fee schedule, the government is able to manage provider behavior as well as national health care spending.

hospital provides "free" care to someone as charity, it must raise charges to those who are insured (and the few people who cover their bills out of their own pockets) to pay for it. Insurance doesn't reduce the cost of medical care; rather, it redistributes costs so that different people end up paying.

Under third-party payment systems, the connection between what the first party (the patient) pays and what the second party (the provider) receives is indirect at best. The "charges billed" for a visit to the emergency room often bear little resemblance to what you have to pay or what the hospital receives. In health economics, one must give up the familiar concept of simple two-party transactions in which "bought" and "sold" happen at the same price. This chapter discusses how much the patient (or his or her family) pays, not how much the doctor or hospital actually receives, which is usually quite different (see Chapters 6 and 8). Insurance breaks the linkage between what the patient pays and the amount the provider is paid.

People pay premiums to be insured but then don't pay directly for the medical care they use. Health insurance is similar to having a credit card that allows you to buy whatever you need, but for which payment is set at $100 per month, regardless of the number of purchases you make. As you might expect, because one doesn't have to pay any extra for more purchases, the amount spent tends to rise uncontrollably. That's why most indemnity insurance plans providing unlimited reimbursements in return for a fixed premium have disappeared from the market. Most people are now covered by **managed care plans** (see Section 5.1.4), in which a manager controls the number and type of services covered in return for more affordable premiums. Managed care plans use their control over purchasing to negotiate lower prices from hospitals, doctors, and drug companies. In a sense, managed care represents the evolution of the insurer from a passive financial inter-mediary to an active purchasing agent.

5.1.3 How Benefits Are Determined

Insurance is a legal contract that specifies three things:

▲ How much will be paid, to which providers, and under what conditions
▲ The types of evidence of loss required
▲ Who will arbitrate disputes

Most people never see the complete contract drawn up between their employer and their insurance company; they only see informational pamphlets, hear descriptions during new employee orientation, and so on. All such descriptions of benefits, even those in an advertisement or a brochure written in Spanish or another language, are legally binding contracts. If a policy states that it covers eye examinations, it covers eye examinations. If a policy states that it will pay $16 for filling a tooth cavity, it will pay $16. The insurance plan must pay any amount that a court decides a reasonable person reading such descriptions would expect the insurance plan to pay. Furthermore, any benefits routinely paid in previous years and not explicitly revoked become a precedent, even if those benefits aren't mentioned in the contract. The use of fine print to leave the insured burdened with thousands of dollars of unexpected bills simply isn't allowed and, in fact, would be self-defeating for an insurance company. Over time, premiums will be adjusted upward to cover whatever medical costs are incurred.

5.1.4 Managed Care Plans

The fundamental difference between traditional indemnity insurance and managed care is that a manager intervenes to monitor and control the transaction between doctor and patient (see Figure 5-2). The management company acts as the patient's agent, trying to get better care and lower prices. An outside party, such as the plan medical director or a software program, identifies medical procedures and services that might not fit with accepted clinical practice. The manager examines the process of care and controls the flow of funds, making payments in some circumstances and holding back in others. Because the **managed care organization (MCO)** accepts risk for and manages medical care, it has an incentive to provide care efficiently. To remain viable, the MCO must compete on the basis of both quality and cost.

MCOs take several forms:

▲ **Preferred provider organizations (PPOs)** or **point-of-service plans (POSs)** are the most loosely organized MCOs. The insuring MCO negotiates contracts with a set of doctors and hospitals (the network) to obtain care at a discount. Patients receiving care within the network pay

Figure 5-2

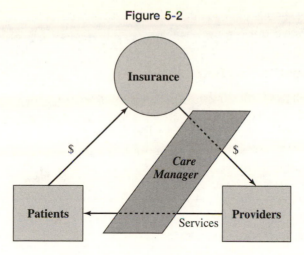

Flow of funds with managed care.

only a small copayment. Patients may obtain care outside the network but may have to pay substantially more or receive a referral from their regular doctor, stating that such specialty care is medically necessary.

▲ **Health maintenance organizations (HMOs)** require referrals for most specialty care. The insurance only pays for care within the network, and the networks are usually more limited than under POS or PPO plans.

▲ **Closed-panel HMOs** provide all care in-house, using their own doctors and hospitals. The largest closed-panel HMO is Kaiser Permanente, which has more than 8 million members, mostly in the western United States.

FOR EXAMPLE

Kaiser Permanente

Kaiser Permanente is the largest not-for-profit HMO in the United States, with revenues of $31.5 billion in 2005. Founded in 1945, this closed-panel HMO is based in Oakland, California, and operates in nine states and Washington, DC. It's actually a consortium of three distinct entities: Kaiser Foundation Health Plans, which offers prepaid not-for-profit health plans; Kaiser Foundation Hospitals, which operates not-for-profit medical centers and outpatient facilities; and the Permanente Medical Groups, which are partnerships of physicians that provide and arrange for medical care for Kaiser Foundation Health Plans members in each respective region. The medical groups are for-profit partnerships and also receive funding from Kaiser Foundation Health Plans. Kaiser has 8.3 million health plan members, 134,000 employees, 11,000 physicians, 30 medical centers, and 431 medical offices.[1]

5.2 Types of Insurance Plans

Most people in the United States (about 60%) have some form of private health insurance, usually through an employer. Government programs, mostly Medicare and Medicaid, cover 30 percent of the population (approximately 87 million people), and about 26 million people, or 9 percent of the population, purchase private insurance individually. That leaves about 46 million people, or 16 percent of the population, uninsured. (See Table 5-1; these statistics are based on a 2004 population estimate of 290 million.)[2]

5.2.1 Employer-Based Group Health Insurance

More than half the U.S. population is covered by employer group health insurance. An employee usually obtains insurance by choosing one of the options

Table 5-1: Health Insurance Coverage of the U.S. Population[3]

	Non-Elderly	Elderly
Total persons	270 million	39 million
Total persons insured	82.2%	99.2%
Employer coverage	32.0%	35.5%
Employer coverage (dependents)	30.4%	N/A
Other private insurance	6.8%	7.1%
Military	2.9%	7.1%
Medicare	2.5%	95%
Medicaid	13.4%	9.4%
Uninsured	17.8%	0.8%

Table 5-2: Annual Premiums for Employee Health Insurance Coverage, 2005[4]

	HMO	PPO	POS	Indemnity	Average
Single					
Total premium	$3,768	$4,152	$3,912	$3,780	$4,020
Amount paid by employee	$564	$600	$732	$492	$612
Family					
Total premium	$10,452	$11,088	$10,800	$9,984	$10,884
Amount paid by employee	$2,604	$2,640	$3,252	$2,316	$2,712

offered through his or her employer, deciding whether to include children and other dependents, and contributing to the total premium (see Table 5-2). Almost all large employers provide health insurance benefits, but fewer than one-third of small employers (those with fewer than 10 employees) do so, and those that do often make the employee pay a large part of the premium so that fewer people choose to participate. The largest employee groups are usually self-insured (i.e., the employer bears the risk, although it may use an insurance company to administer benefits; see Section 5.2.2).

PPOs cover well over half (61 percent) of all insured employees. HMOs cover 21 percent, POSs cover 15 percent, and the remaining 3 percent have traditional indemnity insurance.

5.2.2 Self-Insurance

Self-insurance is another type of insurance that may be offered by a large company or organization. Self-insured companies essentially assume the risk and pick up the health care costs of their employees. Typically, these companies will pay for health care costs as they happen rather than pay an insurance company large premiums on a regular basis. Additionally, a self-insured company will usually set aside a trust or maintain a reserve fund to cover anticipated health care costs for a given amount of time. Self-insured organizations often contract with third-party administrators who handle the administrative duties needed to run the plan, such as claims and billing.

By self-insuring, a company or organization can benefit in terms of reduced costs, tighter management of its health care dollars, and certain tax advantages. Employees can benefit from a self-insurance program by avoiding some of the restrictions many fully insured plans place on them, such as a requirement to obtain in-network coverage.

5.2.3 Self-Paid Private Insurance

Nine percent of the population, mostly people who are self-employed or who work for small companies that don't provide employee benefits, purchase private health insurance individually. Individuals acting on their own behalf lack group purchasing power and often pay significantly increased premiums, even for reduced levels of coverage.

5.2.4 Medicare

Because many elderly people don't belong to employer groups and would be subject to severe adverse selection (see Section 4.4) if they purchased insurance individually, the U.S. government created **Medicare,** a federal insurance program that covers individuals over age 65 and some people with disabilities. A substantial portion of the money for Medicare comes from a tax of 2.9 percent on all wages, half paid by the employer and half paid by the employee, with the remainder coming from general tax revenues and premiums.

As part of the Medicare Prescription Drug, Improvement and Modernization Act of 2003, Congress added a provision for prescription drug (Plan D) coverage to traditional Medicare plans. This law also introduced Medicare Advantage plans, in which the government offers financial incentives to private insurers to take on some of the burden of covering the nation's elderly. Advantage plans, which can be set up in a variety of ways, including HMOs and PPOs, replace traditional Medicare for those who choose to participate in them. However, the vast majority of Americans over age 65 choose to stick with traditional Medicare, which is split into three parts:

▲ **Part A (hospital) coverage:** Part A coverage is provided upon application to people age 65 or older and to those entitled to specified programs, such as Social Security and programs for people with end-stage renal disease.

▲ **Part B (physician and outpatient services) coverage:** To obtain Part B coverage, beneficiaries must pay a premium, which is supposed to cover one-quarter of the actuarial cost but usually falls short and must be subsidized by general tax revenues. Prior to 2007, the monthly premium was the same for all Part B participants, but based on the Medicare Prescription Drug, Improvement and Modernization Act, beneficiaries with higher incomes must pay an income-based surcharge, which is being phased in over a three-year period. In 2007, the standard monthly premium was $98.40. Beneficiaries with incomes of $80,000 to $100,000 paid a 13.3 percent surcharge, for a total monthly premium of $111.50. Beneficiaries with incomes of more than $200,000 paid a surcharge of 73.3 percent, or about $72 per month, for a total monthly premium of about $170.50.[5]

▲ **Part D (prescription drug) coverage:** Part D coverage provides protection for people who have very high drug costs. Everyone who has Medicare is eligible for this coverage. Beneficiaries must pay a monthly premium, which varies by plan, and a yearly deductible; they must also pay a part of the cost of their prescriptions, including a copayment or coinsurance.

While the specifics of coverage can be complex, clear and detailed descriptions of benefits are readily available at www.medicare.gov. Because Part B coverage is so heavily subsidized and Part A beneficiaries are usually enrolled unless they explicitly choose to opt out, almost all individuals insured through Medicare (98 percent) have both Parts A and B. In addition, 88 percent of those with Medicare have supplemental "Medigap" insurance[6] that covers copayments, deductibles, drugs, and some other expenses.

5.2.5 Medicaid

People who are poor can't pay for insurance, and many of them (10 percent of the population) are covered under the **Medicaid** program. This combined federal/state program insures people whose incomes are insufficient to pay for health care, primarily those on welfare, and it also provides supplemental coverage for a substantial number of elderly people, including a majority of those living in nursing homes.

As previously mentioned, Medicaid is funded jointly by the states and the federal government. The federal government may pay as much as 80 percent of the total program cost for low-income states but only half for wealthier states. Program design differs from state to state. Although Medicaid was designed to cover mothers with low incomes and their children, it has become the largest funding mechanism for nursing homes. This has occurred primarily because Medicare has very limited nursing home coverage; therefore, as the elderly incur expenses during long nursing home stays, they become poor enough to qualify for Medicaid.

5.2.6 Other Government and Private Programs and Charity

Besides the forms of insurance discussed so far in this chapter, various other programs also pay for certain health care costs. Charity paid for about $58 billion in health care in 2002. That same year, workers' compensation, automobile accident insurance, and similar programs paid more than $25 billion. The Department of Veterans Affairs received $22 billion in funding, with a somewhat smaller amount being paid for dependents through the Department of Defense. Programs sponsored by the Maternal and Child Health Bureau, Substance Abuse and Mental Health Services Administration, Bureau of Indian Affairs, and a variety of other programs accounted for about another $28 billion in health care.[7]

5.2.7 The Uninsured

Despite the wide variety of health insurance plans available, 45 million Americans have no health insurance. Uninsured individuals who need care must try to pay with their own limited resources, find special government programs, depend on charity, or simply present themselves at hospitals or clinics and ask to be treated free of charge. The percentage of the population without coverage depends significantly on the efforts of local and state governments. States choosing expansive Medicaid programs and broad outreach to the working poor can reduce the number of uninsured individuals substantially.

While some uninsured individuals pay large sums out of pocket when they get sick, a much greater number stay healthy and pocket the cash or, having no resources, depend on charity when they are ill. That is why the problem of so many uninsured individuals is so difficult to solve. For many of the uninsured, not having insurance is the most economical option. Three-fourths of uninsured Americans are under age 35, and people this young tend to be healthy, to be enrolled in college, or to earn low wages. For them, paying $300 a month or even $100 a month for health insurance doesn't make sense.[8] People over age 35 who are working in low-paying jobs often need money to eat and pay rent more than they need it to provide protection from uncertain medical bills that may never materialize. There's also a small number of people who are chronically ill and wouldn't pass even a cursory medical exam and hence can be insured only if they take jobs in companies that provide group coverage.

It would be easy to insure everyone by mandating universal coverage, yet this is unlikely to happen in the United States because it's politically unpopular. Most of the suggested reforms wouldn't have a major impact because those people currently without insurance are often uninsured because of rational economic choices that they have made themselves or that insurance companies have made.

5.2.8 State Children's Health Insurance Program

A 2006 study by the Robert Wood Johnson Foundation found that one in four children without health insurance receives no medical care each year, compared with one in eight children with health insurance.[9] The State Children's Health Insurance Program (SCHIP) was enacted by Congress in 1997 as Title XXI of the Social Security Act to provide $40 billion to increase coverage for the 10 million children under the age of 18 who are uninsured. The program covers children whose parents make too much money to qualify for Medicaid but too little to afford private insurance. The program works through state governments, but some have used available funding for other purposes, leading to unevenness in implementation. However, since the program was first implemented, the percentage of children without health insurance has decreased by more than

> ## FOR EXAMPLE
>
> ### What Do People Buy When They Don't Buy Health Insurance?
>
> Most of the time, being uninsured is a matter of choice. It may not be a sensible choice or may be the result of a choice no one would want to face (either buy food or buy health insurance), but it's a choice nonetheless. Knowing what people buy when they don't buy health insurance provides insight into their choice. One study indicates that what people buy with the money they save from not purchasing health insurance depends significantly on whether they are poor or relatively well off.[10] According to the study, for people in the bottom quartile of the income distribution, the money they didn't spend on health insurance went mostly toward food, rent, and other necessities. For people in the upper income quartile, the spending pattern was quite different: The largest spending increase was for transportation, specifically for expensive used cars. This study indicates that programs that try to help people who are truly needy may inadvertently subsidize people who are uninsured simply because they want to spend money on other things.

20 percent. Unfortunately, almost 8 million children still go without any health insurance, even though about 70% of those children are eligible for SCHIP or Medicaid coverage.

5.2.9 Health Savings Accounts (HSAs)

Insurance provides protection against the cost of medical care. Inevitably, this protection makes people less sensitive to costs; that is, they are more willing to use extra services and less concerned about finding the best price for the services they use.

Health savings accounts (HSAs) are attempts to make patients more aware of costs and force them to act as smart shoppers. In an HSA, a person deposits a set amount of money each year in a tax-advantaged account, which can then be used to purchase medical services. Any money left in the HSA at the end of the year can be rolled over to the next year or eventually used to fund retirement. With an HSA, money in the tax-advantaged account is used until the account is depleted, and every additional dollar of medical care after that takes $1 out of the patient's pocket. This is a high-powered incentive to motivate people to pay attention to costs, shop for the lowest prices, and avoid unnecessary services. To provide protection against substantial losses, HSAs must be packaged together with high-deductible major medical plans (e.g., insurance that pays a specified percentage, such as 90 percent, of all expenses above a limit, perhaps $5,000).

A HEALTH CARE CONUNDRUM

One conundrum of the insurance market is that you tend to get what you pay for: If you only insure catastrophes, you get a lot of catastrophes. If a catastrophic plan provides full coverage above a limit, then patients (and hospitals) have no incentives to control costs. Conversely, trying to get patients to pay more to make them cost-sensitive in this range might seem cruel and not work well in practice; an employee with a disability who must come up with 20 percent of a $450,000 liver transplant bill isn't going to be happy and will find many newspaper reporters sympathetic to his or her complaints that this kind of insurance isn't fair.

Using HSAs to increase patients' incentives to save money may solve some problems but could create others. Because risks are not being pooled in a group, the individual is largely at risk for midrange expenditures (i.e., those between $1,000 and $5,000). This makes HSAs attractive to relatively young and healthy employees who expect to be able to keep total medical spending below the annual HSA contribution amount in most years, but not to older employees or those who have dependents suffering from chronic illnesses. Such adverse selection means that the premiums for employees who don't choose HSAs are almost certain to rise. Also, the bulk of medical costs are not in the low or middle range but attributable to those few unfortunate patients who get very sick and have costs at the high end, where the major medical coverage kicks in and reduces the incentive to save money.

SELF-CHECK

- Explain the difference between **Medicare** and **Medicaid**.
- List three options that people without insurance have for getting medical care.
- Describe how **HSAs** work.

5.3 Incentives for Patients, to Payers, and to Providers

People make medical decisions based on the type of insurance they have. Insurance contracts not only provide coverage for risks, they also structure the incentives. This means that if an insurance policy provides coverage for a certain type of medical service or procedure, it's giving policyholders an incentive to take advantage of that service because the policyholder doesn't have to pay money out of pocket to use it. Similarly, if the policy doesn't cover a service, it's giving policyholders a disincentive to use the service because the patient will have to pay for the service with private funds. For example, consider the difference between Policy A, which provides three days of hospital coverage for a mother and her newborn child, and Policy B, which covers only two days in the hospital. Mothers with Policy A have an incentive to stay three days, whereas those with Policy B have an incentive to limit their stay to two days because they would have to pay for the third day out of their own pocket.

HMO and PPO contracts use reduced deductibles and copayments to provide incentives for patients to use only hospitals for which the HMO or PPO has negotiated volume discounts—and it's the promise of additional volume that makes hospitals offer discounts. Most drug reimbursement is now of the "triple-tier" form: a low per-prescription fee for generic drugs, a moderate per-prescription fee or percentage for drugs on an approved list (formulary), and a higher per-prescription fee or percentage for "off-list" drugs. Indeed, oftentimes, a physician must write a letter (a significant disincentive) for the patient to get any reimbursement at all if the prescribed drug is not on the list. By structuring incentives this way, insurance contracts achieve the following goals:

▲ They reduce or increase the use of certain services.
▲ They steer patients to approved providers.
▲ They affect the sort of price negotiations that take place.

Insurance, like many other business arrangements, tends to serve the interests of those who write the contracts. In the long run, contracts must meet the needs of all parties, but it can take a long time to get there. Also, it's possible to structure contracts so that the interests of some parties are ignored. For example, a corporation might be willing to eliminate coverage for alcoholism because it could just fire an employee rather than rehabilitate him or her, or it might be willing to put an annual maximum on the number of days of hospital treatment to discourage people with HIV/AIDS from taking jobs there. Universal national health insurance coverage would put everyone under the same contract so that no one could be excluded. However, if everyone is insured under the same plan, no one has incentives to shop around for better prices, there is no ability to pick and choose which coverage is or isn't worthwhile, and there is no chance to go somewhere else if the service provided by the insurer is unsatisfactory. Insurance contracts in the real world represent a balancing of incentives and interests, a balance that is changing all the time.

FOR EXAMPLE

Disincentives for Using Birth Control

Women of childbearing age spend approximately 68 percent more out-of-pocket on health care costs than males of the same age, mostly because of costs associated with reproductive health, such as gynecological exams and birth control. Prescription contraceptives can be expensive—approximately $360 per year for oral contraceptives, $180 per year for Depo-Provera, $450 for Norplant, and $240 per year for an intrauterine device. Although federal and state legislation requiring insurance companies to cover prescription contraceptives has dramatically increased the number of insurance companies covering prescription birth control, some insurance policies don't fall under these laws and don't cover this expense. Insurance policies that don't cover contraceptives for their policyholders create a disincentive to use birth control to prevent unwanted pregnancies. As noted by *Healthy People 2010,* a statement of national health objectives published by the U.S. Department of Health and Human Services, "in the absence of comprehensive [contraception] coverage, many women may opt for whatever method may be covered by their health plan rather than the method most appropriate for their individual needs and circumstances. Other women may opt not to use contraception if it is not covered under their insurance plan."[11]

SELF-CHECK

- Describe how an insurance policy creates incentives for some medical services and disincentives for others.
- What is a triple-tier formulary? Why do insurance companies use these formularies?

SUMMARY

Paying medical bills with insurance makes health care a third-party transaction. All three parties—patients, providers, and insurers—must benefit from the transaction. It is important to keep in mind that health care is paid for by people (as patients, taxpayers, or employees giving up some wages to get health benefits), not by corporations.

Insurance comes in a range of contractual forms, from pure insurance with fixed premiums, to various forms of risk sharing, to administered services only, to self-insurance plans in which the employer bears all the risk. Insurance contracts create incentives for patients, providers, and insurance companies to behave in ways that affect the market. Almost any contract favors some interests and harms others.

KEY TERMS

Closed-panel HMO	A managed care plan that provides all care in-house, using its own doctors and hospitals.
Health maintenance organization (HMO)	An organization that contracts to provide comprehensive medical services (not reimbursement) for a specified fee each month.
Health savings account (HSA)	A tax status given to a variety of savings and investment vehicles that allows tax deferred deposits up to stated yearly limits, tax-deferred interest, and tax-free withdrawals for qualified medical expenses.
Managed care organization (MCO)	An HMO, a PPO, or another organization that accepts financial risk for and manages medical care.
Managed care plan	A type of insurance plan in which a manager controls the number and type of services covered in return for more affordable premiums.
Medicaid	A combined state/federal program that insures people whose incomes are insufficient to pay for health care, primarily those individuals on welfare and elderly people in nursing homes.
Medicare	A federal government insurance program that provides hospital (Part A), medical (Part B), and prescription drug (Part D) benefits to persons over age 65 and some qualified people with disabilities.
Preferred provider organization (PPO)/point-of-service plan (POS)	A managed care plan that offers enrollees a discount for using hospitals and physicians within an approved network of contracted providers.

ASSESS YOUR UNDERSTANDING

Go to www.wiley.com/college/getzen to evaluate your knowledge of insurance contracts and the flow of funds in the insurance industry.
Measure your learning by comparing pre-test and post-test results.

Summary Questions

1. An insurance company may still be profitable even if underwriting gains are negative because:
   (a) underwriting gains fail to account for the positive impacts of moral hazards.
   (b) administrative costs are included in underwriting but have nothing to do with profitability.
   (c) investment income on premiums held before payment of benefits may offset underwriting losses.
   (d) under managed care, the insurance company can expect steadily declining claims.

2. The U.S. tax system creates an incentive:
   (a) to provide health insurance to employees because it is nontaxable compensation to employees and a deductible expense for employers.
   (b) to pay for health care with after-tax dollars because that is the only way the employee will get the advantage of the tax deduction.
   (c) to minimize health insurance coverage because it is an expense to the employer, and the employees would prefer to receive higher wages and pay for their own health insurance.
   (d) to consume less medical care because the more one spends, the more likely it is that the dollars are from income taxed at a high marginal rate.

3. The funds to pay providers:
   (a) ultimately come from households, except when they come from a government program.
   (b) ultimately come from households, except when they come from employer-provided health insurance.
   (c) ultimately come from households, except when they come from private health insurance.
   (d) always ultimately come from households.

4. Medicare is a state- and federally funded program that provides health coverage for the nation's poor. True or False?

5. Which of the following is *not* well covered by Medicare?
   (a) Hospitalization expense
   (b) Nursing home care
   (c) Clinical laboratory services
   (d) Home health care
   (e) Physician expense

6. Individuals purchasing their own insurance often pay significantly higher premiums than those who get insurance through an employer. True or False?

7. Insurance companies use incentives such as lower copayments and deductibles to encourage patients to use certain hospitals and physicians. True or False?

Review Questions

1. Who benefits from a three-party insurance transaction?

2. Which government insurance program is more affected by adverse selection, Medicare or Medicaid?

3. HSAs are sometimes touted as reducing the inefficiencies in the health care system, motivating people to pay attention to costs, shop for the lowest prices, and avoid unnecessary services. However, HSAs haven't eliminated all market inefficiencies. Identify inefficiencies associated with these accounts.

4. It is often said that for many of the uninsured, not having insurance is a rational economic decision. Explain.

5. Explain how an insurance contract can provide more or fewer incentives to do the following:
   (a) Choose a higher-quality (more expensive) hospital
   (b) Spend more days in the hospital
   (c) Use more drugs
   (d) Choose a higher-quality (more expensive) surgeon

Applying This Chapter

1. If the funds to pay for health care always eventually come from households, what difference does it make whether health care coverage is expanded by mandated private benefits or government programs? (In answering this question, try to deal with issues other than simply support for or opposition of government spending.)

2. Federal law gives a worker who becomes unemployed the right to buy continuing health insurance coverage through the employer after leaving the company. Why might it be rational for a factory worker who loses his or her job to give up this legal right to purchase coverage and become uninsured, even if he or she knows that he or she is at risk for high medical expenditures?

3. How might an insurance company structure incentives in such a way as to discourage people from seeking mental health services? How might it structure incentives to encourage people to seek mental health services?

YOU TRY IT

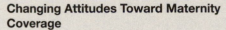

Changing Attitudes Toward Maternity Coverage

Prior to 1970, maternity was usually treated differently from other medical expenses, either excluded entirely from coverage or subject to a flat lump-sum cash (indemnity) benefit. Why? During the 1970s, 23 states mandated that treatment related to pregnancy be covered the same as any other type of treatment, and in 1978, such coverage became uniform throughout the United States. Would mandated maternity benefits make working in a salaried position more or less attractive to women? Would they make women of childbearing age more or less attractive as employees? Would they increase or decrease the number of births performed by Cesarean section? Who do you think bore the expense of implementing this mandate? Write a paper indicating the rationale for your answers to these questions. (For a discussion of these issues, see Gruber, Jonathan, "The Incidence of Mandated Maternity Benefits," *American Economic Review* 84(3): 622–641, April 1994.)

Comparing Insurance Policies

Insurance policies vary widely, even when issued by the same company. For instance, even BlueCross coverage differs, depending on the employer. Obtain at least two insurance policy contracts or brochures that explain coverage for different policies. Write a paper comparing the policies, considering the types of benefits offered and the incentives and disincentives each type of coverage creates.

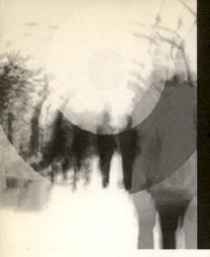

6

PHYSICIANS
The Economics of Practicing Medicine

Starting Point

Go to www.wiley.com/college/getzen to assess your knowledge of the role of physicians in the health care system.
Determine where you need to concentrate your effort.

What You'll Learn in This Chapter

▲ How physicians are paid
▲ How physician incomes are based on specialty
▲ How much it costs to run a practice
▲ How doctors act as patients' agents
▲ The role of licensure in the supply and demand for medical care

After Studying This Chapter You'll Be Able To

▲ Evaluate the physician payment system
▲ Analyze the role of physician specialty in determining physician pay
▲ Calculate the cost of running a physician practice
▲ Assess the role of agency and insurance in transferring responsibility from patients
▲ Critique the practice of medical licensure

INTRODUCTION

At the center of medical practice stands the physician. Physicians direct the flow of patients by controlling admissions, referrals, regulations, insurance reimbursements, and prescriptions. Physicians earn high incomes, partially in compensation for their extensive investment in their education. However, the value placed on this investment is a result of market forces rather than any intrinsic feature of practicing medicine.

A very powerful and special bond exists between doctor and patient. This relationship is based on medical science—and ethics and emotions—as well as economics.[1] The bond is supported by the practice of physician licensing, which protects patients while at the same time limiting the supply of physicians and, thereby, ensuring that physicians are well paid.

6.1 Physician Payment: How Funds Flow In

While most of the labor force is employed and paid a salary by large organizations, most physicians are independent entrepreneurs or partners running what are, in effect, small businesses.[2] The income of physicians in solo or group private practices mostly comes from **fee-for-service payments,** or payment of a specified amount for each visit or procedure, although an increasing amount is coming from complex, negotiated third-party contracts. In the 1930s, physicians were essentially free to charge whatever they decided was appropriate but often collected much less than what they charged. Today, 88 percent of physician revenues come from third-party payments,[3] and most fees are subject to some form of external review or control (see Table 6-1).

It's important to distinguish between what the physician charges (i.e., the amount that appears on the bill) and the actual payments made by the insurance company, which may be considerably less. One of the initial steps in the evolution of physician payment in the United States was the development of usual, customary, and reasonable (UCR) fee schedules. The BlueShield plans, which provided the largest portion of physician insurance and operated with the support of local medical societies, collected information on what each physician charged for each service in a local area during the previous year. When a physician submitted a bill, it was checked to determine whether it was above his or her median charge for the same service the previous year (usual), above the 75th percentile of charges by all doctors in the area (customary), or justifiably higher because of a patient's complicating secondary illness or another acceptable reason (reasonable). When Medicare was implemented in 1966, it adopted the BlueShield UCR method of paying physicians.

An effort to reduce payments, particularly for certain services, led insurers to begin using **fee schedules.** A fee schedule is a list that specifies how much

Table 6-1: Types of Physician Payment

Charges:	The amount appearing on a bill, without insurance.
Fee-for-service:	A specified payment for each unit of service provided.
Fee schedule:	A set "menu" of prices for each service that is agreed upon in advance.
UCR:	A method for denying bills that are out of line with the "usual, customary, and reasonable charges" made by this and other physicians for the same service last year.
RVS:	A schedule based on objective standards showing relative value points for each service compared to a common unit (i.e., regular office visit). Deciding a dollar value per point converts it into a fee schedule.
RBRVS:	The relative value schedule set by Medicare for physician fees.
Capitation:	A set payment per person per month regardless of the number of services used.
Salary:	A paycheck from an employer.

the insurance company will pay physicians for particular services. Fee schedules can be proposed by the sellers (i.e., physicians) to try to keep prices up or by the buyers (i.e., Medicare, insurance companies) to try to keep prices down. A major difficulty with fee schedules is the amazingly large number of services that must be priced. It's easy to come up with a reasonable price for a coronary bypass operation or services associated with a normal birth, but what about for oblique lateral pelvic X-rays, measurement of bilirubin or potassium levels, management of schizophrenia, and a host of other medical services?

To bring order to fee schedules, organizations have devised **relative value scales,** which give each service a point value. A common service (e.g., standard office visit, hernia repair surgery) is usually given a weight of 1 point, and all other services are given point values relative to that standard unit of service (e.g., 5 points, 0.2 points). After the physician and insurance company agree on the value per point, payment for each service is determined (e.g., if value per point is $20, a physician providing a 3.5-point service is paid 3.5 × $20 = $70). In 1992, the **Medicare resource-based relative value scale (RBRVS)** was implemented. A team of health economists and health services researchers studied the resources used in providing physician care to estimate a point value for each service, based on (1) physician time, (2) intensity of effort, (3) practice costs, and (4) costs of advanced specialty training.[4] The Centers for Medicare and Medicaid Services (CMS) of the U.S. Department of Health and Human Services, which administers the

Medicare program, set the dollars per point for 2006 at $37.90, with adjustments for geographic variation in practice costs and for malpractice insurance.

The Medicare physician reimbursement system provides a kind of "public good" for other insurance programs; that is, it offers a universally understood and practiced standard fee schedule that insurance companies can adopt or easily modify by changing the dollar conversion factor or separating certain categories. Medicaid, BlueCross, and commercial insurance contracts that cover the 87 percent of the population under age 65 often base their payments on a modified form of the Medicare RBRVS or use Medicare payment levels as a benchmark.

6.1.1 Copayments, Assignment, and Balance Billing

Medicare and other insurers' contracts often require patients to cover part of their medical expenses. The most common patient expenses are as follows:

▲ Patients in managed care plans are typically required to make **copayments**, or payments of a specified amount for each service rendered. For example, a copayment of $10 or $20 per office visit may be required, both to reduce premiums and, by forcing the patient to bear some costs, to reduce the number of services utilized.

▲ Most patients must also meet certain **deductibles**; in other words, they must pay a certain amount out of their own pocket before the insurance company begins to pay their medical bills. A deductible requires the patient to pay, say, the first $100 or $500 out of pocket per year or per illness. Some insurance policies, called high-deductible policies, require the patient to pay anywhere from the first $1,500 to $7,500, depending on the policy.

▲ **Coinsurance,** in which patients must pay a certain amount or percentage or a medical bill that insurance does not pay for, may also be part of an insurance agreement. Requiring patients to pay coinsurance of, say, 10 percent or 20 percent of the bill, is a common part of major medical benefits.

Insurance contracts are so complex that it's often difficult for either the patient or the physician to know exactly who is responsible for which part of the bill. Two forms of payment can be distinguished, however:

▲ **Individual reimbursement:** Under **individual reimbursement**, the patient pays all the charges, sends copies of the bills to the insurer, and is reimbursed for the medical expenses that are covered.

▲ **Assignment:** Under **assignment**, the physician sends the bill to the insurer. The patient is charged for the copayment and may be balance billed for the difference if the physician's charges exceed the maximum fee allowed by the insurance contract.

Under the Medicare participation agreement, a physician who accepts assignment agrees not to **balance bill** for any charges over the Medicare payment, meaning that he or she will not bill the patient over and above what Medicare pays for any particular service. Patients like assignment because they don't have to handle paperwork and aren't stuck with additional fees. Physicians like the fact that they're paid directly and more rapidly, but they don't like being denied the right to charge as much as they believe their services are worth. Indeed, the prohibition of balance billing in Canada led to a national physician's strike when the rule was first imposed.

Under current U.S. Medicare rules, physicians are limited to an additional 15 percent above the Medicare fee for balance billing if they choose not to accept assignment and are penalized by receiving only 95 percent of the regular fee schedule for services. In effect, Medicare has ruled out balance billing by making it economically unattractive. Medicaid rules are often more stringent and have significantly lower payment rates, which is why many physicians choose not to participate in the Medicaid program. Some physicians choose not to participate in Medicare to avoid the payment limits imposed by the RBRVS system, but because 20 percent of all physician bills are paid for by Medicare, this is difficult for physicians to do unless their practice is mostly obstetrics, sports medicine, or another specialty in which they treat few elderly clients.

6.1.2 Physician Payment in Managed Care Plans

As insurance companies have tried to control their costs by exercising market power, they have refused to passively pay whatever physicians charge them and instead have instituted a system of negotiated fees. For some common and easily specified services purchased in large volume (e.g., intraocular lens implants, psychiatric evaluations for drug abuse), an insurance company can often obtain a low fixed price, set in advance, in return for guaranteeing the physician a certain number of patients or procedures. When individual fees aren't negotiated, it's common for managed care contracts to specify discounted fees, offering perhaps 75 percent of what the physician would ordinarily bill other patients.

The complexities of per-unit service pricing are bypassed completely under **capitation,** or payment of a fixed amount per person per month, regardless of the number of services used (see Chapter 10). A health maintenance organization (HMO) using a capitation rate of $30 per month pays that amount to the physician for each of the HMO members enrolled with that physician, whether the members visit the doctor's office once, twice, 10 times, or not at all. **Independent practice association (IPA) HMOs** that contract with many physicians use capitation rates to pay physicians, but a **staff HMO** hires physicians to work exclusively in the HMO's facility and pays physicians a salary, with perhaps some bonus based on productivity or on the profitability of the HMO. With this arrangement, the physician, in effect, becomes an employee of a large medical care firm. Salaried physicians are also found in administrative posts and in research and teaching organizations. About 42 percent of physicians are now salaried employees, and the number continues to grow as health care organizations become larger and more complex. Chapter 10 presents a more extensive discussion of managed care contracting.

6.1.3 Incentives: Why Differences in the Type of Payment Matter

How physicians are paid determines the incentives they face to work harder, raise prices, or admit patients to the hospital:

▲ Under fee-for-service insurance, a physician gets paid more for doing more.

▲ Under capitation, the payment is the same, regardless of the number of services provided; therefore, a physician may do less.

▲ Under a relative value scale, payment is based on the number of points; therefore, physicians may push to classify a service in a higher point category.

Payment type may affect patients' access to physician care as well. The Medicaid program has come under severe budgetary constraints and thus tends to pay physicians less than BlueShield, HMOs, and commercial insurance. Although physicians are constrained by ethics and law to provide high-quality care to all who need it, economic theory predicts that government imposition of mandatory price controls leads to shortages. For instance, a group of experimenters called 300 physician offices and requested appointments, identifying their type of insurance as Medicaid.[5] Almost half the physician offices said that they were not accepting new patients, and when the experimenters did get appointments, the average wait was two weeks. The experimenters then called back, identifying themselves as having commercial insurance, and 78 percent of the doctors' offices gave them appointments within two days. As this study illustrates, physicians try hard to provide adequate care to the poor, but if the payment levels are consistently lower, the level of service will be lower.

6.1.4 A Progression: From Prices to Reimbursement Mechanisms

As the medical care system has moved away from fee-for-service arrangements and closer to salaried arrangements, the linkage between the flow of funds from patients and the flow of funds to physicians has been severed. Although there may be some "price" attached to each service under Medicare RBRVS, the price bears almost no resemblance to what it would be in a normal market: The patient doesn't pay the price, nor does the price allow the supplier to match output to demand because it's imposed externally. Who is paid and how much is determined, in part, by concerns about how the elderly will vote in the next election, the effectiveness of insurance lobbies, or a need to find the least difficult way of balancing the budget. Tracking the flow of funds to and from physicians is further obscured by referring

FOR EXAMPLE

Physician Incentives: Fee-for-Service Care vs. Salary Care

In an intriguing experiment, half the doctors in a pediatric clinic were randomly selected to be paid on a fee-for-service basis and half were selected to be paid a salary.[6] The fees were set so that the average doctor seeing the average number of patients would earn the same on either a fee-for-service or salary basis. The fee-for-service doctors saw more patients, recalled them for more visits, and generally exceeded the normal guidelines for the amount of services, while the doctors who were on salary saw fewer patients, had them return less frequently, and more often provided fewer services than indicated by standard guidelines. This experiment demonstrates that economic predictions regarding the incentive effects of different types of payment are borne out in a practice setting.

to all payments as *reimbursement,* even though insurance companies don't "reimburse" physician costs (physician time is the bulk of the expense), so payments are more accurately termed physician *fees, revenues,* or *salary.*

SELF-CHECK

- Explain the difference between UCR **fee schedules** and the **Medicare RBRVS.**
- Explain how **copayments** differ from **deductibles** and **coinsurance.**
- What does it mean when a physician accepts **assignment?** What does it mean when a physician **balance bills?** Can a physician who accepts assignment balance bill?
- List some pros and cons of **capitation.**

6.2 Physician Incomes

Physicians are among the most highly trained and well-compensated workers in the United States. The average pretax income for a primary care physician in 2003 was $146,405,[7] about four times the average worker's salary. The wage gap between physicians and other professionals seems to be closing, however. Although physician earnings grew more rapidly than average workers' earnings for most of the twentieth century, during the period from 1995 to 2003, they experienced a sharp decline. Physician earnings decreased about 7 percent after accounting for inflation, while earnings for other professionals increased by 7 percent.[8]

Table 6-2: Physician Characteristics[9]

Total number of U.S. physicians	884,974
Physicians active in patient care	700,287
Residents in training programs	102,563
International medical graduates	224,043

To a large extent, physicians' high earnings were attributable to the quality of those who entered the profession (almost all were in the top quarter of their college graduating classes), the long years of postcollege training required, the extra effort (most physicians worked about 50 percent more hours than the average salaried worker), and compensation for having to act as entrepreneurs and manage medical businesses (self-employed physicians earned 50 percent more than those who chose to work on salaries). However, even after adjusting for all these factors, an individual still obtains a premium for becoming a physician. Perhaps even more important than higher incomes is the implied "floor"; physicians virtually never face unemployment, and many are able to accept "low-paid" positions (i.e., those that pay less than $100,000 per year) to follow their own interests in helping the poor, working with children, traveling to exotic locations, or studying interesting diseases.

Even during training in residency programs, physicians earn about $35,000 per year, which is about the same as the average worker, although certainly less than the opportunity cost of the doctor's time (see the discussion of the costs of time and returns in Section 7.1). As with most other workers, physicians' earnings grow rapidly early in their careers, rise to a peak around age 50, and decline thereafter (see Tables 6-2 through 6-5).

Table 6-3: Physician Incomes Based on Specialty

Median Income	Specialty	Percentage of Physician Population
$180,000	All physicians	100%
$148,000	Pediatrics	8%
$145,000	Psychiatry	5%
$145,000	General/family practice	11%
$150,000	General internal medicine	17%
$222,000	Allergy/immunology	1%
$224,000	Pulmonology	1%
$282,000	Dermatology	1%

(continued)

Table 6-3: Physician Incomes Based on Specialty *(continued)*

Median Income	Specialty	*Percentage of* Physician Population
$350,000	Cardiovascular practice	3%
$205,000	Emergency medicine	3%
$215,000	Obstetrics/gynecology	5%
$234,000	General surgery	5%
$300,000	Orthopedic surgery	3%
$400,000	Plastic surgery	1%

Table 6-4: Physician Income Based on Practice Size/Type

Median Income	Practice Type	*Percentage of* Physician Population
$154,000	Employee or contractor	42%
$155,000	Self-employed solo	25%
$240,000	Self-employed group	33%
$200,000	2 physician partners	
$217,000	3-physician group	
$220,000	4-physician group	
$250,000	5- to 25-physician group	
$240,000	25+physician group	

Table 6-5: Physician Income by Age

Median Income	Age	*Percentage of* Physician Population
$140,000	Under 35 years	16%
$174,000	35–44	24%
$198,000	45–54	25%
$180,000	55–64	17%
$150,000	65 or older	18%

There is a marked difference in earnings by specialty. Generalists and family practitioners are at the low end, with pediatricians and psychiatrists only slightly above. The high end is made up of surgeons, radiologists, and anesthesiologists. Much of the difference in incomes among specialties is attributable to the reimbursement system: Physicians get paid more for doing something (e.g., reading an x-ray, performing an operation) than for caring or thinking (e.g., listening to a patient's history, deciding which path of treatment to follow, helping the family of a dying person). The reimbursement system is driven by "billable events." A physician always finds it easier to get paid for a procedure, because it is observable and has a standard billing code, than for a personal interaction or conceptual effort. The bottom line for a physician is that the income potential from choosing a particular specialty has more to do with how the services of that specialty are treated by insurance than with the work or training involved.

The Medicare RBRVS system was designed to rebalance incomes across specialties and provide more payment for thinking and caring, but this system is only partially successful. Health insurance is designed to protect individuals against potentially large but infrequent losses while minimizing excess purchase of discretionary services. While this makes sense from a risk management perspective, in practice, it means that fees for some specialties are almost fully covered (e.g., surgery, anesthesia), leading to increased demand for those procedures and higher incomes for the physicians offering such services, while other specialties are subject to copayments and deductibles that limit demand and incomes (e.g., pediatrics, psychiatry).

FOR EXAMPLE

Physician Incomes: More Cuts on the Way?

In 2006, CMS announced plans to cut payments to physicians by 5.1 percent, with projected cuts totaling 34 percent over the following nine years. The cuts will affect the approximately 875,000 physicians who see elderly and disabled patients. CMS justifies the cuts based on the fact that spending on physician-related services such as lab work, imaging, and physician-administered drugs has increased at faster-than-expected rates. How do physicians plan to respond to such cuts? According to a survey of physicians by the American Medical Association,[10] 71 percent of surveyed physicians said they'll make one or more changes in their practice, such as reducing time spent with Medicare patients. Forty-two percent said they'll no longer visit nursing homes to see patients.

SELF-CHECK

- Indicate the median income for physicians.
- List two of the highest-paid physician specialties.
- List two of the lowest-paid physician specialties.

6.3 Physician Costs: How Funds Flow Out

Because physicians are usually small business owners running their own practices, they have startup costs, labor costs, insurance costs, and other small businesses expenses.

6.3.1 Physician Practice Expenses

The expenses of maintaining a practice take up almost half of all the funds flowing into physician offices (see Table 6-6). Physicians must pay for other medical professionals and assistants who help them take care of patients, as well as taxes, rent, utilities, supplies, malpractice insurance, and so on. In addition to all these ongoing expenses, it usually takes at least $100,000 in startup capital to equip even the most basic office, and an elaborate suite housing an active practice in specialties such as plastic surgery could cost several million dollars. One reason for physicians to work together in group practices is to obtain economies of scale from sharing office space, equipment, information systems, assistants who specialize in support functions (e.g., laboratory technicians, billing and appointment clerks, physical therapists), and so on.

Physicians worked an average of 57 hours per week, seeing 105 patients, and giving 4 hours of charity/uncompensated care. The average charge for a patient visit was about $100 in 2006.

6.3.2 The Labor–Leisure Choice

Most of a physician's income is compensation for all the hours of work put in. How should this time be valued? What is its opportunity cost? For a young physician starting out with relatively few patients, it's common to take on a temporary part-time moonlighting job in a hospital emergency room or in a well-established senior practice that sees many patients for wages of $75 to $150 per hour. Because doctors give up those jobs as their practices become established, their time must be worth more than that, but what forgone opportunity defines this higher hourly rate? What a busy physician gives up is leisure: time to be with family, time to run and swim and watch television, and even time to sleep.

Table 6-6: Physician's Office Practice Revenues and Expenses[11]

Revenues		
Private insurance	$198,000	45%
Medicare	$123,200	28%
Medicaid	$ 57,200	13%
Patient paid	$ 61,600	14%
Total gross revenues	*$ 440,000*	*100%*
Expenses		
Net income	$195,000	52%
Non-physician employee wages (3.5 full-time equivalents per physician)	$ 61,500	16%
Wages for employee physicians (fill-in physicians used on an as-needed basis)	$ 9,000	2%
Office rent and expenses	$ 45,000	12%
Medical supplies	$ 15,750	4%
Malpractice liability insurance	$ 17,250	5%
Equipment	$ 6,750	2%
Other expenses	$ 24,750	7%
Total expenses	*$ 375,000*	*100%*

The more lucrative each hour of practice is and the more hours the physician puts in, the more each hour of forgone leisure is worth. Most doctors work very hard, averaging more than 50 hours per week. Furthermore, once they make $150,000 or $250,000 per year, a little time off may well be worth more to them than earning an extra $5,000 by working late. This is one reason the supply of physician time isn't very elastic; even doubling or quadrupling physicians' income couldn't get physicians to double the number of hours worked. For some physicians, supply is "backward bending"—that is, higher income per hour may make them feel sufficiently rich that they work fewer rather than more hours.[12]

6.3.3 The "Doctor's Workshop" and Unpaid Hospital Inputs

Almost every doctor needs to use a hospital to provide patient care. Some specialties (e.g., anesthesiology, thoracic surgery, pathology) are practiced almost entirely inside hospitals. Yet physicians don't pay the hospital for the privilege of working there and usually aren't employees of the hospital. The hospital functions as the

> ## FOR EXAMPLE
>
> ### Backward-Bending Supply
>
> If backward-bending supply seems difficult to understand, think about how much you would work if I paid you $100 per hour, $1,000 per hour, or $100,000 per hour. Eventually, you would decide to work less and enjoy leisure more because additional money simply wouldn't mean that much to you.

"doctor's workshop." Because the efforts of hospital nurses, laboratory technicians, and record-keeping professionals don't "cost" the physician anything, physicians tend to overuse these efforts instead of using similar inputs in their offices. It's easy to see how doctors might favor a system of not-for-profit hospitals supported by the community and government subsidy. The value added to their practices by these hospitals far exceeds the hours physicians are expected to "give" to hospital educational and administrative functions.

6.3.4 Malpractice

One of the most contentious physician practice expenses is malpractice insurance. **Malpractice** is physician failure to meet professional standards; malpractice insurance protects physicians in the event that they are sued for malpractice. The rationale for allowing medical malpractice suits is that they improve incentives for safety by forcing doctors to behave more carefully when treating patients. About 1 in 20 physicians will incur a malpractice claim in any given year, and 2 in 5 will be sued at least once during their careers. The premium for a physician's malpractice insurance averages about $20,000 (or 5 percent of gross revenues) but ranges from $5,000 or less for family practitioners to $100,000 or more for orthopedic surgeons and neurosurgeons. While malpractice premiums have risen rapidly in some years, virtually all the additional costs are quickly passed on to patients and their insurance companies in the form of higher fees.

Malpractice is a real problem, but the current malpractice system may not be the best solution. The randomness of the legal process, as well as the fact that most physicians are almost fully insured for losses due to malpractice, limits the effectiveness of the system to change behavior. However, being sued is costly in terms of lost time and increased anxiety, and most physicians exercise extraordinary care in treating patients. Some physicians have claimed that the fear of being sued has raised medical costs by forcing them to practice "defensive medicine."

Does the malpractice system deter negligence by physicians? Only to a limited extent—and at considerable cost. Yet while the ability of malpractice suits to compensate patients for damages or to force doctors to practice better medicine has been roundly criticized with good reason, it hasn't been easy to find a solution that is clearly more efficient or acceptable to both doctors and patients.

SELF-CHECK

- List two physician expenses.
- Explain the concept of backward-bending supply as it applies to the number of hours physicians work.
- What is malpractice insurance?

6.4 The Transaction Between Doctor and Patient

The bond of trust between doctor and patient is one of the strongest professional relationships in society. When patients show up at a doctor's office, they are apt to ask two questions: "What is wrong with me?" and "What should I do about it?"

If told that they have a disease, most patients trust the doctor to perform the right diagnostic and therapeutic procedures, with little idea of what those might be or what the charges will add up to.[13] If a surgeon is called in, he or she is likely to be a complete stranger who asks for thousands of dollars to make an evaluation and incision. Patients who agree to surgery can only hope that in the long run, it will do some good. Unlike a person shopping for a car, a suit, or a haircut, patients don't know what they need, what it should cost, and even, once paid for, how much good the treatment actually did. Instead of having a clear specification of what is to be expected from both parties, the patient must

FOR EXAMPLE

Patient Knowledge: Shopping for Health Care

According to a 2006 Great-West Healthcare survey on consumer attitudes toward health care, 79 percent of those surveyed never learned the cost of a medical service or learned it only after they paid for it.[14] Consumers are far better at guessing the cost of nonmedical products and services than medical ones. In the Great-West Healthcare survey, they could guess the cost of a new Honda Accord within 5 percent, the cost of a Bose Wave music system within 6 percent, and the average cost of a car oil change within 11 percent, but they were much farther off the mark when it came to guessing medical costs. They overestimated the cost of an emergency room visit by 70 percent, underestimated the cost of a routine doctor visit by 52 percent, and low-balled the cost of an average four-day hospital stay by 61 percent. (Consumers estimated the cost of the average four-day hospital stay to be $7,762, but it is actually approximately $20,000.)

trust the doctor to do what is right and to bill fairly for the necessary care (which will, in most cases, mainly be paid for by insurance).

6.4.1 Physicians as Patients' Agents

It's the superior ability of the physician to answer the "What is wrong with me?" and "What should I do about it?" questions that tends to make the doctor–patient relationship so much different from an ordinary commercial transaction. While the physician's information isn't perfect, it's much better than that of the patient, and the physician is able to seek additional information required for treating an illness, at much lower cost. When it's necessary to decide which test to perform, which drug to prescribe, and whether to perform surgery, all these choices can be made better and at lower cost by a physician. An exchange relationship in which one party makes choices on behalf of the other is known as **agency.**[15] Just as a purchasing agent buys supplies for a company and an actor's agent represents the actor in negotiations, a physician is the patient's agent in deciding which treatment is appropriate and which medical services to buy. The reason an agent acts on behalf of another person is that the agent's information and transaction costs are lower. It's cheaper for a physician to make medical choices on behalf of a patient than for the patient to go to medical school to make his or her own decisions.

While many goods and services are exchanged under conditions of less-than-perfect information, it's the importance of our health that sets medical care apart. For example, although I may not know what my mechanic is doing, I can readily observe whether my automobile is working better when it comes back from the shop. Poor-quality parts can be repaired or replaced. At most, I might ask for my money back. Not only is bad surgery difficult to detect, but it can be disabling or even fatal. Once you're dead, repairs, replacements, and even outrageously large malpractice settlements are irrelevant.

SELF-CHECK

- Explain how physicians act as patients' agents.
- What does it mean to say that a physician's information and transaction costs are lower than a patient's?

6.5 Licensure: Quality or Profits?

Licensure is an extension of the agency relationship between doctors and patients to society as a whole. Medical licensure is the establishment of legal restrictions that specify which individuals and firms have rights to provide medical services. Not only do individual patients trust their physicians to act as their personal agents, all of us together have collectively chosen to let the medical profession act as our public agent, deciding who is qualified to practice medicine. Through the institution of licensure, the medical profession serves as a sort of quasi-governmental body, making decisions on behalf of all consumers.[16] Consumers don't examine each doctor's credentials and legal records; they turn that responsibility over to licensure boards. It's less expensive for knowledgeable professionals to do this once for all consumers than to have each patient individually try to determine whether the person listed as a "doctor" in the phone book is qualified to practice medicine. The government doesn't make laws regarding the practice of medicine, but it uses laws to enforce the decisions made by voluntary and independent professional boards.

It's often debated in the media and among economists whether licensure serves the interests of patients (by improving the quality of care) or of physicians (by raising prices and incomes).[17] Such a debate, framed in terms of one side or the other, misses the point: Any public policy in a democracy is, in fact, a form of trade that must serve the interests of both parties if the policy is to be upheld. By the fundamental theorem of exchange, both physicians and patients must be made better off by licensure.

FOR EXAMPLE

The American Board of Medical Specialties

The American Board of Medical Specialties (ABMS) is a not-for-profit agency responsible for physician certification in 24 medical specialties in the United States. Physicians who are candidates for certification are evaluated by member boards of the ABMS. ABMS member boards include the American Board of Anesthesiology, the American Board of Family Medicine, and the American Board of Neurological Surgery. These medical specialty boards review physician educational preparation; assess physician knowledge, skills, and experience in their specialties; and certify all candidates who have satisfied the requirements. Many boards require physicians to become recertified at periodic intervals, thus ensuring that they keep up with advances in their field.[18]

6.5.1 How Licensure Increases Physician Profits

Licensure radically changes the market structure by putting artificial constraints on the supply of physicians. This means that the quantity of physicians doesn't rise or fall depending on the price. Licensure affects physician supply, and thus physician profits, in a number of ways, including the following:

▲ **Limiting who can become a physician:** To the extent that the supply of doctor services is reduced under licensure, prices are higher so that all doctors enjoy higher incomes. (Of course, this means that some people who wished to become doctors aren't allowed to do so.) These profits are maximized if the profession acts as a monopoly in determining how many doctors are allowed to practice.

▲ **Limiting physician productivity:** Supply can also be reduced by work rules that control total productivity. For example, it's common for dental practice regulations to determine how many assistants each dentist can supervise (and therefore the number of total patients who can be seen). Extending the physician's training period also serves to reduce the effective doctor supply because each graduate has fewer remaining years of productivity.

▲ **Increasing the price of substitutes such as chiropractors, nurse practitioners, midwives, and other nontraditional healers:** The effective price of many physician substitutes can be made prohibitively large by prohibiting them from performing some acts (e.g., prescribing drugs, performing surgery, admitting a patient to the hospital). Less extreme, but also effective, are rules that limit health insurance to reimbursement for services performed by or under the supervision of a physician. Even if a substitute provider is willing to provide services at a much lower price than a physician, those services will still cost patients more because they will have to paid for entirely out of pocket.

6.5.2 How Licensure Improves Quality

It's possible to improve quality by revoking the licenses of physicians whose medical practices are shown to be inferior, but such removals are rare.[19] The quality of physicians in practice depends much more on the initial selection of who is allowed to enter the profession, the training they receive, and efforts by practicing physicians to monitor one another and impose informal sanctions (e.g., ostracism from professional groups, denial of hospital privileges, refusal to refer new patients or share business opportunities).[20] Because licensure restrictions guarantee successful applicants a career with high income and prestige, many outstanding students seek admission to medical school. After becoming doctors, they work very hard not to lose that title. The opportunity cost of losing a license is so significant that the threat of losing a license is enough to make it rarely necessary for the profession to actually revoke a license and terminate a physician's right to practice. The threat of losing these extraordinary returns provides an incentive to maintain competency and support licensing boards.

6.5.3 Strong vs. Weak Licensure

The strength of licensure is related to the increased danger posed by the use of surgery and powerful drugs. Some types of medical care, such as cardiac surgery, are inherently dangerous and demand great skill. Bad heart surgeons may have a mortality rate five times higher than good heart surgeons.[21] Given the great impact of measurable physician quality indicators (e.g., training, medical practice records, opinions of peers), we would expect licensure to be very strong for heart surgery. That is the case. Although legally one need only be licensed as a physician in order to perform heart surgery, in practice, doctors are virtually prohibited from doing so unless they have completed a residency, completed a fellowship in the specialty, and been given special hospital privileges after a review by peers who have observed them acting as assistants on a number of operations. These additional mandatory checks make it evident that heart surgery has strong licensure restrictions.

Conversely, other types of medical care are much less dangerous and demanding, such as surgery to remove corns from the foot. Although such surgery can be practiced with greater or lesser skill, it's not likely to cost a life. One doesn't need a residency or hospital medical staff review to remove corns, and indeed corns are often removed by podiatrists, who are not licensed doctors of medicine (MDs), although they are usually licensed doctors of podiatric medicine (DPMs). The lack of special medical staff restrictions and the existence of alternative professional certification show that care of the foot has weak licensure.

As the extent and value of the information gap between patients and professionals increases, licensure becomes stronger. In types of care in which the difference is small, licensure is weak. For heart surgery, technical quality is paramount and well evaluated by professional standards. Medical licensure is supplemented by hospital privilege reviews, insurance restrictions, and so on.

SELF-CHECK

- Explain the role of **licensure** in medical care.
- List two ways that licensure might increase physician income.
- Describe a medical specialty in which strong licensure is warranted. Explain why.

SUMMARY

Over time, physician payment has changed from fee-for-service prices similar to prices of most other economic goods and services to complex reimbursement plans based on administrative formulas and negotiation. Increasingly, physicians are involved with managed care plans that pay a capitation rate or discounted fee schedules based on relative value scales. Most physicians are owners or partners in small businesses rather than employees. They work long hours, but they don't face much business risk. Physicians who practice in cognitive and caring specialties (e.g., family practice, psychiatry, pediatrics, internal medicine) tend to earn less than those who practice in procedure-oriented specialties (e.g., surgery, obstetrics/gynecology, radiology).

Because physicians have greater knowledge of medical treatments than patients, patients must trust physicians to act as their agents and make decisions on their behalf. Licensure is a collective extension of the doctor–patient relationship of agency. It helps solve the problems caused by uncertainty and the information gap between physicians and patients, and it is also intended to increase profits and quality.

KEY TERMS

Agency	An exchange relationship in which one party (the agent) make decisions on behalf of another.
Assignment	An agreement by a physician to take payment directly from Medicare and to accept the amount as payment in full.
Balance bill	The practice of billing a patient for the amount over and above what Medicare pays for a particular service.
Capitation	Payment of a fixed amount per enrolled insurance plan member per month, regardless of the number of services each member uses.
Coinsurance	The amount of a medical bill not paid for by insurance but by the patient.
Copayment	A specified amount a patient must pay for each service received.
Deductible	An amount that must be paid by the patient out of his or her own pocket before the insurance company begins to pay.
Fee-for-service payment	Payment of a specified amount for each health care visit or procedure.
Fee schedule	A list that specifies how much an insurance company will pay physicians for particular services.
Independent practice association (IPA) HMO	An HMO formed by non-exclusive contracts with many providers who operate independently.
Individual reimbursement	A reimbursement system in which the patient pays all the charges, sends copies of the bills to the insurer, and is reimbursed for the medical expenses that are covered.
Licensure	The establishment of legal restrictions specifying which individuals or firms have the rights to provide services or goods.
Malpractice	Physician failure to meet professional standards.
Medicare resource-based relative value scale (RBRVS)	A Medicare-established point value system for services, based on physician time, intensity of effort, practice costs, and costs of advanced specialty training.
Relative value scale	A fee schedule that gives medical services unique point values.
Staff HMO	An HMO in which physicians work exclusively for the HMO and are often on salary.

ASSESS YOUR UNDERSTANDING

Go to www.wiley.com/college/getzen to evaluate your knowledge of the role of physicians in the health care system.
Measure your learning by comparing pre-test and post-test results.

Summary Questions

1. Fee-for-service payments give each service a point value. True or False?

2. In a typical private health insurance program, a participant might be required to meet the first $300 of medical bills each year before the insurance begins to pay. This is best described as:
   (a) a copayment requirement.
   (b) a coinsurance requirement.
   (c) a capitation requirement.
   (d) a deductible requirement.

3. When a physician is under assignment with Medicare, he or she cannot balance bill the patient for any charges over the Medicare-approved amount. True or False?

4. Among the principal ways of paying physicians in the United States, the *strongest* incentive to reduce the volume of services provided is produced by:
   (a) fee for service.
   (b) salary.
   (c) capitation.
   (d) RBRVS.

5. Salary as a payment method for physicians is most likely to create a concern about:
   (a) waste of resources.
   (b) underutilization of needed services.
   (c) low productivity by physicians.
   (d) unnecessary surgeries.

6. Historically, the highest-paid physicians have been:
   (a) salaried primary care physicians.
   (b) solo practitioners who can claim the entire income of the practice.
   (c) primary care physicians paid on a fee-for-service basis.
   (d) procedure-oriented specialists paid on a fee-for-service basis.

7. The malpractice system is an efficient means of deterring negligence by physicians. True or False?

8. "Consumer ignorance" (i.e., a lack of information) is particularly related to which of the following characteristics of the health services industry?
   (a) Agency role of the physician
   (b) Merit good status of health
   (c) Existence of externalities in consumption of health services
   (d) Uncertain incidence of illness
9. The weaker the licensure, the more dangerous the type of medicine practiced. True or False?
10. Licensure increases physician profits by:
    (a) limiting the supply of physicians.
    (b) setting relative value scales.
    (c) increasing the number of physician substitutes.
    (d) determining capitation payments.

Review Questions

1. Which type of payment gives a physician the most incentive to:
   (a) Spend more time with each patient? Spend less?
   (b) Provide more laboratory services to each patient? Provide less?
   (c) Modify the listing of diagnoses to increase revenues? Be objective?
   (d) Reduce hospital utilization? Increase hospital utilization?
   (e) Ask patients to return frequently? Try to handle problems once and for all?
2. Which organization provides the largest amount of payment to physicians in the United States? How does this organization choose to make these payments? Has the form of payment changed over time? Why?
3. What are some of the reasons that most pediatricians earn less than most neurosurgeons?
4. How are the values determined in setting up a relative value scale?
5. What are the objectives of the current medical malpractice system in the United States? How well does it work in achieving these objectives?
6. What is an agent? How does employing an agent reduce the costs of making a transaction? Does employing an agent create any problems that wouldn't occur if the consumer acted alone?
7. How do agency and the information gap between physicians and patients lead to licensure? Do agents get more or less of the gains from trade as the gap increases? Explain why and how the strength of licensure is related to the extent of the information gap.

Applying This Chapter

1. In many European countries (e.g., Germany), all care of hospitalized inpatients is overseen by physicians who are salaried employees of the hospital. Most community physicians are primary care providers; if they refer a patient to the hospital, a salaried specialist will be the attending physician. Analyze the likely economic effects of such a system replacing the current typical hospital–physician relationship in the United States.

2. The relationship of principal and agent is pervasive in our economy—for example, stockholder and manager of a company, seller (or buyer) and real-estate broker, client and lawyer, etc. To what extent is the principal–agent relationship different in health care than in other realms?

3. It is widely acknowledged that there's an information gap between physicians and patients regarding medical care. Yet the trend in health insurance is toward consumer-driven health insurance (such as high-deductible health insurance combined with HSAs), in which consumers are expected to take a more active role in purchasing medical care and services and, as a consequence, reduce health care costs. Consider how the information gap between physicians and patients might affect these consumer-driven plans.

4. Often, when people switch from a traditional insurance plan to an HMO, they must change physicians. That's because HMO members must see physicians who are on a preapproved list; if they go to a doctor not on the list, they must pay significantly more. This rule has come under heavy criticism by patients and patient advocacy groups. Given what you've learned about physician agency in this chapter, explain why changing physicians is such a big deal to many people.

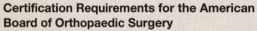

Certification Requirements for the American Board of Orthopaedic Surgery

Go to the Web site of the American Board of Orthopaedic Surgery (ABOS), at www.abos.org, and review the training requirements to be certified in orthopedic medicine. (Click on the "Exam Info" link, then on "Part I," and then on "Rules and Procedures.") Next, go to the Web site for the American Board of Pediatrics, www.abp.org, and review the training requirements to be certified as a pediatrician. (Click "General Pediatric Certification," and then choose "Training" under the drop-down menu labeled "Exam Admission Requirements.") Write a report comparing the residency requirements and the length of time required before becoming fully certified for these two specialties. Explain whether the requirements seem justified, given the risks involved in each field.

Do Your Own Health Care Costs Survey

Call the offices of at least three physicians in different specialties, including one general practice/family physician, and find out the cost of a typical office visit. Prepare a brief report, comparing the costs, being sure to try to account for the differences in price. Next, survey at least five people and ask them to guess the cost of visiting the physicians. How close are their guesses?

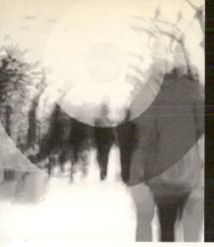

7

PHYSICIAN ORGANIZATION AND BUSINESS PRACTICE
The Physician Marketplace

Starting Point

Go to www.wiley.com/college/getzen to assess your knowledge of physician organization and business practices.
Determine where you need to concentrate your effort.

What You'll Learn in This Chapter

▲ The value of a medical education
▲ The role of licensing boards and the federal government in limiting physician supply
▲ The economic benefits of group practices
▲ The role of kickbacks in the flow of funds
▲ The unique role of price discrimination in the medical market

After Studying This Chapter, You'll Be Able To

▲ Evaluate how physician supply affects the cost and quality of medical care
▲ Analyze physician practice organizations and the role of economies of scale
▲ Determine whether more regulations are needed to reduce physician kickbacks
▲ Assess the factors that result in price discrimination

INTRODUCTION

Physicians are highly paid professionals who invest several years of their lives and thousands of dollars in their education. Yet high physician income is at least in part due to artificial limits on the supply of physicians. Limits on supply include the restrictions on the number of students allowed to enter medical school, caps on the immigration of foreign-trained physicians, and requirements that anyone practicing medicine be licensed. In addition to limiting supply, these restrictions also serve to ensure the quality of medical care provided by physicians. Physicians can also increase their income by forming and/or joining group practices with other physicians. Doing so creates economies of scale and spreads risk among several physicians. A final way that physicians can see increased income is through kickbacks and side dealing, although such practices are considered unethical and, in some instances, illegal.

7.1 Medical Education as an Investment

A select and hard-working group of 16,000 students will graduate with doctor of medicine (MD) degrees from a total of 126 U.S. medical schools this year.[1] And although much has been made of the cost of medical education, most of that cost is borne indirectly by the government and the health insurance system. Just 4 percent of medical school costs are covered by tuition payments from

---

FOR EXAMPLE

Getting Into Medical School

Many physicians first think about becoming doctors in elementary school, but some decide to become physicians after pursuing other careers. All people entering medical school have to take premed courses in chemistry, biology, and so on and must do rather well; almost half of all medical students have an "A" average (i.e., a grade point average of 3.6 or higher) as undergraduates. Getting into medical school is serious business that takes substantial effort, and many students apply to 10 or more medical schools. Much of the selection, however, is self-selection. Weaker students generally choose not to apply. Fewer than half of applicants to medical school are rejected. Of those who are admitted, 98 percent choose to enroll, and of those, 95 percent will graduate, almost all of whom will then enter hospital-based residency training programs lasting three years or more before becoming generalist family practitioners or specialists in any of the other 22 recognized areas of medical practice eligible for board certification.

Table 7-1: Returns to Professional Education

	Business (2 years)	Law (3 years)	Dentistry (4 years)	Primary Medicine (4 years)	Specialty Medicine (4 years)
Tuition	$ 34,452	$ 32,317	$ 70,620	$ 74,504	$ 74,504
Annual income (age 40)	$135,579	$139,616	$133,050	$132,592	$219,733
Hours worked (age 40)	2,448	1,959	1,781	2,565	2,707
Internal rate of return	**26%**	**23%**	**22%**	**16%**	**18%**

students, whereas 46 percent come from patient fees, 30 percent from research funds, and 20 percent from government appropriations and gifts.[2] Although tuition might run as high as $50,000 per year, and most medical students (83 percent) are left with debts from student loans when they graduate, the amount of those loans (which averaged $120,000 in 2005[3]) isn't very large in relationship to the income a physician can expect; the loans typically amount to less than 1 percent of lifetime earnings. Far more onerous than the monetary obligations are the years of toil spent in learning the practice of medicine.

The returns on medical education are the increased annual earnings, relative to a person's opportunity cost, that flow from the decision to go to medical school. Also important is the fact that the returns from a medical education are much less risky than from a bachelor of arts (BA), master of business administration (MBA), or doctor of law (JD) degree (see Table 7-1). In addition, becoming a medical doctor confers prestige and other valuable privileges.

SELF-CHECK

- List three reasons why medical school is considered a good investment.
- Indicate why the returns on the investment in medical school are less risky than the returns on the investment in a graduate degree in literature.

7.2 Physician Supply

Legal control over physicians resides with state licensure boards, yet supply is actually determined by control over the number of students allowed to enter medical school, as well as the number of foreign medical graduates allowed to come to the United States for training, many of whom stay to practice. Unlike law school, from which many students fail to graduate, graduate and fail the bar exam, or pass the bar exam but can't find a job, almost all medical students graduate and practice medicine. There are exams in school and afterward, but almost everyone passes, and the limitation of numbers is sufficient to ensure that everyone who wants to can find a position practicing medicine.

In 1900, the U.S. supply of physicians was 1.73 MDs per 1,000 people. That number declined to 1.33 MDs per 1,000 people in 1930 (see Figure 7-1). The supply of physicians held constant at that level for the next 35 years, yet improvements in medicine greatly increased public demand, as did the rise in personal income over those four decades. With supply constant and demand increasing, earnings of physicians rose. Concern was voiced that not enough physicians were available and that a shortage had arisen.[4]

7.2.1 The Great Medical Student Expansion

As the benefits of modern medicine became more evident, access to care was increasingly seen as a necessity in the rising American standard of living, one that workers had already paid for through their health insurance premiums. The constraints on supply caused longer waits for appointments, less time for patients to talk with increasingly rushed physicians, fewer old-style general practitioners willing to make house calls, and other deteriorations in service. The public was unhappy, and the politicians, who now provided most of the financing for medical schools, were willing to do something to fix the imbalance.

Figure 7-1

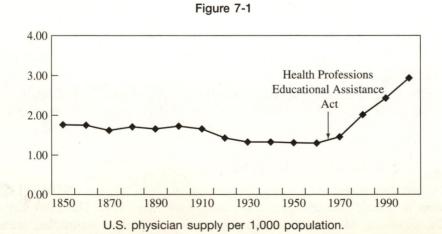

U.S. physician supply per 1,000 population.

Figure 7-2

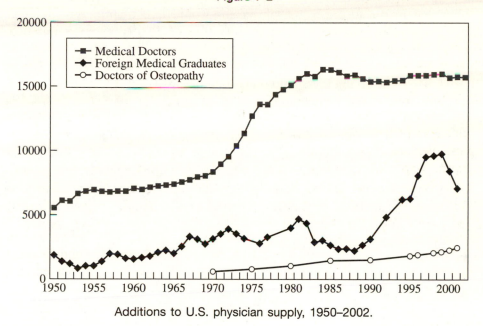

Additions to U.S. physician supply, 1950–2002.

Congress passed the Health Professions Educational Assistance Act of 1963, forcing medical schools to admit more students and allowing more foreign physicians to immigrate to the United States. In response to the act and subsequent amendments, physician supply rose steadily to 1.61 physicians per 1,000 population in 1970, 2.02 in 1980, 2.44 in 1990, and 2.94 in 2000—more than twice the level of supply that prevailed from 1930 through 1965 (see Figures 7-1 and 7-2). The number of entering students almost doubled in 10 years, from 8,759 in 1965 to 15,351 in 1975. The government did three things that brought about this increase[5]:

▲ It built more medical schools.
▲ It offered additional funding, on the condition that existing schools increase the number of students enrolled by at least 5 percent each year.
▲ It changed immigration rules to favor "shortage" occupations, including physicians. Foreign graduates made up just 6 percent of all physicians in practice in 1960, but by 1965, that had doubled to 12 percent, and it further increased to 17 percent in 1970 and 20 percent in 1980.

7.2.2 Restriction of Physician Supply

As the number of residents in training grew rapidly during the 1970s, it began to seem as though there were already plenty of physicians. The 1981 Report of the Graduate Medical Education National Advisory Committee, widely known as the GMENAC Report, projected a growing surplus, raising the possibility that in the future, some physicians would face unemployment.[6] The American Medical Association (AMA) complained loudly about a potential surplus, commissioning several studies to show that the United States was training an excess of physicians and that foreign graduates were no longer needed. Moves were made to reduce the rate of growth in the number of U.S. physicians. No more new schools were to be built. Class sizes were fixed at existing levels.

The number of first-year MD students peaked at 17,320 in 1981 and has been held below that number since then (it was 17,109 in 2005).[7] Because the number of U.S. medical graduates hasn't kept pace with the growth in U.S. population, much less the growth in technology and incomes that raised demand in the first place, all the expansion in supply over the past 20 years has had to come from three other sources:

▲ The delayed effect of the 1965–1975 "physician boom"
▲ Increased immigration of non-U.S. physicians
▲ Increased production of non-MD physicians

7.2.3 Balancing Physician Supply and Incomes: Projecting the Future

The development of scientific medicine created the need for a new type of doctor in the twentieth century. To raise the quality of the individuals in the profession (as well as their prestige and incomes), reforms required that most of the inadequately trained practitioners be forced out, thus reducing physician supply between 1900 and 1930. From then until 1965, the number of new MDs graduating each year was held steady, at about 4 percent of the total physician stock, numbers just sufficient to offset the 3 percent who retired each year and a 1 percent growth in the U.S. population, so that the physician-to-population ratio remained constant, at about 1.33 per 1,000.

The 1 percent growth in physicians set to match the 1 percent increase in population wasn't enough to address three key factors increasing demand for medical care:

▲ People's changing expectations about access to medical care
▲ New technology
▲ A rising standard of living

Today, becoming a doctor still offers above-average rates of return on post-college education. However, the very high earnings growth that physicians enjoyed during the 1960s and 1970s was a temporary historical aberration, brought about by rapid growth in demand due to new technology in the context

> ## FOR EXAMPLE
>
> ### Chiropractors as a Substitute for MDs
>
> Chiropractors, who often rely exclusively on spinal manipulation to treat disease and still train some practitioners in for-profit schools, have been severely and relentlessly attacked by the AMA.[8] Licensure acts explicitly exclude chiropractors from the practice of medicine, and this opposition hasn't changed, even though the AMA hasn't been able to ban chiropractic practice, nor indeed prevent some of its own members from referring patients to chiropractors. While some of the AMA opposition to chiropractic care is based on the lack of scientific foundation for manipulative treatments, much of it is motivated by economic concerns.

of fixed supply. In the future, doctors will have high but not such extraordinarily high earnings. While still doing much better than most graduates from other fields, new physicians will face more competition as they enter the market and thus will be more likely to become employees holding salaried jobs and to hold on to such positions longer during their careers.

SELF-CHECK

- Indicate how physician supply is usually regulated in the United States.
- List three things the U.S. federal government did that increased the supply of physicians in the early 1960s.
- List three reasons demand for physicians increased between 1931 and 1965, even though there was a consistent physician-to-population ratio.

7.3 Group Practice

Physicians who join together in groups have higher net earnings than those who practice alone, as evidenced by the following salaries:

▲ $155,000 for solo doctors

▲ $200,000 for those in 2-physician partnerships

▲ $217,000 for those in 3-physician groups

▲ $220,000 for those in 4-physician groups

▲ $250,000 for those in groups of 5 to 25

▲ $240,000 for those in groups of more than 25 physicians[9]

In addition, physicians in group practices usually have better lifestyles, including more interaction with colleagues, more support services, and fewer nights spent handling patient emergencies.[10]

Group practices serve to increase net income through **economies of scale**, in which the average cost per unit decreases as output increases, raising the productivity of inputs and hence lowering costs. What does it mean to have economies of scale that make larger practices more efficient in the use of inputs? To a physician owner, it could mean two things:

1. The cost of the inputs required to produce a given amount of output has been reduced.
2. Visits per hour of physician time (outputs) have been increased.

In reality, some of both occurs.[11] Equipment and office space come in discrete units and therefore are inefficiently used in small practices. For example, an x-ray machine that can handle 10,000 patients may cost only 50 percent more than one that can handle 2,000, and even the smaller one is frequently idle for a doctor practicing alone. A large group can match equipment needs to the total patient volume of the group as a whole and thereby achieve economies of scale. Similarly, each physician may need from one to four exam rooms at a time to maximize patient flow and from two to six assistants. A solo doctor may compromise by having an office with three exam rooms and four assistants, and thus sometimes the rooms will be overcrowded and the assistants overworked, while at other times both rooms and assistants sit idle, wasting money. A group can plan for an average because it's unlikely that all the physicians will be busy or inactive at the same time, and thus the group can achieve a better match. Office rent takes up 12 percent of the gross revenues for solo practices, 10 percent for two-physician partnerships, and just 7 percent for large group practices.

A large group can also allow for more specialization in the use of labor, so that a 10-physician group can have a laboratory technician, a billing specialists, a receptionist, an intake nurse, an exam room assistant, and so on, while a solo practice must make do with a general-purpose medical assistant or nurse. In a large group, assistants' labor can more easily be substituted for physician time, and as this labor becomes more productive, physicians can use more employees rather than fewer. It's worth paying more for assistants to save the physicians' time because the physicians' net profit per hour of work increases.

FOR EXAMPLE

Comparative Advantage and Physician Assistants

Suppose that a physician takes 15 minutes to do an intake examination and 5 minutes to do a follow-up. A physician assistant (PA) takes 40 minutes to do an intake examination and 30 minutes to do a follow-up. Even though the PA is less efficient at both tasks, the medical group makes the PAs do intakes but not follow-ups. Why? Because in 8 hours, a PA could do 12 intakes, freeing up 3 hours of physician time to do high-value surgery, while having the PA do 16 follow-ups would free up just 1 hour and 20 minutes of physician time. It's not the "cost" of using the PA to provide services that matters; it's the value of the additional services that the physician can provide. The principle that people and firms should produce the things at which they are *relatively* more efficient and use others to produce the things at which they are relatively less efficient is known as comparative advantage. There are gains from trade when relative costs differ, even if one party is better at everything. That's why investment bankers let someone else balance their checkbooks, great artists let helpers fill in the background scenery, and great athletes let someone else play on punt returns.

Physicians in group practice also spread risk across the members of the group, which creates economies of scale. The group can collectively enjoy a smoother and more certain income stream. Perhaps even more importantly, the emergency calls that interrupt the home life of every doctor are much less disruptive when combined and redistributed in a group. A solo practitioner must be "on call" every night or find someone else who is willing to cover. On Sunday, one emergency call could interrupt a football game, and there could be no more calls until a sleep-shattering call at 3 a.m. For a group, it's usual for each doctor to accept all the calls for a single day. A group doctor might handle seven emergencies on a Sunday but know that Friday night and Saturday are free because any patients who need assistance will be handled by one of the partners. The burden of emergencies isn't the time spent in caring for patients but the uneven spacing. This is a risk that is shared, and thus effectively reduced, in a group.

Because it is obviously so much more efficient for a doctor to handle 10 patients in one night than 1 to 3 patients each night per week, why don't solo doctors contract with each other to do just that? For that matter, why can't independent physicians arrange to share office space or nurses? To some extent they do, and to that extent, they start to become a group. As the contracts and sharing become more complete and cover more aspects of practice, the doctors who trade with each other become a single firm—that is, a group practice. But it's difficult to share. All the doctors must agree to standardize certain practices, coordinate efforts, choose a leader, accept the leader's ruling on disputes, and so on—in short, to be managed. Sharing means being an employee or partner rather than the boss. Management is costly, and good physician managers, like all other good managers, are rare and valuable commodities. For some physicians, it's cheaper (and more fun) to put up with some inefficiencies and lack of specialized inputs to be their own bosses and not have to listen to, or give orders to, anyone else.

For a group to act as a collective, the guarantee of quality must extend to all the physicians in the group. Just as all licensed physicians benefit from monitoring the quality of care provided by the profession and eliminating or reforming bad doctors, a medical group practice benefits from increased demand to the extent that it can closely monitor and control the quality of all its members.[12] The Mayo Clinic is a premier example of a medical group practice that acts as a "brand-name firm" and gains a marketing and revenue advantage from being perceived as a group with identifiable quality rather than just a random collection of individual physicians who happen to work in the same building.[13]

SELF-CHECK

- List two ways that **economies of scale** make larger practices more efficient than smaller practices in the use of inputs.
- What is the risk that is shared when a group assigns all emergencies each day to a single physician on a rotating basis?

7.4 Kickbacks

". . . and if a doctor shall cheat his patient by overcharging for medicaments, then shall a finger of his left hand be cut off."

—*Code of Hammurabi, 2300 B.C.*

From the beginning, the AMA code of medical ethics has dealt with economic issues, rightfully noting that doctors must put the health of patients above profits if people are to trust them. The physician–patient agency relationship is most threatened in day-to-day business by the practice of paying "referral fees," or **kickbacks,** which are surreptitious payments in order to obtain business. The agent is supposed to be, and is, paid for acting in the principal's (i.e., the patient's) best interest. When doctors accept a fee for referring patients to one hospital rather than another, or for giving a surgical case to Dr. B instead of Dr. A, they may be tempted to go with the one who will pay them the most, not the one who will provide the best care. In ordinary business dealings, such a payment would be termed a bribe.

Before medicine became established as a profession, kickbacks were common. Surgeons in large cities would advertise in rural newspapers their willingness to pay $100 or more for each case sent to them. While such behavior seems unthinkable now, kickbacks keep cropping up. For example, what was once the country's largest chain of psychiatric hospitals was investigated and convicted for paying physicians and social workers who sent in clients. The kickback scheme had become so well established that there was a standard going rate of $70 for each patient day.[14]

Why do kickbacks continue to occur if everyone knows that they are bad and they are condemned by all the official governing organizations? Because in the short run, it's easy to profit by betraying a patient's trust to make a dollar. Acting ethically and following professional standards, which put the interests of patients first, forces a doctor to put aside his or her own narrow self-interest. The violator hopes not to get caught. Even if an unethical physician does get caught, much of the punishment actually falls on other doctors because the profession as a whole gets blamed for a lack of standards and suffers from a reduced demand and falling prices for services. Trust and agency build professional value, and taking a kickback is one way for a member to steal part of that value, benefiting personally while harming others.

One of the major activities of physicians is prescribing drugs. If drug companies made payments to physicians, those dollars could distort the physicians' choices on behalf of their patients, perhaps encouraging physicians to prescribe a drug that is less effective or one that is effective but three times as expensive as substitute drugs that would work just as well. An even more difficult problem arises when the physician isn't just prescribing the drug but also selling it. Knowing that a patient is in pain and that he or she trusts the physician, a physician could fatten his or her profit margins by overcharging for drugs. The potential for abuse is so high that physicians in this country have been legally prohibited from selling drugs or owning pharmacies since 1934. Even a pharmacy in a medical clinic must be run as a separate business to avoid conflicts of interest.

FOR EXAMPLE

Prescribing for Profit

In Japan, where physicians are allowed to sell drugs and own pharmacies, the government sets price controls to keep physicians from overcharging, but that doesn't stop physicians from overprescribing. General practice physicians in Japan get about one-third of their net income from sales of pharmacy items, and their patients are prescribed twice as many drugs as similar patients in the United States.

The issue with kickbacks isn't price; it's deceit. If Dr. Arnold says, "I am better than the others, and I want $20 more for each visit," that's her privilege. Patients can agree or go somewhere else. There is no fraud. On the other hand, to prescribe a drug and accept a $20 rebate from the manufacturer, or to send a surgical case to Dr. Jones, knowing that he will send a case of wine in return, is fraud. The patient is unknowingly paying (somebody has to pay for the wine— to Dr. Jones, it's just a cost of doing business that he adds into the overhead for the surgical bill) and has an agent whose decisions may be based on maximizing kickbacks rather than the patient's welfare. Note that if Dr. Arnold and Dr. Jones were partners in a large group practice, a patient would expect to be sent to one of the surgeons in the group (e.g., Dr. Jones), and there would be no fraud. Also, Dr. Jones would expect Dr. Arnold to send the patient to him as a matter of routine, and there would be no kickback payment. The amount of money changing hands in the transaction might be the same, but the ethical and economic considerations would be quite different. In essence, a patient of the group would be buying "the group" and wouldn't care how Dr. Arnold and Dr. Jones split the money. However, the patient who goes to Dr. Arnold and who is unaware that Dr. Arnold has any business arrangement with another doctor has a right to expect Dr. Arnold to objectively choose the surgeon who is best and to negotiate the lowest price.

As medicine has become more complex, with more transactions involved in each episode of patient care, it has become increasingly difficult to avoid such conflicts of interest. Of particular concern in recent years have been incidences in which for-profit companies providing ancillary services (e.g., diagnostic radiology, home intravenous therapy) offer physicians "investments" in these businesses in return for sending patients.[15] So many such abuses took place that in 1976 that federal anti-kickback laws were passed, prohibiting any Medicare or Medicaid payment from companies to physicians based on the volume of patient referrals. Later, the 1989 "Stark law" (named after its sponsor, U.S. Representative Fortney Stark of California) banned physicians from referring patients to clinical laboratories in which they have a financial interest. The 1993 "Stark II" law widened the ban to prohibit self-referrals to hospitals or radiology laboratories in which physicians are invested. The law also prohibits bonus plans within group practices, based on the volume of laboratory referrals. Only a minority (fewer than 10 percent) of physicians invest in businesses that raise conflict-of-interest issues from self-referral, and only a few engage in profiteering at the expense of the government and patients.[16] Yet the actions of these few are troubling to a public already dismayed at the high cost of health care, and it is likely that further restrictions will be placed on specialized hospitals and other facilities owned by physicians. Eventually, physician ownership or partnership in hospitals and other diagnostic or therapeutic facilities may be banned entirely, as ownership of pharmacies has been.

SELF-CHECK

- Explain what a **kickback** is and give two examples of kickbacks in the medical field.
- How do kickbacks affect the trust between physicians and patients?
- What did the Stark and Stark II laws ban?

7.5 Price Discrimination

One of the characteristics of medical markets first noted by economists was that different patients pay different prices for the same service.[17] Some price differences are simply due to differences in cost or value (e.g., surgery by an experienced, board-certified specialist vs. surgery by a new resident still in training, midnight treatment in the emergency room vs. a routine visit to a doctor's office). However, even after these factors are taken into account, there's still a sizable variation in charges. For example, people who are well insured or who have high incomes frequently pay more than uninsured or poor people; laboratory and other small-ticket items are often overpriced; and services for which patients can "shop around" (e.g., eye exams, normal births, physical therapy) show less price variation than emergency medical care, where immediate treatment is required.

A major reason for such **price discrimination**—which is the practice of charging different prices for the same service to different types of patients or to patients in different types of care—is that it increases total revenue.

To maximize revenues when providing two different types of care, physicians should charge different prices, even if their costs are the same for each service, and they should charge a higher price where demand is least price sensitive. Conversely, where demand is very price sensitive, a reduction in price brings in many more patients and increases revenues (see Figure 7-3). Pain, fear of dying, and wealth all serve to reduce price sensitivity. However, the most important factor in making medical consumers less price sensitive is insurance (see Figure 7-4). Therefore, we would generally expect physicians to charge more for services that are more fully covered by insurance, more life-threatening, more painful, and for which patients have the least ability to shop around.

When asked about charging different prices for the same service, some physicians respond angrily to the suggestion that they are maximizing profits and assert that they act from a benevolent impulse, charging high prices to those who can afford to pay (or are well insured) so that they can take care of the destitute. Under closer examination, however, it becomes evident that there is a mixture of motivations that includes both charity and higher incomes in a blend

Figure 7-3

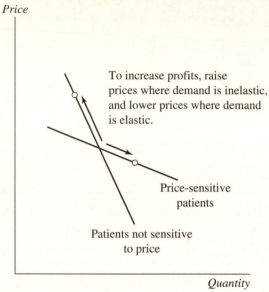

Price

To increase profits, raise prices where demand is inelastic, and lower prices where demand is elastic.

Price-sensitive patients

Patients not sensitive to price

Quantity

Price discrimination, by patient type.

that is not always clearly separable. Charging students less helps a group that is usually poor and might not get care if they had to pay full price—and brings in more revenue for exactly the same reason. (Why do you think movie theaters and airlines give student discounts? Is it a charitable impulse or a smart business

Figure 7-4

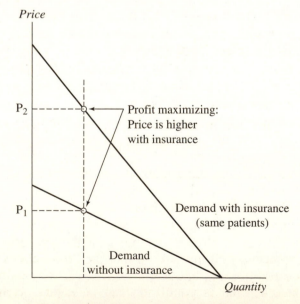

Price

P_2

Profit maximizing: Price is higher with insurance

P_1

Demand with insurance (same patients)

Demand without insurance

Quantity

Price discrimination, by insurance status.

FOR EXAMPLE

Discriminating Against the Uninsured

Critics of discriminatory pricing policies often complain that self-pay patients—those who don't have insurance—are typically charged anywhere from two to five times what insured patients are charged for the same service. For instance, according to a report on hospital pricing policies in Ohio, self-pay hospital patients in that state are charged twice as much as patients with insurance.[18] In 2003, the estimated cost of the average hospital stay was $5,040. Medicare and Medicaid paid a discounted rate that was actually *below* the estimated cost—$4,939 for Medicare and $4,838 for Medicaid. Private insurance companies paid $6,040 for the same care. Ohio's uninsured patients, however, were charged the hospital's full "sticker price" of $12,852.

practice to raise revenues because they know students have little discretionary money and wouldn't come to the theater or fly as often otherwise?) Price discrimination is pervasive in medicine and well accepted by patients, the government, and insurance companies. If two people come into a shop, and one is charged twice as much as the other for oil, food, or rent, the person charged extra will complain or threaten to sue. The unusual willingness of people to accept or even praise price discrimination in medicine is one of the factors that has convinced economists that health care markets differ in significant ways from markets for most other goods and services.

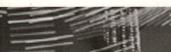

SELF-CHECK

- Explain what **price discrimination is.**
- List two reasons that physicians engage in price discrimination.
- In what situations are physicians most likely to charge patients more for a service?

SUMMARY

Control over physician supply and licensure in the United States is actually exercised by control over medical education. Since 1980, physician graduate rates have stayed constant, even as population and per-capita income have grown, increasing demand and pushing physician incomes upward.

Group practice, increasing the scale of physician operations, increases output per physician. The ability to trade patients more efficiently is a major function of such economic organizations.

Price discrimination is common in medicine, although much of the motivation seems to be purely charitable and is officially sanctioned by the public. Unlike price discrimination, kickback payments on referrals are considered unethical. Similarly, physician ownership of hospitals, laboratories, physical therapy clinics, and diagnostic radiology facilities has been shown to lead to abuses of trust and is increasingly being discouraged and regulated by government payers.

KEY TERMS

Economies of scale   A situation in which the average cost per unit decreases as output increases.

Kickback   A surreptitious payment in order to obtain business.

Price discrimination   The practice of charging different people different prices for the same good or service.

ASSESS YOUR UNDERSTANDING

Go to www.wiley.com/college/getzen to assess your knowledge of physician organization and business practices.
Measure your learning by comparing pre-test and post-test results.

Summary Questions

1. The majority of the cost of medical education is paid for through medical student tuition. True or False?

2. The return on an individual's investment in medical education:
   (a) is likely to be higher than the return on high school but lower than investment in shorter forms of education, such as a bachelor's degree.
   (b) is about the same as the long-run average return on investment in financial assets after inflation.
   (c) is much riskier than the return on other professional education, such as law, because of the rise of managed care.
   (d) exceeds the return on most higher education, including the doctorate level in most academic fields.

3. The licensing of physicians should increase the derived demand for physician services because it:
   (a) effectively raises the price of substitutes if they cannot be paid by insurance unless they work with or are supervised by a physician.
   (b) raises the price of physician services because of the cost of administering the licensing system.
   (c) increases the cost of complementary goods, such as prescription drugs.
   (d) means that physician productivity becomes irrelevant to demand.

4. In the United States, effective control over supply and licensure of physicians has generally been exercised by:
   (a) essentially unregulated free-market response to economic opportunity in medicine.
   (b) control of access to and content of medical education.
   (c) governmental control over the number and distribution of residency training positions.
   (d) the federal government in order to ensure standardization.

5. When a physician refers a patient to another physician within the same group practice, the referring physician benefits by keeping business within the practice. Such referrals are considered to be kickbacks and are unethical. True or False?

6. If a physician can price discriminate between two markets, the lower price will be charged in the market in which:

   (a) demand is greater.

   (b) demand is smaller.

   (c) demand is more price elastic.

   (d) demand is less price elastic.

7. Which of the following is *not* an example of genuine price discrimination?

   (a) A hospital supply company charging a different price to a group of hospitals purchasing large quantities collectively and a single hospital buying smaller amounts of the same items

   (b) A hospital charging a different price for treating HMO patients and traditionally insured patients with the same condition

   (c) A physician charging a wealthier patient more in order to cover the cost of treating a poor patient with the same condition who cannot pay

   (d) An HMO offering more attractive rates to a company in a more competitive market than to a company in a market in which the HMO is dominant

8. The text describes kickbacks and similar practices as an abuse of the principal–agent relationship because:

   (a) health care providers should never be concerned with earning a profit.

   (b) they may deceive the patient concerning the physician's possible motive for an action.

   (c) it is better that patients not know about any financial relationships among providers.

   (d) most patients can't afford to pay these extra fees.

Review Questions

1. Do medical licenses raise the quality of medical care, or do they just raise the profitability of medical practice?

2. Who pays the costs of medical education: the student, the patients, the insurance companies, or the taxpayers?

3. What controls the supply of physicians in the United States? Distinguish between short- and long-term supply and between the actual decision-making individuals and organizations vs. the underlying economic and political forces.

4. Do physicians pay each other for patient referrals? If so, explain how.

5. Why do physicians choose to practice together in groups? Is assembling physicians into groups any different from assembling employees into a

manufacturing firm, lawyers into a legal firm, or baseball players into a team?

6. What advantages does a large physician group have over a solo physician? What disadvantages?

7. When physicians choose to give a discount on fees, does this raise or lower their income? Will a profit-maximizing physician charge higher prices for services or groups of patients for which demand is more elastic or less elastic? Explain why.

8. Why are kickbacks illegal?

9. Has the growth of third-party payment systems in health care affected the ability of physicians to practice price discrimination?

Applying This Chapter

1. Several politicians have proposed that the United States become more restrictive regarding immigration, allowing fewer foreign-educated physicians to undergo training or establish practices in the United States. Would this increase or decrease the earning power of U.S.-educated physicians? Which specialties do you think would be most affected?

2. Are chiropractors substitutes or complements for physicians in the production of medical services? What about podiatrists? Psychologists? Which professions are more competitive and which are more cooperative? Why?

3. Give some examples of how physicians in a group practice might benefit from economies of scale when it comes to marketing their practice.

4. Besides financial "referral fees," or kickbacks, how else might physicians benefit by referring their patients to other physicians? Indicate whether the benefits you identify are ethical.

Medicare Assignment

Some states have mandated Medicare assignment. Assignment means that the doctor agrees to treat a patient and accept the fee Medicare sends as payment in full. Doctors not accepting assignment bill the patient (almost always for more than Medicare would pay), and the patient pays the doctor, sends in the bill, and gets reimbursed by Medicare. Typically 20 percent to 60 percent of physicians in an area accept Medicare assignment because patients prefer it and payment is assured. Other physicians want to bill for the extra money. The number of doctors accepting assignment depends on the rates Medicare is currently paying, local market conditions, how full the doctor's practice is, and other factors. Assume that a new state law mandates that all physicians accept Medicare assignment. In a brief essay, consider what would happen to price, quantity, demand, and supply. Distinguish between short-term and long-term effects. Describe other effects you might expect.

Physician-Owned Hospitals vs. Not-for-Profit Hospitals

The health care industry has been plagued by scandals in recent years, including those at Tenet, HCA, Health-South, and other companies. There have been numerous allegations of improper activity, but just as damaging have been the reports of intense pressure to produce results for the bottom line, using methods that may not be illegal but certainly stretch the boundaries. Among these concerns is the widespread ownership of stock by physicians who practice in the hospitals and the impact this may have had on their practice patterns. In a brief essay, consider whether physician ownership of hospitals is any different than the shared interest that the medical staff of a not-for-profit hospital has in the success of the hospital, especially if they are linked to it in some sort of joint venture for managed care contracting.

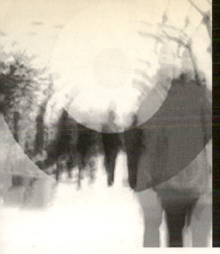

8

HOSPITALS
Sources and Uses of Funds

Starting Point

Go to www.wiley.com/college/getzen to assess your knowledge of hospitals.
Determine where you need to concentrate your effort.

What You'll Learn in This Chapter

▲ Where hospitals get their income
▲ What major hospital expenses are common
▲ What the practice of cost shifting entails
▲ How hospital financing works
▲ Who controls hospitals

After Studying This Chapter, You'll Be Able To

▲ Evaluate how Medicare and managed care affect hospital decision making
▲ Argue why labor makes up the majority of hospital costs
▲ Evaluate whether cost shifting is a fair practice
▲ Assess the impact of an "I'll pay for mine, and you pay for yours" attitude in health care reimbursement
▲ Assess the role of physicians in hospital management

INTRODUCTION

When hospitals were first formed, they relied almost entirely on charitable donations, serving poor populations that had few other options for health care. Advances in technology and better physician training made hospitals more desirable, attracting patients who could afford to pay their bills out of pocket. The advent of insurance and Medicare had a dramatic impact on the economic structure of hospitals. An early reimbursement structure that covered patient expenses as well as the cost of indigent care allowed hospitals to flourish, and at the same time, this general reimbursement system offered hospitals little incentive to contain costs. Rising costs led Medicare and insurance companies to tighten reimbursement practices, however, leaving hospitals with the burden of finding new ways to cover indigent care. Today, hospitals are usually reimbursed a flat rate based on patient diagnosis, with the rate being determined by Medicare and insurance companies rather than the hospitals themselves.

Labor expenses, such as those for nurses, aides, administrators, and sanitation maintenance staff, constitute approximately 75 percent of hospital costs. This puts hospitals in a bind when it comes to cutting costs because society frowns on layoffs and wage cuts.

Hospitals have unique and fascinating organization and decision structures. In a typical market, firms would be very sensitive to consumer demands. However, because insurance covers the cost of most hospital care, hospitals must respond to insurers. At the same time, physicians, who usually aren't employees of hospitals, play a unique decision-making role in hospitals: They make most of the decisions regarding patient care, including those regarding diagnoses, the services required, and the length of hospital stay, and patients expect them to make these decisions based on patient needs rather than the cost of care.

This chapter examines many issues related to hospital funding. It begins with a look at how funds flow into and out of hospitals and then examines how hospitals can manage their finances, including using cost shifting. Finally, the chapter concludes by exploring the ways hospitals obtain financing and by describing some of the typical organizational structures used within these complex institutions.

8.1 Revenues: The Flow of Funds into the Hospital

From the founding of the first hospital in the American colonies in 1751 until the beginnings of BlueCross in 1929, the primary source of hospital funding was philanthropy from the community, supplemented by patient fees. Since 1940, hospital revenues have grown rapidly, but philanthropy and patient fees have decreased drastically as a percentage of the total. Now the largest sources of payment are Medicare and managed care firms:

▲ Medicare provides government funding for the 60 percent of patient days used by the elderly.

▲ Managed care firms shop for low prices and good information systems to control costs.

8.1.1 Creating New Ways to Pay for Hospital Care

Around 1960, the dominant payers for hospital care in the United States were nonprofit BlueCross plans. At that time, these plans were affiliated with various hospital associations. They were designed to reimburse the full cost of patient care, thus allowing hospitals to break even while taking care of the indigent and undertaking whichever new treatments, diagnostic technology, or research they wanted. By 1995, several BlueCross plans had fallen into bankruptcy. The surviving plans all started managed care plans to compete with (or complement) their traditional insurance plans. Some, such as the giant BlueCross of California, turned themselves into billion-dollar private for-profit firms.[1]

A new financing system had to be created—and re-created again and again—to provide all the new technology and services that Americans wanted in hospital care. By 2002, 200 times more money was transferred from the pockets of the public into hospital expenses than had been paid at the end of World War II, with an average increase of more than 10 percent per year. However, hospital revenue growth has slowed substantially since 1990 as managed care has taken hold, and more revenues are now coming from outside hospitals, in the form of outpatient services and new business ventures (e.g., ambulance, nutrition counseling, home health care services). In 2006, the average community hospital's inpatient revenues were around $65.3 million, with about $12,448 received for each patient admitted ($2,223 per day for an average 5.6-day stay). These hospitals typically received another $36 million for outpatient services. Table 8-1 lists the current sources of hospital revenues.[2]

As you review Table 8-1, keep in mind that these numbers are related to complex contracts for hundreds of thousands, or even millions, of dollars. For example, a hospital chief financial officer (CFO) has to enter into an intricate legal relationship with Medicare or a joint venture with a group of radiologists, or structure a risk-sharing arrangement with a consortium of community physicians. Such deals are quite different from retail sales added up at a cash register.

We can learn some important details from Table 8-1:

▲ Unlike in most markets, consumers' decisions based on price will likely have an insignificant impact on hospital behavior. That's because more than 95 percent of hospital revenues come from someone other than the recipient of services.[3]

▲ The government accounts for 56 percent of all hospital revenues.

Table 8-1: Hospital Characteristics

Total number of hospitals	5,795
Community hospitals	4,919
Average number of beds per hospital	152 beds
Occupancy rate	67%
Admissions per 100 population	12.0
Average length of hospital stay	5.6 days
Number of emergency room visits per day	63
Number of outpatient visits per day	256
Number of employees	836
Number of registered nurses	214
Average cost per outpatient visit	$303
Percentage of revenues from outpatients	36%
Average cost per patient day	$2,223
Average revenue per hospital	$102 million
Average profit margin	5.4%

Sources of Funds		*Uses of Funds*	
Patient self-pay	3%	Labor	53%
Private insurance	36%	Professional fees	5%
Philanthropy, other private funding	5%	Supplies, other	34%
Medicare	29%	Depreciation and interest	<u>8%</u>
Medicaid	20%		
Other government	<u>7%</u>		
Total	*100%*		*100%*

8.1.2 Sources of Revenues

Although a complete picture is beyond the scope of this book, an overview of the major ways in which revenues currently flow into hospitals is helpful in grasping the financial incentives hospitals face (see Figure 8-1).

Figure 8-1

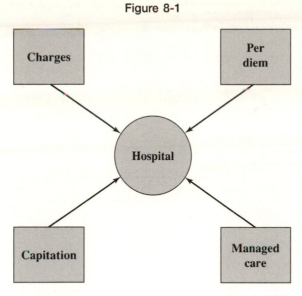

Major sources of hospital revenue.

Philanthropy and Grants

Grants are donated funds that are intended for a specific purpose, such as to conduct cancer research, build a new operating pavilion, provide outreach programs for prenatal care, and so on. Donors want to make sure that these funds are used for the purpose intended, but grants and charitable donations put little direct pressure on hospitals to compete on price or to control costs. Instead, this revenue flows from the belief of the donor that the task facing the hospital is important and socially valuable and isn't to make profits or even necessarily to show measurable effects.

Global Budgets

A hospital operates under a **global budget** when it receives a fixed grant amount to cover all its costs. This form of payment is typical for state mental hospitals, military hospitals, and hospitals run by the Department of Veterans Affairs and other government entities, as well as a few specialized private institutions. Because global budgets are fixed, they provide few incentives either to attract more patients or to reduce costs. In Canada, England, and much of the developed world outside the United States, global budgets are the most common form of hospital payment.

Charges

Hospital charges are like what are known as "list prices" in most industries. A hospital, like a flower shop, can set its charges at whatever level it likes. However, it's rare for a patient or an insurance company to actually pay what is "charged." Still, these paper charges often form the basis for reimbursement under a system of "discounted charges" (e.g., an insurance company agrees to pay 60 percent of list price) or under a cost reimbursement system, such as that described later in this chapter.

Per Diem

Latin for "per day," **per diems,** or per-day payments for services, were common when hospitals originated and are increasingly favored in managed care contracts today. Originally, per diems were charges set by the hospital, and they usually exceeded costs to help subsidize nonpaying patients. Today, per diems are often negotiated with managed care firms under very competitive conditions and are sometimes set below average costs per day in order for a hospital to maintain or increase its market share.

Cost Reimbursement

Cost reimbursement sets the payment levels equal to the hospital's actual costs. Because the hospital's output is so difficult to define and measure, it may be more equitable and easier to reimburse for incurred costs rather than try to set appropriate prices. The BlueCross plans wrote manuals describing how not-for-profit hospitals can break even by setting charges to cover costs (including costs for treating nonpaying patients and setting aside money for a prudent reserve) and designed a method of cost reimbursement to break even. This method is known as ratio of cost to charges applied to charges (RCCAC). When Medicare was created in 1965, it adopted the RCCAC method, and this form of cost reimbursement became the dominant method by which funds flowed into hospitals from the 1960s until the mid-1980s. The RCCAC method is still used to determine most hospital unit costs today.

The RCCAC method worked very well for a number of years to reimburse hospitals for all their costs. Indeed, it worked so well that costs rose explosively. Costs rose so much that cutbacks became inevitable, causing arguments between hospitals and Medicare over money. Medicare initially accommodated the needs of hospitals by covering the cost of caring for patients who didn't pay. In a subsequent interpretation of the rules, Medicare in effect began to say, "Because we pay all our bills in full and on time, we're not responsible for those who don't." This helps the Medicare budget but not the hospital, which must then increase charges to other payers to make up the difference.

Diagnosis-Related Groups

Diagnosis-related group (DRG) payments are reimbursements that compensate by the case (rather than per day or per charged item), based on the diagnosis of the treatment. DRG payments cover the complete hospital stay, including all ancillary services, but not surgery and other physician fees. The government created this prospective payment system for Medicare payments by splitting all illnesses into DRGs and estimating the cost per case within each group. Adjustments were then made for factors such as local wages in the area in which the hospital is located, extremely long or short stays, hospitals with large teaching programs, and hospitals with a large proportion of indigent patients. In essence, DRGs are prices set by the government at what it believes is a fair rate.

The DRG system is called a prospective payment system because DRG rates are set in advance, which is not the case with retrospective cost reimbursement payments, which are continually adjusted to match any change in costs. Under a charge system such as the DRG system, the sellers (i.e., hospitals) have the power to set rates arbitrarily; however, the market has the power to refuse to buy. On the other hand, under a retrospective cost system, there is no set rate but rather reimbursement of actual costs incurred, perhaps subject to some review. Thus, with a DRG prospective payment system, the buyer (i.e., Medicare) really has all the rate-setting power.

In the first year that Medicare used the DRG system (1983), it did little to force rates down, but in the years since, reimbursement has become progressively tighter; therefore, Medicare patients have become less and less profitable to treat. After Medicare's DRG system was put in place, it was adopted by many other payers, including private insurance companies.[4]

FOR EXAMPLE

Revamping DRGs

In July 2006, the George W. Bush administration proposed revising the Medicare DRG payment system. Under the existing system, Medicare was reimbursing hospitals for patients with certain conditions, such as pneumonia, no matter how severe or mild the illness, as long as the illness fit one of the DRG categories. In its initial version of the revamped DRG plan, the Bush administration wanted to replace the existing 526 DRG categories with 861 categories, in large part to account for levels of illness severity, and thereby reduce the payout for many procedures. The U.S. secretary of health and human services said that the existing system encouraged hospitals to provide "treatments that happen to be the most profitable." Among the proposed cuts was a 33 percent reduction in the payout for surgery to open clogged arteries by inserting stents. Similarly, the payment for hip and knee replacements would have been reduced 10 percent, to $14,500. After this plan came under severe attack from hospitals and health care advocates, the government scaled back its plans in August 2006. For instance, instead of a 33 percent reduction in payment for a stent, it called for a 2 percent cut. However, the government threatened additional cuts in 2007.

Capitation

As discussed in Chapter 6, capitation refers to the payment of a fixed amount per person per month for a defined set of services; this payment doesn't vary based on a patient's actual use of the services. When an organization agrees to accept payment on a capitation basis, it in effect becomes a risk-bearing insurer.

Capitation can be both beneficial and harmful to revenues depending on the type of health care organizations and services involved. With capitation, an organization has a definite amount of revenue coming in. If an organization's services are lean and costs are very low, capitation might have a positive impact on the organization's revenue. This type of capitated arrangement would most likely have a positive influence on revenues for a single organization providing a single service with low costs. If an organization has many services and is spread out too thinly in terms of costs, then capitation could be very harmful to revenues because costs could outweigh any possible revenues from capitation agreements. This latter situation has been the case with many health care organizations, causing them to abandon capitation and move toward fee-for-service plans that offer greater chances at positive revenue streams. Under capitation, many health care organizations assumed too much risk compared to the capitation fees and therefore lost revenue.

When a hospital sets up a capitation arrangement, some larger organization, such as a corporation that controls a number of hospitals, is creating an insurance company/health maintenance organization (HMO) to provide services on a capitated basis. When the contract extends to multiple institutions and different kinds of care, the hospital becomes a health system rather than a traditional community hospital. Again, this may have an impact on revenue due to the spreading of costs over a greater number of hospitals, services, and capitation fees for each area and institution.

Managed Care Contracts

In today's health care environment, BlueCross and most other private insurance companies are increasingly shifting to managed care contracts with hospitals (see Chapter 10). In these arrangements, payment is usually made on the basis of per diems, discounted charges, or a negotiated fee schedule. The crucial difference that sets managed care contracts apart from cost reimbursement or payment of charges is the role of the care manager. Rather than just paying the bills, the insurance company has a specialized nurse or physician critically examine each case to determine, for example, whether hospitalization was justified, whether a lower-cost alternative (such as outpatient surgery) was available, and whether adequate documentation was provided for all laboratory tests. By negotiating discounts, discouraging use, and denying payment for disallowed or undocumented charges, managed care firms can usually obtain medical care for their clients at a lower cost than traditional indemnity or cost reimbursement insurers; they are, therefore, taking over the market. Being constantly questioned and audited hasn't been easy or pleasant for the doctors who admit patients enrolled in these plans or for those working in hospital financial departments. Patients also dislike having to justify and obtain approval for every additional service or extra day in the hospital, but they are willing to put up with these problems if their insurance premiums are sufficiently reduced.

SELF-CHECK

- List the two largest sources of hospital payments in the United States.
- List two forms of hospital funding that don't pressure hospitals to contain costs.
- List two forms of hospital funding that do pressure hospitals to contain costs.
- Explain how **DRG** payment works.

8.2 Costs: The Flow of Funds Out of the Hospital

Hospitals are personal care institutions, and labor accounts for the bulk of their costs (refer to Table 8-1). In the early days, food and housing took up most of a hospital's budget, but today such "hotel functions" are relatively minor in comparison with the provision of medical care. Similarly, energy, raw materials, and other goods are relatively unimportant in a hospital's budget. Few physicians are employees of the hospital; physician care is paid for separately and is usually not included in the hospital budget. The services of contracted pathologists, radiologists, and emergency room doctors do show up under the category "professional fees."

It might be thought that the acquisition of lithotripters, magnetic resonance imaging (MRI) scanners, and other expensive medical technology devices would make "equipment" a large expense category for hospitals, yet the wages of the skilled people required to operate each new piece of equipment usually runs two or three times the cost of the machinery itself.

When payroll, professional fees, and local services, such as lab work, are added together, these labor expenses account for about 75% of a hospital's overall costs. This fact makes it politically difficult to cut costs because the most effective way to do so is to cut people by reducing wages or laying off employees.

FOR EXAMPLE

Hospital Salary Samplings

Here's a sample of typical hospital position salaries for Long Beach, California:

Position	Average Salary
CCU nurse	$61,385
Hospital administrator	$298,670
Neonatologist	$300,461
Nurse anesthetist	$132,180
Nurse practitioner	$83,941
Registered nurse	$58,912

SELF-CHECK

- What is the largest category of expenses for hospitals?
- List two other types of hospital expenses.

8.3 Financial Management and Cost Shifting

Revenues must exceed expenses for an organization to survive, but there's no reason the people incurring the expenses must be the ones who pay the bills. While in most consumer markets, it's typical for people to pay out of pocket for the goods and services they receive, in health care, this almost never takes place.

8.3.1 Cost Shifting

In the first part of the twentieth century, when hospitals took care of the poor who couldn't help themselves, it was obvious and necessary that the burden of financing would fall primarily on a different group of people who did have money: philanthropists and taxpayers. As technology advanced and hospital services became more desirable to all people, it was inevitable that there would be a great increase in hospital expenditures and that there would be more discrepancy between the people who received care and paid for that care and the people who received care but couldn't pay. Insurance, pooling funds from the many so that a few could receive care, was a significant extension of financing that furthered the ability of the market to transfer the burden of payment away from individuals who were sick. One of the expenses that was factored into private insurance premiums was charity care; thus, insured patients were also paying for those who had no insurance.

The process of using excess revenues from one group of services or patients to subsidize other services or patient groups is known in health care as **cost shifting.** Under philanthropic funding, all revenues are cost shifted—they are intended as donations to benefit others, not the giver. With insurance and cost reimbursement, the flows are more complex, but it's clear that somebody else is paying for nonpaying patients because they don't bring any revenues into the hospital. Several other functions, such as medical education, research, and community outreach, are also usually supported through cost shifting because they bring in very little revenue—certainly less than what they cost to provide.

Cost shifting is a pervasive and long-standing feature of medical care reimbursement. In general, hospitals have had public support for taking revenues from a variety of sources and using them to fund not just basic care but outreach to indigent people, community prevention programs, research, teaching, and other activities that were seen as being in the public interest.

8.3.2 Changes in Cost Shifting

A number of forces have interacted over the past twenty years to cause this once solid consensus on cost shifting within hospitals to crumble. A tremendous and unanticipated rise in expenditures for Medicare and Medicaid began to force the government to modify the reimbursement system to cut costs. This had a dramatic impact on the practice of cost shifting in health care. After a series of legislative cost controls attempting to maintain the solvency of the Medicare program failed to work, unpopular premium and tax increases had to be pushed through Congress. Medicare, forced into a corner, began to refuse to pay for the cost of indigent care. Medicare claimed that it needed to be a "prudent buyer" and therefore reneged on the fundamental cost-shifting premise.

On one hand, Medicare's decision not to fund charity care and bad debt made sense. The bills of all Medicare patients were being paid in full and on time. Acting as an insurer of people 65 and older, Medicare was certainly fulfilling its financial obligation to hospitals. On the other hand, hospitals had always charged everybody extra to make up for losses on charity care. Furthermore, it appeared that if anyone should be taking responsibility for the poor, it should be the government. Medicare, by taking a narrow interpretation of its contractual responsibilities to hospitals, broke up the larger social contract based on cost shifting, which had been fundamental to hospitals as caring community institutions.

8.3.3 Effects of Cost-Shifting Changes

As Medicare ratcheted down its rates, hospitals had to look elsewhere to make up the difference. And so, whereas charges to commercial insurance companies had been 10 to 15 percent above average cost, the breakdown of cost shifting pushed these "overcharges" up to 20 to 30 percent above cost. The private insurance companies howled in protest as they were forced to pick up what previously had been paid for through general tax funds. The university hospitals, with large indigent populations and big research programs, were in even worse shape than the community hospitals. They had a much smaller fraction of revenues coming from commercial insurance and, to make up for losses, had to raise their commercial rates 50 to 100 percent. The federal and state governments argued that the provision of Medicare and Medicaid had reduced the hospitals' burden of bad debt and charity care, but the large number of people seeking care who were still uninsured made hospitals skeptical.

Small price differences and a shared sense of purpose were sufficient to allow the cost shifting that made up a social contract for hospitals to continue. Big price differences and a hostile, "I'll pay for mine, and you pay for yours" attitude ruined this system. Market forces came into play.

8.3.4 Cream Skimming

The outrageously high prices for tests done in hospital laboratories created a profit opportunity for commercial companies, which started providing services through independent doctor-entrepreneurs, cut prices in half, and still had large profit margins. For example, specialized psychiatric hospitals that treated only mild cases of mental disorder sprang up, able to make money at a pier diem far below that of the inner city psychiatric wards filled with violent and chronically disturbed individuals. Whenever prices are distorted by cross subsidy, there is an opportunity for a firm to make extraordinary profits by what is called **cream skimming.** Cream skimming is providing only one or two services that are overpriced and not providing services that are more costly and subsidized.

Tradition and expressions of disapproval were able to limit the extent to which profits were drained from the system by cream skimming prior to 1970. Since then, however, the margins have become too large, and the ideology of health care too fragmented, to keep the old system afloat.

It has become clear that hospital financial managers (by taking advantage of the system) and Medicare (by refusing to take responsibility for all of America's needy) contributed to the demise of cost shifting and the increase in the practice of cream skimming.

The collapse of cost shifting forces us now to confront the question of who will pay for the indigent and who will pay for medical research. Although there is a general recognition that caring for the indigent and paying for research will cost something, the public seriously underestimates how large that bill will be because of the cost-shifting practices that have gone on for so many years. Most of the income in the United States is earned by employed people between the ages of 30 and 60. This generally healthy group, whose wealth is increasing, makes up less than a third of the population. Paying for the other two-thirds of the population, and for all the medical advances working people want, will require transfers of billions and billions of dollars. From where will this money come? We are in the process of giving up on the old system of transferring funds but have not been able to find and agree on a new one.[5]

FOR EXAMPLE

Government Spending on Health Care

Spending on health care makes up 20 percent of the federal budget and a similar percentage of most state budgets as well. What does this mean for you? For one, it means that if you paid $5,000 in taxes last year, around $1,000 of your tax money went to health care programs.[6]

SELF-CHECK

- Define **cost shifting** and **cream skimming**.
- List two factors that contributed to the end of the cost-shifting system.
- Now that Medicare refuses to cover the cost of nonpaying patients, who covers these costs?

8.4 Hospital Financing

Revenues for an organization must not only exceed current expenses, they must also be sufficiently above operating costs to compensate those who have invested money in the organization. For example, if a hospital borrows $10 million for construction, it must pay back the principal over time and pay interest on the loan each year. For a philanthropist making a donation, the returns on his or her investment take the form of social services rather than interest or dividends.

8.4.1 The History of Hospital Financing

The startup funds for most hospitals came from a combination of philanthropy and local governments. Land and buildings were often donated. At the beginning of the twentieth century, there were also a number of doctors' hospitals, usually started in a portion of a doctor's house or in a converted dwelling nearby. The financing for the construction of these small, private hospitals came from the doctor's own savings or from family members.

In 1946, the Hill-Burton Act was passed, making construction funds available to new hospitals in areas that had fewer than four beds per 1,000 people. As a form of repayment, hospitals receiving these funds were to give an equal or greater value in free care to indigent people. Subsequent changes were made to allow Hill-Burton Act funds to be used for expansion and renovation projects as well as new construction.

8.4.2 The Impact of Medicare and Medicaid on Hospital Financing

The Hill-Burton Act, retained earnings, and philanthropic fund drives provided most financing for hospital construction and renovation until the enactment of Medicare and Medicaid in 1965. Upon the introduction of these government programs, hospitals, which had chronically suffered operating losses, suddenly had steady revenue streams guaranteed by the government. They could meet the demand for new construction by borrowing against the promise of government funding, and they proceeded to do so with a vengeance.

The impact of Medicare and Medicaid on the finances of hospitals can't be overstated. Hospitals went from social organizations that had to beg for money each year to solidly funded services backed by the government. For a time, it was virtually impossible for most hospitals to go bankrupt and hence for investors not to get repaid. In this environment, hospitals went on a borrowing spree, loading up with more than $10 billion in debt by 1980. However, any business that takes on lots of debt is likely to come under financial pressure. Despite being organized as nonprofit organizations, hospitals were no exception. With millions of dollars of interest payments to make each year, hospital managers had to become more and more bottom-line oriented. As the threat of bankruptcy became real, the social welfare and community benefit orientation that had prevailed since the turn of the century increasingly gave way to a business orientation.

Hospital borrowing rose so rapidly that it had to lose steam eventually. Too many new beds were added, and many hospitals became unable to pay their monthly debt payments. Also, pressures on the Medicare budget led to tighter and tighter reimbursement. In 1985, the first bond defaults began to occur. Investors quickly revised their expectations and treated hospital debt as risky and hence required a higher rate of interest. Access to financing became more difficult. Old and decrepit facilities couldn't tap the bond market and were acquired by for-profit hospital chains (discussed in section 8.4.4) that could use the stock market to quickly raise money, refurbish the facilities, and make money. Many towns were willing to sell their hospitals for nothing—even providing special subsidies and tax breaks—rather than let them go bankrupt and disappear. The environment also had changed so that more hospitals felt it necessary to become part of systems covering all types of care over a broad geographic area. To do so, strong hospitals wanted to merge with or buy weaker ones and to buy nursing homes, home health agencies, physician practices, and medical office buildings.

8.4.3 The Decline of the Stand-Alone Community Hospital

The stand-alone community hospital was a good structure for creating a social contract.[7] Business leaders, citizens of the town, and the poor all participated in a visible symbol of community responsibility that was governed by a local board of directors. The move toward larger and more integrated health care systems has shown that the stand-alone structure is inflexible and increasingly outmoded. People no longer identify primarily with a community or look to voluntary action to provide health care, and the solo hospital has no way to move money from where the funds are (e.g., in wealthy suburbs) to where the needs are (e.g., in distressed urban and rural areas, in providing assistance to elderly people with disabilities). Creating a chain of hospitals is one way to regionalize and rationalize the allocation of funds. Recently, there has been a spurt of acquisitions and conversions of hospitals to for-profit status, although it's still unclear how far this trend will go and to what extent the government, as the primary payer for hospital care, will let it go. What has become clear is that private equity markets have far outstripped private philanthropy as a source of capital for meeting the demands for new health care services and new health care facility construction in the twenty-first century.

FOR EXAMPLE

The Allegheny Bankruptcy[8]

Allegheny General Hospital was at one time one of the largest hospitals in the Pittsburgh area.[9] It provided a broad range of services, had high occupancy, and generated large cash flows. In 1987, it merged with the cash-poor Medical College of Pennsylvania in Philadelphia to form the Allegheny Health and Education Research Foundation (AHERF). From 1990 to 1996, AHERF went on a hospital-buying spree. It acquired a children's hospital, another Philadelphia medical college, and a number of community hospitals in the Philadelphia and Pittsburgh markets. Along the way, AHERF was leveraging the strong cash flows from its Allegheny General Hospital to buy up financially troubled hospitals.

During the 1990s, many hospitals, fearful of the advent of managed care, began purchasing physician practices to make sure they would not lose admissions. AHERF was aggressive in doing so, trying to increase market share, and rapidly increasing the price paid for practices in the Philadelphia area. In the end, much money was spent, and few new admissions were gained. AHERF also began competing aggressively for managed care business during the 1990s, including entering into "full-risk" contracts, under which the hospital agrees to take care of all HMO member health care needs for a percentage of that member's HMO policy premium. Competition with other hospital networks bid down the prices paid, and inexperience with full-risk management caused expenses to rise, resulting in substantial losses.

By 1996, AHERF was beginning to suffer serious financial losses. To hide poor financial performance, AHERF executives transferred funds from one

(continued)

division to another to make each appear profitable at the time of the division's audit. Some transfers included restricted funds intended for use at one institution only or for a specific purpose (i.e., cancer research, nursing education); such transfers are illegal. Lack of diligence by both AHERF's board of directors and auditors left these transfers hidden. As happened with Enron, this financial shell game eventually unraveled. In 1997, AHERF became the largest not-for-profit bankruptcy in U.S. history, and its CEO was eventually sent to prison.

8.4.4 For-Profit Hospitals

For-profit hospitals are owned by a group of investors or shareholders and have many of the characteristics of the standard model firm. As the name indicates, these hospitals are out to make a profit for their owners, shareholders, and other related parties. Oftentimes, the physicians in these hospitals are investors or owners in the hospitals themselves. Efficiency is usually high in for-profit hospitals while costs are low. These hospitals normally take the form of specialized facilities that only provide in-demand, elective types of services to people who can afford them and typically do not offer loss-producing services like emergency care. There are several for-profit hospital systems in the U.S. that have become quite large corporations on the business stage. For-profit hospitals, if they so choose, can become leaders in particular fields because they have the money, efficiency, and ability to adapt in a fast-changing health care environment.

SELF-CHECK

- List the three primary sources of capital financing for hospitals prior to Medicare and Medicaid.
- Explain what the Hill-Burton Act did for hospitals.
- What has replaced philanthropy as a major source of capital financing today?

8.5 Hospital Organization

From an economic viewpoint, the standard-model firm is an organization created by the owners, who invest time and money to make a profit. To turn a profit, the firm must meet the needs of customers who pay for the firm's products as well as the needs of employees and other vendors. Each party must benefit in order for the organization to continue to exist. A firm operates as a rational economic organization because the owners who make the decisions must bear the consequences, whether good (i.e., profits) or bad (i.e., losses).

Hospitals, however, differ from the standard firm in three significant ways:

1. Because of insurance or charity, patients typically don't pay hospitals directly.
2. Ownership of hospitals is usually unclear because of not-for-profit voluntary or governmental organization.
3. Medical care is largely controlled by doctors, who generally neither pay nor receive any money from hospitals and, therefore, have no direct connection from a flow-of-funds perspective.

Doctors are not customers, employees, or owners of a hospital, but in practice, they are the dominant voice in hospital operations; therefore, they sometimes look like they are all three. This structure—combining power, money, and service with no direct line of control or financial accountability—is a unique form of economic organization that makes it difficult to model or predict the behavior of hospitals. A hospital doesn't do anything without directions from a physician; only physicians are allowed to admit patients, perform surgery, or prescribe drugs. A hospital organizes a medical staff, but some claim that the reality is the other way around—that the medical staff organizes the hospital as its workshop.[10]

An exception to this, however, is privately owned hospitals. Owners of these types of hospitals may be physicians, investment groups, or shareholders. In these types of hospitals, the structure is much more like the standard model firm.

The American Hospital Association maintains that hospitals are, in essence, public institutions whose purpose is to benefit the community. From a flow-of-funds perspective, this makes sense because most of the capital investment in a voluntary hospital comes from the community, in the form of charitable donations and taxes. The problem is, how is community benefit defined and who, exactly, exercises control?[11] The hospital board, although in theory representing the community, is often deferential to the medical staff and depends on the information provided by the administration to make decisions.

FOR EXAMPLE

Looking to the VA for Hospital Leadership

The U.S. Department of Veterans Affairs (VA) runs 154 hospitals and 875 clinics throughout the country for active-duty and retired military personnel. It's the largest health care network in the United States, serving 5.4 million patients, all of whom qualify for free or low-cost care. In the past

(continued)

10 years, VA hospitals have gone from the worst hospital system in the nation to the best. A RAND Corporation study reported that VA patients are more likely to receive recommended care than patients in the national sample. In addition, the quality of care was better for VA patients on all measures except acute care, on which the VA fared on par with other hospitals. Several factors contributed to the dramatic improvements, but one key factor was the implementation of a sophisticated electronic medical records system that allows instant communication among providers across the country and reminds providers of patients' clinical needs; in contrast, only 20% of civilian hospitals have computerized medical records systems. VA leadership has also established a quality measurement program that holds regional managers accountable for essential processes in preventive care and in the management of common chronic conditions.

The VA is in a better position than other systems to make these sorts of top-down changes for a variety of reasons. It gets its funding from a single payer (the federal government); in contrast, private-sector hospitals receive payment from third-party insurers who set the prices they will pay. And because the VA system is committed to treating patients throughout their lives, it can justify spending money on preventive care such as weight-loss programs. The VA is also in a unique position to control costs. All its physicians are salaried employees, and the VA is allowed to negotiate prices with drug companies and other suppliers, which it does aggressively. The bottom line: The VA spends an average of $1,300 *less* per patient than other hospitals while providing superior care.[12]

SELF-CHECK

- List three ways that hospitals differ from standard firms.
- Who controls not-for-profit hospitals? How?

SUMMARY

Most early hospitals were funded primarily by charitable donations and government tax appropriations. Today, more than 95 percent of all hospital revenues come from third parties, with more than half coming from government through the Medicare and Medicaid programs. Patients pay so little of hospital bills that charges are virtually irrelevant in decision making.

Labor is the largest category of health care expenditure. When employees of local service firms are included, personnel accounts for more than 75 percent of a hospital's costs. Therefore, the only way to cut costs is to reduce wages or reduce employment, neither of which is politically popular.

Cost shifting is the process of charging one group (e.g., commercially insured patients) more to cover the loss due to undercharging another group (e.g., indigent patients, Medicaid patients). The pervasiveness of cost shifting and insurance coverage gave hospital managers room to raise revenues as a means of supporting the hospital and little incentive to find efficiencies that would reduce costs. However, changes in Medicare reimbursement and the advent of managed care firms that shop to obtain hospital services at the lowest possible price have eroded the ability of hospitals to shift costs.

Although accounting for just 8 percent of operating costs, access to capital has been crucial in shaping the growth of hospitals. Philanthropy was first replaced by government construction grants through the Hill-Burton Act of 1946, which were replaced by tax-exempt municipal revenue bonds in the 1970s and subsequently by equity financing through the stock market.

Hospitals differ from most other firms in that they are largely paid for by third parties, most commonly not-for-profit organizations directed by volunteer boards rather than owners and dominated by doctors, who are independent professionals who work for themselves and have no direct financial ties to the hospital.

KEY TERMS

Cost reimbursement	Payment for services based upon a hospital's actual costs.
Cost shifting	The process of using excess revenues from one set of services or patients to subsidize other services or patient groups.
Cream skimming	The process of providing only the services that are overpriced, not the ones that are more costly and subsidized.
Diagnosis related group (DRG)	A system of reimbursement that compensates by the case (rather than per day or per charged item) based on the diagnosis of the treatment.
Global budget	A fixed grant amount intended to cover all of a hospital's costs.
Grant	Donated funds that are intended for a specific purpose.
Per diem	Per-day payment for services.

ASSESS YOUR UNDERSTANDING

Go to www.wiley.com/college/getzen to evaluate your knowledge of hospital systems. *Measure your learning by comparing pre-test and post-test results.*

Summary Questions

1. Labor constitutes the largest category of expenses for hospitals. True or False?
2. The largest single source of revenue for U.S. hospitals in the aggregate is:
   (a) Medicare.
   (b) Medicaid.
   (c) private health insurance, including HMOs.
   (d) philanthropy.
3. The process of using excess revenues from one group of services or patients to subsidize other services or patient groups is known in health care as:
   (a) cream skimming.
   (b) cost shifting.
   (c) capitation.
   (d) cost reimbursement.
4. Since the introduction of managed care plans in the 1990s, the rate of hospital revenue growth has:
   (a) increased.
   (b) decreased.
   (c) stayed the same.
   (d) doubled.
5. The DRG system in hospitals:
   (a) is another name for per diem payment, in which a hospital receives a fixed payment per patient day.
   (b) refers to drug rehabilitation groups, organized by managed care to save expense on behavioral/mental health services.
   (c) is a retrospective payment system based on what costs were incurred in treating patients in certain disease groups.
   (d) is used by Medicare to set fixed-case payment levels based on the patient's diagnosis at the time of discharge.
6. During the period from the implementation of Medicare and Medicaid until approximately the end of the 1980s, the dominant form of capital financing in hospitals was:
   (a) the Hill-Burton Act.
   (b) debt.

(c) equity in the form of stock.

(d) retained earnings used as reserves for depreciation.

7. Cream skimming is the practice of reaping extraordinary profits by providing only services that are overpriced. True or False?

8. Who controls not-for-profit hospitals?

(a) Doctors and administrators

(b) Administrators and the community

(c) Patients and administrators

(d) Doctors, administrators, patients, and the community

9. Private philanthropy is the largest source of capital for funding the construction and expansion of hospitals. True or False?

Review Questions

1. Who pays for most of the care in hospitals? Are the people who pay the bills the same as the people who receive the care?

2. What accounts for the largest portion of hospital costs?

3. Over the past 100 years, the major source of hospital revenues has changed three times. Name these types of payments, and explain why each one gave way to the next.

4. How do hospitals pay for medical research?

5. Are doctors usually employees, owners, or managers of hospitals?

6. What does it mean for Medicare to act as a "prudent buyer" of hospital services? Does its doing so strengthen or weaken Medicare as a social insurance program?

7. Who benefits from cost shifting—the poor or the rich? Do any health care workers benefit from cost shifting?

8. What kind of impact did the Hill-Burton Act have on hospitals?

Applying This Chapter

1. If a hospital decides to raise prices because it needs more money, what effect does this have on:

(a) Patients who pay their own bills?

(b) Patients whose bills are paid by an insurance company?

(c) Insurance contracts reimbursed on the basis of costs?

(d) Previously negotiated per diem contracts with HMOs?

2. U.S. Secretary of Health and Human Services Mike Leavitt has said, "Every American should have access to a full range of information about

the quality and cost of their health care options." What hospital practices might he be referring in this statement?

3. As noted in this chapter, VA hospitals average $1,300 less per patient than other hospitals while providing superior care. What sets VA hospitals apart from other hospitals? Why might they be in a better position to contain costs? What features of VA hospitals could other hospitals adopt in order to provide superior care at a lower cost?

YOU TRY IT

Specialty Hospital "Cream Skimming"

According to the Centers for Medicare and Medicaid Services, the current system of DRG payments provides incentives to hospitals for providing certain types of services and treating certain types of patients. For instance, the DRG overpayment for cardiovascular care has led to the creation of specialty hospitals that exclusively treat patients with cardiovascular problems. Because these hospitals don't provide services for less profitable illnesses, they can reap the profits rather than engage in cost shifting to cover the costs of less profitable services. One of the results of this cream skimming is that community hospitals, which provide a full spectrum of care, get fewer high-profit cardiac patients and are left to provide all the less profitable services.

Write an essay in which you consider the long-term consequences for patients and community hospitals if specialty hospitals are allowed to continue cream skimming. What would be the effects of revising the DRG payment system to make the payments more equitable for all services?

Reviewing Hospital Finances

Go to the website of a hospital in your area and prepare a report about the hospital. In your report, be sure to address the following questions: How many beds does the hospital have? How many physicians does it work with? Is it a not-for-profit or for-profit hospital? What is its operating budget for the year? How much charity or uncompensated care does it provide?

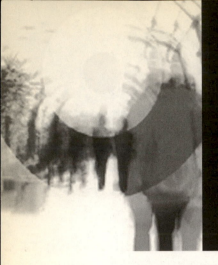

9

HOSPITAL COSTS
Management and Regulation

Starting Point

Go to www.wiley.com/college/getzen to assess your knowledge of hospital cost management and regulation.
Determine where you need to concentrate your effort.

What You'll Learn in This Chapter

▲ Factors contributing to wide variations in hospital costs
▲ How hospitals manage their budgets
▲ How hospitals can use economies of scale to run more efficiently
▲ The importance of quality in assessing hospital care
▲ How hospitals compete for patients
▲ Controlling hospital costs through regulation

After Studying This Chapter, You'll Be Able To

▲ Assess whether a hospital that charges more is worth the higher price
▲ Evaluate known short-run and long-run variations in hospital expenses
▲ Estimate a hospital's efficiency based on its size
▲ Assess hospital care based on quality
▲ Evaluate the value of competition among hospitals
▲ Critique the effectiveness of government regulation of hospital costs

INTRODUCTION

The cost of a hospital stay can vary significantly from one hospital to the next, and it's often difficult to compare hospital costs in any meaningful way. The easiest way to compare hospital costs is to look at the cost of each unit of service individually, but that doesn't account for the quality of care received.

Hospital administrators face the daunting task of controlling costs in the face of a lot of unknowns. They use a budget process to control costs, building in flexibility to account for uncertainty and changes. They also rely on economies of scale to smooth out the flow of fluctuations in patient admissions, although very small hospitals and very large hospitals don't benefit from economies of scale.

Obviously, hospitals need patients in order to stay in business. But because physicians and insurance companies, not the patients themselves, control the flow of patients, hospitals must compete for those entities that have the power to make the revenue come.

In the face of spiraling hospitals costs, the government has imposed regulations on hospitals over the years. It seems, though, that any attempt on the part of the government to cut costs in one area of hospital care has lead to increases in costs in other areas.

This chapter takes a closer look at these various issues related to hospital costs. It begins by considering why some hospitals cost more than others and how a hospital's management team can work to control costs through the budgeting process. Various issues related to economies of scale, hospital quality, and competition among hospitals are then examined. Finally, the chapter closes with a look at some of the government actions undertaken in the past in an attempt to control hospital costs.

9.1 Why Do Some Hospitals Cost More Than Others?

The cost of a day in the hospital can be as little as $300 or more than $2,000. It's not surprising if a day in the hospital costs $2,000 for a critically wounded trauma patient in an intensive care unit (ICU) and just $300 for a patient resting after breaking a leg while skiing.[1] The ICU patient is much sicker and requires more complex services. It's also understandable that staying in one of the nation's top research and teaching hospitals under the care of famous doctors can cost more than staying in a small rural facility with limited equipment and staff.[2] The hospital bill can be a misleading guide to costs. One hospital may charge more but give every patient a discount, while another sticks to list prices. Or, one hospital could charge $400 for a bed, with extra charges for medication, laboratory tests, physical therapy, and so on, while another hospital could charge $500 for a bed and all other services, making it less expensive.

FOR EXAMPLE

Comparing Sticker Prices for Chest Pain Care

Chest pain is one of the most commonly treated ailments in hospitals. Yet, the average price (based on the Medicare-based DRG for chest pain) varies considerably from hospital to hospital. Consider two hospitals in northern Ohio. St. Vincent Mercy Medical Center in Toledo, which has approximately 17,000 inpatient admissions a year and is an accredited Chest Pain Center, charged a sticker price of $12,467 in 2004. The estimated cost to the hospital for treating chest pain was $4,415. Defiance Regional Medical Center, 60 miles southwest of Toledo, which wasn't an accredited chest pain center at the time of the survey, charged a sticker price of $3,848. The average cost to the hospital was $2,376.[3]

A number of factors account for such a wide variation, including the following:

▲ Severity of patient's illness

▲ Quality of care

▲ Intensity of services (e.g., number of nursing hours or lab tests)

▲ Cost shifting

▲ Differences in billing

▲ Prices of labor and other inputs

▲ Efficiency

It's often assumed that a hospital with a lower cost per patient day is more efficient, but such a conclusion is only justified if the hospitals being compared provide the same services to similar patients under similar conditions. Since it's rarely the case that two hospitals are the same, efforts must be made to adjust for all the other factors listed earlier in this section to compare costs. If all factors are not the same, the more relevant question is: Is a hospital that costs 10 percent more (or 20 percent, or 400 percent) really worth that much more? While this question is more meaningful, it's also much more difficult to answer, and the answer depends on the patient's values as well as calculations of technical efficiency. Therefore, it's useful to look first at the simpler and more standard question of variations in costs for the same unit of service.

SELF-CHECK

- List two reasons why a hospital bill can be a misleading guide to costs.
- List at least three reasons why hospital bills for the same types of treatments may differ in price among facilities.

9.2 How Management Controls Costs

Hospital management can do a number of things to control costs, depending on the time frame involved and what it knows about future patient needs.

9.2.1 Short-Run vs. Long-Run Costs

If a hospital receives fewer admissions than expected this morning and wants to reduce its costs by the afternoon, not much can be done. People have already shown up for work, meals have been prepared, and so on. In the short run, almost all costs are fixed. Any reduction in the number of patients will, therefore, cause the average cost per patient to be higher than usual. If the reduction in admissions continues and management is given enough time to respond, the hospital may shut down a wing, refrain from hiring, and perhaps lay off some employees. This demonstrates a general rule: As more time is allowed for adjustment, more changes can be made, and as more changes are made, costs per unit become lower.

Thus, in the very long run, almost all costs become variable. A hospital director can train new management, hire clinical staff, replace an existing building with a new one, pave some grounds for parking, and even move the facility. If management expects to average only 100 patients per day, it would build a smaller hospital, hire fewer people, and incur lower fixed costs. If management expects 175 patients a day, it would build a medium-sized hospital. If 300 patients a day are expected, management would build a large hospital. For any expected level of output, management would choose a building size and number of permanent employees that would minimize costs.

9.2.2 Uncertainty and Budgeting

Over both the long and the short run, a manager must deal with two kinds of changes that affect the hospital's costs: foreseeable variations and unknown variations.

Foreseeable Variations

Expansion to accommodate a growing population in the suburbs, eliminating maternity beds in response to declining fertility, and opening a cardiac rehabilitation unit to serve an aging community are all examples of foreseeable long-run changes. A lower number of hospital admissions on Saturday and Sunday and on Christmas and New Year's Day are examples of foreseeable short-run changes. Adjustment to foreseeable changes can be planned in advance. For example, hiring, training, and space and building modifications can be accomplished on a schedule so that the pace of adjustment reflect conscious decisions by management to minimize costs.

Unknown Variations

Random variations must also be accommodated in the operations of the organization, but unlike foreseeable variations, these are not known in advance. For example, there may be sixteen admissions on Monday, twelve on Tuesday,

Figure 9-1

	Planned (known)	**Random** (uncertain)
Short Run	Scheduling Weekly budget Part-timers	Overtime, temps Inventory Maintain excess capacity
Long Run	Capital budgeting Change plant size Facility conversion	Hold financial reserves Encroachment by or on competitors Bankruptcy

How hospitals deal with change.

and twenty-two on Wednesday, and there may be twice as much work for the admitting office to do on Wednesday as on Tuesday, with the same amount of staff and equipment. Staff members are likely to do only what is necessary on a particular day, and perhaps even work late, while putting off until the next day some routine tasks, such as filing charts, checking documentation, and entering data into forms. Long-run unknown changes might occur because a new factory is built nearby, resulting in many new families moving to the area; an epidemic such as AIDS increases the demand for care; or a competing hospital is built, reducing demand. Such major changes often force a hospital to change its long-run strategy (see Figure 9-1).

9.2.3 Developing a Budget

How do managers control costs? Primarily through the use of a budget, a plan stated in dollars. A budget that doesn't change with volume is called a **fixed budget** (also known as a standard budget), and a budget that changes with volume is called a **flexible budget.** Typically, a hospital or medical group practice creates an **operating budget** that projects all anticipated expenses for the next year. For example, if labor expenses rose 7 percent in 2005 and 9 percent in 2006, management may project an increase of 8 percent in labor costs for 2007.[4] Managers usually define short-run changes as those that occur during the current budget period. Long-run changes and plans are incorporated in a **strategic budget** (also known as a long-run capital budget) that focuses on trends in the number of patients and capital renovations and expansions (new buildings and equipment, adding partners). These budgets often are accompanied by *pro forma* **financial statements,** or projections of incomes, assets and fund balances for a period of three, five, or even twenty years in summary format. Only infrequently are detailed budgets prepared for more than one year in advance. This discussion of common budgeting practices illustrates two important points:

1. Short-run adjustment is always more costly than long-run adjustment.
2. As the time perspective changes, so does the focus of management attention on cost control.

   To illustrate these points, consider how managers handle a variety of different variations. Known short-run variations are dealt with by making limited changes in the number of staff scheduled. For example, fewer nurses may work at 3 a.m. and on Sundays. However, the percentage change in staff is less than the percentage change in patient load, because all units must still have a head nurse, technical support, and so on, even though they are only partially full. Changes in plant capacity are prohibitively expensive in the short run. For example, although fifty beds may be empty in the hospital on Sunday night, not all of them would be in unit 7-East. To close that unit down, many patients would have to be transferred out of that unit on Sunday and transferred back in on Monday when patient occupancy increased again. The savings from not having a head nurse on 7-East on Sunday would be more than offset by all the transfers; thus, it would actually cost more to shut down one unit for the sake of "efficiency." Therefore, most units are underutilized on weekends and most staff members usually have an easy day.

   A known long-run change, such as a declining trend in admissions due to the closure of a local manufacturing plant, calls for a permanent reduction in capacity. Unit 7-East can be converted into storage or nursing home beds, or leased to a group of physical therapists. Furthermore, staffing should be reduced proportionately to the long-run decline in patients, so that every employee carries a regular workload, rather than making partial staff adjustments on nights and weekends.

   Random short-run fluctuations are dealt with primarily by building in some excess reserve capacity, making the staff work faster or slower, and allocating less immediate tasks to the slower days. Suppose that admissions are as suggested earlier: sixteen people are admitted on Monday, twelve on Tuesday, and twenty-two on Wednesday. Management might be able to get staff members to work extra hard and put in overtime on Wednesday to accommodate the influx of patients, but the staff won't stay if they are abused with continual overloads. They will quit and go to work at another hospital, raising labor costs at the first hospital, because the manager would have to use temporary employees and retrain new staff members frequently. If the hospital has a range of ten to twenty-five admissions per day, with an average of sixteen, it can staff for sixteen admissions plus a bit of reserve. However, if another hospital had less random variation and always had fourteen to eighteen admissions per day, it could match staffing more exactly to the number of patients, would need less reserve capacity, and have a lower average cost per unit for the same average number of patients. This is but one example of the general principle that dealing with uncertainty is costly, and the greater the range of uncertainty, the greater the cost.

   Unforeseen long-run changes test the organization's ability to control costs. The hospital must make a strategic gamble based on a specific expectation of the

FOR EXAMPLE

What's Behind the Increasing Demand for Hospital Care?

Hospitals often justify expansion by citing the need to care for the aging baby boomer population. However, a study published in *Health Affairs* found that advances in medical technology will have a much larger impact on demand for hospital capacity than the graying of the population. Between 2005 and 2015, researchers estimate that population aging will raise use of inpatient services by only 0.74 percent per year—or 7.6 percent over the entire decade, compared with a projected overall 64.8 percent increase in inpatient use during the same period. Aging will play a bigger role in increased inpatient use between 2005 and 2015 than in the previous decade, but the overall impact of aging will still be relatively small. The study also found that the consequences of aging vary widely across medical conditions treated in an inpatient setting. Population aging will have a relatively large effect on increased use for some conditions, especially certain cardiovascular and orthopedic services. But aging also has the opposite effect on other conditions, including stagnant or declining use for certain care related to childbirth and mental illnesses. "Although aging will likely have an important impact on spending, its magnitude will be dwarfed by the impact of advances in technology that affect medical practice patterns," the study concludes.[5]

future (e.g., the population will grow older and increase demand, or people will move to Florida, reducing demand; a major competitor will go bankrupt, giving the hospital a great opportunity, or perhaps the competitor will go all out trying to survive by stealing the hospital's patients). The hospital could build in flexibility by making investments to cover both alternatives, but it would then incur higher costs per unit, no matter what happens.

SELF-CHECK

- List two examples of short-run hospital costs.
- List two examples of long-run hospital costs.
- Explain why short-run costs are less variable than long-run costs.
- Distinguish between a **fixed budget** and a **flexible budget**.
- Explain the purpose of a **strategic budget** and *pro forma* financial documents.

9.3 Economies of Scale

Hospitals exist to allow a large number of doctors to share expensive capital equipment and cooperate in the care of many patients. Since many of these costs are fixed, hospitals should show economies of scale (i.e., the average cost per patient day should fall as more patients are treated). It appears that basic hospital services for routine care are most efficiently delivered when organized and staffed in units of twenty to forty beds, usually known as a floor or wing. The need to accommodate random fluctuations in the number of admissions and to preserve a buffer of empty beds for emergencies creates economies of scale. Admissions to a forty-bed hospital might fluctuate by ± 10, or 25 percent; therefore, only thirty beds might be occupied on average. In a 400-bed hospital, excess admissions to one unit are likely to offset a lack of admissions in another; therefore, the overall fluctuation might be ± 25, or 6.25 percent, which is larger in absolute numbers but much smaller as a percentage. Thus, percentage occupancy rates can be higher, and per unit costs lower, in a large facility that is more able to smooth out patient flow. The greater division of labor in a large hospital that allows staff to become more specialized and efficient at a particular function also creates economies of scale.[6]

There is good evidence that economies of scale are important in hospital services. Hospitals with fewer than one hundred beds are usually too small to offer a full range of services; are unable to fully utilize operating suites, computed tomography (CT) scanners, and other diagnostic equipment; and can't allow staff to specialize. Very small hospitals clearly have higher costs per day, although this is somewhat obscured because they tend to offer fewer expensive and technologically advanced services. A better indication of the fact that hospitals with fewer than one hundred beds suffer from a lack of economies of scale is that a disproportionate number of them have gone bankrupt or been absorbed by larger institutions over the past twenty years. Only in rural areas have small general hospitals been able to thrive, and even their numbers are falling as better highways and helicopter transport have reduced the time required to travel to large urban medical centers.

Diseconomies of scale, in which the average cost per unit rises as the quantity produced increases, arise from the difficulties of coordinating and managing a larger and larger institution. Relatively few hospitals have more than 500 beds, evidence that costly administrative and transportation difficulties arise when this number of beds is exceeded. Patients increasingly complain about "getting lost in the system" and being part of a "factory" rather than a caring institution. Table 9-1 shows that costs per day rise long before the 500-bed size limit is reached.

9.3.1 Different Products Have Different Economies of Scale

Hospitals are complex institutions, and different parts of a hospital actually produce very different products. The "average" is made up of units for routine care, along

**Table 9-1: Average Cost per Patient
Day by Hospital Size**

6–24 beds	$ 896
25–49	891
50–99	744
100–199	925
200–299	1,122
300–399	1,277
400–499	1,353
500 or more	1,468

Source: American Hospital Association, *Hospital Statistics 2002,* Table 2.

care, along with some very specialized units, such as heart transplant, oncology, and respiratory intensive care. Although it might take only twenty beds to create an efficient-size cardiac-care unit, only a large hospital has enough cardiac admissions to fill such a specialized unit. Most 400-bed university hospitals are, in fact, composites, with perhaps one hundred beds providing general care, with twenty dedicated to oncology, fifteen to nephrology and kidney transplant, twenty to cardiology, forty to pediatrics, and so on. Thus, although the efficient size of a unit that produces one product is just twenty beds, the more specialized types of care a hospital provides, the larger it must be to reach efficient scale. Indeed, a hospital large enough to produce heart transplants and nuclear medicine efficiently is too large to produce routine care for broken bones and pneumonia and, therefore, suffers from diseconomies of scale with regard to these less-specialized services.

One solution to the conflict between economies and diseconomies of scale is to treat patients with uncomplicated illnesses at local community hospitals of relatively modest size (100 to 150 beds) with few specialized services, while referring patients whose treatment demands sophisticated technology and expertise to large institutions usually affiliated with universities. However, just as increasing hospital size causes diseconomies of scale by making management communication and coordination more difficult, so does the process of transferring patients back and forth between community and specialty hospitals. The savings from triaging patients so that their illnesses are treated in the most efficient size hospital are to some extent offset and eventually reversed by the increase in the number of transfers required, since each transfer requires some extra documentation, management oversight, duplication of tests, and so on.

FOR EXAMPLE

Massive Mass General

World-renowned Massachusetts General Hospital ("Mass General" or MGH) was founded in 1811 and is the oldest and largest hospital in New England. The 898-bed medical center has an occupancy rate of 92.92 percent and offers sophisticated diagnostic and therapeutic care in virtually every specialty and subspecialty of medicine and surgery. MGH admits approximately 45,000 inpatients annually and handles almost 1.5 million outpatient visits. Its emergency services handles over 76,000 visits annually. Each year the surgical staff performs more than 34,000 operations, and the MGH Vincent Obstetrics Service delivers more than 3,500 babies. Mass General has an annual operating revenue of approximately $1.7 billion dollars.

9.3.2 Contracting Out

It must be noted that some services show economies of scale at sizes far larger than any hospital in existence. Laboratory testing, for example, has become so automated that costs are minimized in facilities that process hundreds of thousands of tests per day. To take advantage of such economies of scale, many hospitals contract out such services. Rather than having their own laboratories for conducting routine tests, they use a laboratory that may service hundreds of hospitals. Food services, security, and even emergency rooms are now contracted out to allow hospitals access to economies of scale through contractual relationships.

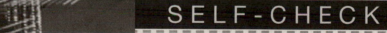

SELF-CHECK

- Explain how hospitals can benefit from economies of scale.
- What factors contribute to **diseconomies of scale** in hospitals?

9.4 Quality and Cost

What does it mean when someone says that technological improvements have made the production process better? It may mean that the identical product can now be produced at a lower cost per unit. It may also mean that a better product can be produced, regardless of cost. Medicine has been dominated by the latter type of technological change. The tremendous value of any increase in cure rates is one factor biasing researchers toward discoveries that have the effect of increasing costs. Yet quality enhancements have occurred rapidly in other areas of technology, such as computing, while still reducing unit costs. Why have such developments been so notably absent in medicine? Quite simply, it has been much more profitable to discover a new cure than to find a method to cut costs.

Insurance and cost reimbursement virtually eliminated price competition in hospital care. Without this competition, there was no incentive for research laboratories to seek innovations that reduced costs or for hospitals to switch to cheaper versions of existing equipment. The process of trading off a small reduction in speed or accuracy for a large reduction in price that occurs in most markets has rarely taken place in health care.

High quality is much more affordable than before. Suppose, for example, that in 1964 a person had a heart attack (myocardial infarction, or MI) and faced the choice of (a) taking medication costing $150 that gave a 30 percent chance of having a fatal MI within five years (70 percent mortality), or (b) undergoing a new, experimental operation costing $25,000 that gave a slightly better chance of survival, with 68 percent mortality. It would be rational for one to take the medication rather than to give up $24,850 additional dollars for such a slight improvement in one's chances. Let's also suppose that in 2002, much better medication more than doubled the chance of survival, with only 29 percent mortality, and cost only $75. In addition, research and practice improved surgery to the point where it had only a 14 percent five-year mortality and a reduced cost of $15,000. The 2002 option of giving up $14,925 to cut the risk of dying in half is very attractive. Thus, even though technological advances reduced the cost of both options, the amount spent on medical care would rise. Improvements in medical production frequently create this type of response. Even though 1960s medicine can be produced now for less than it cost in 1960, patients choose to spend more to get high-quality modern medicine that would have been impossible or prohibitively expensive to obtain in 1960.

Quality costs money, and the drive for higher quality is one of the defining characteristics of modern medicine. While we can't always agree on what quality is, we know that more quality is always preferred to less and that the cost-quality trade-off is extremely important in understanding the economics of medical practice.

FOR EXAMPLE

Health Care Is a Good Value

According to a study published in the *New England Journal of Medicine,* the U.S. health care system is a good value despite high costs. Even though health care spending has increased dramatically since 1960, people are living longer as a result. Whereas a baby born in 1960 had a life expectancy of 69.9 years, the study notes that a baby born in 2000 can expect to live for 76.9 years. The researchers acknowledge that some of this gain is due to declines in the rates of smoking and fatal accidents, but they attribute at least half of the gain to more and better health care.[7]

9.5 Competition Among Hospitals

The flow of revenues into a hospital follows the flow of patients. In some cases, such as emergency room or outpatient clinic visits, patients themselves decide where to go, and for these types of care, hospitals compete directly by trying to attract patients. However, for most care the decision regarding hospitalization is made by the physician. The patient follows the advice of the physician and, therefore, the hospitals compete for doctors.[8] If the ability to decide on hospitalization is taken out of the doctor's hands by the insurance company, as it increasingly is under managed care (see Chapter 10), then hospitals must compete for contracts and appeal to payers, which usually forces the hospital to put more emphasis on lowering prices. The important point is that the hospital must compete for the contracting party that has the power to make the revenues come to them, not necessarily for the patient.

Quality is the most important aspect of medical care, and hospitals such as Johns Hopkins and the Mayo Clinic have an edge over the competition because of their reputation for outstanding care and scientific prowess. Regardless of whether the final decision-making power lies in the hands of the patient, the physician, or the payer, all of these parties must be satisfied with the hospital, and quality is usually the most important concern (see Table 9-2).

9.5.1 Competing for Patients

The types of care for which patients make their own decisions are those in which they are able to judge important aspects of quality and in which they pay a large share of cost directly out of their own pockets. Maternity care is a good example.

Table 9-2: Competition Between Hospitals

Hospitals Compete for:	On the Basis of Quality and:
Patients	Amenities, out-of-pocket money
Doctors	Technology, practice assistance
Contracts	Price, information systems

> ## FOR EXAMPLE
>
> ### Do Hospital Patients Value Inefficiency?
>
> One obvious way to lower hospital costs is to run hospitals more efficiently. One study of American hospitals concluded that inefficiency accounts for almost fourteen percent of total industry costs. However, as pointed out by an ongoing RAND Health Center study, hospitals offer many health services or amenities, such as private rooms, good food, and attentive nurses due to low staff/patient ratios, that economists would consider inefficient but that are highly valued by patients.[9]

Many mothers want to have their babies close to home, have strong preferences regarding patient services (natural childbirth, religious orientation, attitude of staff), and can get good information for comparing hospitals by talking to other mothers in the neighborhood. Since the need for care is known months in advance, potential parents can do the kind of comparison shopping which is impossible to do after accidents or heart attacks. For these reasons, hospitals must actively compete for patients on the basis of price and service. Casual investigation reveals a number of special deals, from free baby clothes, gourmet meals, and a post-partum vacation to cut-rate "fixed-price packages," not unlike the competition for selling cars and houses. Outpatient clinics, where patients are more likely to self-refer and where cost-sharing is usually higher, also use marketing strategies such as nice waiting rooms, receptionists who call to make or remind patients about appointments, free transportation to the clinic, and deductible or co-payment waivers. The rise of "preferred provider" plans (see Chapter 10) that provide full coverage only for a limited group of hospitals has also increased the importance of direct marketing to patients.

> ## FOR EXAMPLE
>
> ### The (Luxury) Center for Maternity Care
>
> Advertising brochures for the Center for Maternity Care at the Mount Sinai Medical Center in New York City make the center sound more like a spa than a hospital. The center offers rooms in which wood panels conceal medical equipment, so that the rooms feel more like home. Partners are encouraged to stay the night in luxury sleeper chairs, check the Internet via special in-room ports, and take in the view of Central Park. Baths feature Italian glass tile, luxury fixtures, and spa-like bath and shower facilities.

9.5.2 Competing for Physicians

The physician-patient agency relationship and control over admissions means that most hospital competition is over doctors rather than patients. Recruitment incentives are a very visible sign of such competition. Income guarantees (e.g., if you come to hospital X, and your income in the first year is less than $125,000, we will make up the difference), relocation assistance, and promises of referrals from other doctors on the medical staff are common contractual provisions. Sometimes there is even a "signing bonus" similar to what a professional athlete might receive. Hospitals also compete by helping physicians earn more money in their private practices by providing free or subsidized office space; providing secretarial, phone, and billing services; setting aside ten beds for nephrology or another specialty so that the specialist will always be able to admit a patient; and so on.[10] Reducing practice costs or work effort is a limited competitive tool. Far more important is helping a physician build his or her practice by a hospital's reputation for quality and the technological sophistication of services offered.[11] A cardiologist is able to attract more patients if he or she is the only cardiologist in town who has access to a catheterization lab that does stent, or percutaneous transluminal coronary angioplasty (PTCA), or a newer development in vein obstruction removal. In some instances, such competition can lead to a sort of "medical arms race," in which nearby hospitals each try to be the first with the most, and respond strategically. For example, if one hospital gets an MRI scanner, the other one gets one that is bigger; if one gets a lithotripter, the other gets one that has more settings and finer resolution; and so on. It's possible that competing on the basis of which hospital has the most new technology can lead to inefficiencies and escalating costs, with the two scanners and two lithotripters empty half the time because there are only enough patients in the market to keep one piece of equipment operating at full capacity. This points out one of the major problems of hospital markets structured on the basis of competing for physicians to increase patient flow: A hospital has an incentive to subsidize office space to attract physicians, not to reduce charges to patients, change billing practices, or make trade-offs that lead to overall reductions in the cost of medical care. The competition for physicians doesn't necessarily push hospitals toward an efficient use of inputs or mix of services.

9.5.3 Competing for Contracts

It has become more and more common for insurance companies to make contracts directly with hospitals, negotiating a fixed or discounted price, and limiting patients to hospitals with which the insurance company has a contract. Payers can direct patient flow even when contracts are not fully binding. Although Medicare has a contract with every hospital, it will allow heart transplants only in certain approved facilities, and in a request for proposals to become an approved provider, price is a factor. Health maintenance organizations (HMOs) can be even more aggressive, sometimes threatening to transfer a large group of patients to a rival facility unless negotiations result in a substantial discount or making approval conditional on assurances that the HMO will receive the lowest price the hospital gives to any contractor.

Such large-scale arrangements are inevitably less accommodating to the needs of individual patients and the professional autonomy of physicians. However, any attempt to implement public accountability and successful cost control involves trade-offs.

9.5.4 Measuring Competitive Success

How can it be determined which hospitals are more successful in the competition for patients? A hospital that has failed by going out of business is clearly not successful. Analysis shows that hospitals with fewer than 100 or more than 500 beds appear to be inefficient and less able to compete.[12] Analysis has also shown that for-profit hospitals are not necessarily more efficient or better competitors than nonprofits (the number of for-profit hospitals has fluctuated, but these hospitals accounted for around 10 to 20 percent of total bed supply throughout the twentieth century, indicating competitive performance that is about average). Such traditional measures as total assets, market share, and geographic spread have been used as indicators. With 90 percent of hospitals operated by either voluntary (charitable and/or religious) or government organizations, profits are less useful as a measure of success than they are in other industries. However, the excess of revenues over expenditures is available to fund growth and is necessary to avoid bankruptcy, and thus can be a useful indicator.

What has proven almost impossible to measure is the success of a hospital in achieving its goals as a provider of health care to the community. Although charity care, participation in outreach programs, and mortality rates are often monitored and commented on, there is general agreement that these are incomplete and inadequate measures at best, and are frequently misleading. Economists and other policy makers are in the awkward position of recognizing that they know which dimensions are most important (quality, compassion, technological advances), but they don't know how to gauge them numerically or even how to make a fair comparison between hospitals.

9.5.5 Measuring the Competitiveness of Markets

Competition can be a significant factor in forcing hospitals to become more efficient and provide better services. However, a single hospital in a rural area or a chain that controls almost all the hospitals in an urban market, isn't constrained by competition. Mergers or acquisitions that reduce the amount of competition are the central concern of the Federal Trade Commission (FTC) and a source of much litigation under antitrust law. Competition is usually measured by the number of hospitals in a geographic area (e.g., within a 15-mile radius; within a city, county, or metropolitan statistical area) or by the overlap between hospital services (how many patients use several hospitals). The relevant market for services such as liver transplant, residential psychiatric care, and abortion covers a large area because patients are willing to travel hundreds of miles for treatment, whereas the market for other services such as kidney dialysis, outpatient psychiatry, and prenatal care depend on patients living nearby, and hence are much smaller. After decades of being exempt or ignored, hospitals have come under increasing scrutiny by the FTC, and antitrust enforcement is now considered an important alternative to regulation as a means of controlling costs.

SELF-CHECK

- How do hospitals compete for business when the payer is a managed care organization?
- Indicate the kinds of hospital services for which patients comparison shop.
- List two ways that hospitals compete for physicians.

9.6 Controlling Hospital Costs Through Regulation

Hospital costs have grown about 10 percent a year over the past fifty years. Even after adjusting for inflation, the increase in cost per day is still an astounding 1,790 percent from 1946 to 2002 (an average of 5 percent above inflation each year).[13] By and large, the public has wanted the additional care and new technology and hasn't been displeased with the billions of dollars expended. However, after the passage of Medicare and Medicaid in 1965, costs became a problem for public policy for two reasons:

1. The influx of government money caused costs to rise much more rapidly than before.
2. The costs were now being paid by the government (i.e., taxpayers) rather than through the mutually agreed-upon private transactions of individuals or employer-paid insurance, and thus caused state and federal budget deficits (see Figure 9-2).

In the immediate postwar period, the Hill-Burton Act of 1946 funded the building of more hospitals, and the Health Professions Educational Assistance Act of 1963 increased the number of doctors. The early 1960s were boom years when it seemed that the economy would continue to grow robustly "forever." This desire to continue spending enabled Congress to create Medicare and Medicaid as entitlement programs in 1965. However, by 1975, the United States was trapped in a global recession, federal and state expenditures had escalated far beyond even the most outlandish budget projections, and the need for cost-cutting was clear.

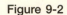

Figure 9-2

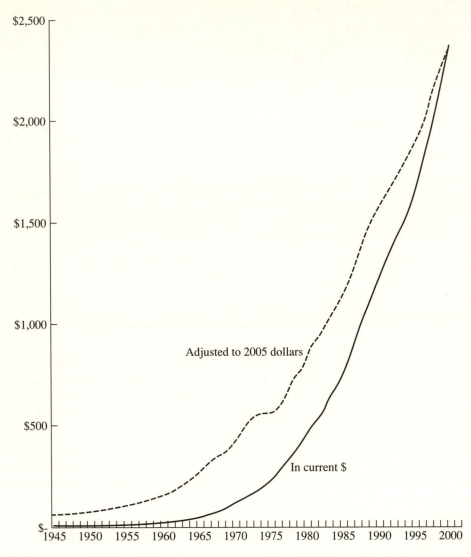

Hospital costs per patient per day, 1950–2005.

A number of initiatives were funded to promote "regional medical programs" and create planning boards for oversight. Evaluations showing that planning alone couldn't cut costs, and the obvious excess capacity created by the Hill-Burton construction boom, led to the idea that a forced reduction in the growth of hospital beds could reduce the rate of growth in hospital costs.

Certificate-of-need (CON) legislation required that a planning body conduct a study and approve any capital project that would increase the number of hospital beds in the region.[14] Although CON legislation reduced the number of

FOR EXAMPLE

Conning the System?

An unintended side effect of CON and most other regulations is that they create barriers, making it harder for new organizations to enter the market, thus protecting existing hospitals and retarding the evolution of the health care system toward more efficient configurations. Studies of CON in operation confirmed the economists' version of the golden rule ("they that have the gold make the rules"): almost every well-established, wealthy, and politically connected hospital that applied for certification eventually got it, while denials fell disproportionately on outsiders that threatened the status quo or weaker institutions that lacked a constituency. The death knell for CON came in the form of a Supreme Court ruling that discriminatory reimbursement of a hospital chain that refused to apply for a CON (which the chain knew would be denied because of opposition from existing local hospitals) constituted an illegal restraint of trade under antitrust laws and harmed consumers by restricting competition.

new beds built, hospitals increased the amount of capital equipment for each bed; thus, capital spending continued to rise at the same rate. CON was eventually determined by the Supreme Court to represent an illegal restraint of trade.

The attempt to impose controls moved on to utilization review (UR), a process to eliminate unnecessary surgery and other services by having a panel of doctors and nurses in a professional standards review organization (PSRO) review patients' charts to find cases of inappropriate care. The PSRO or other agency would be empowered to order the doctor to change improper behavior and, failing that, to deny payment. In practice, the process proved cumbersome and ineffective, although the current managed care review, which does appear to work better (see Chapter 10), developed from the experience with UR.

Perhaps the most far-reaching cost-control regulation was the replacement of Medicare's open-ended system of retrospective cost reimbursement by the prospective payment system (PPS) in 1984, in which diagnosis-related groups (DRGs) were used for setting federally administered prices per discharge covering the entire patient stay. However, the reductions in cost per inpatient admission were more than offset by rapid increases in outpatient charges; therefore, overall Medicare costs have continued to rise as rapidly as before.[15]

The Balanced Budget Act of 1997 (BBA) was successful in cutting costs, at least in the short run. It directly reduced Medicare payments to physicians, hospitals and home-health agencies. Altogether, these reductions were able to save more than $100 billion over five years. However, as the curbs put in place by BBA really began to bite, protests from hospitals and physician groups have grown louder, and politicians more sympathetic. By early 2003, a consensus had arisen that some release from the stringent constraints imposed on Medicare payment increases would have to be implemented soon.

Whatever successes might be attributed to cost-control regulation have been limited and short lived.[16] The unique aspects of the health care market, such as the nonprofit status of hospitals and the agency relationships between physicians and patients, make any attempts to set prices or to quantify quality and other important attributes exercises in futility. A government official in a state capital, or in Washington, D.C., isn't going to be able to specify a detailed contract in advance to purchase something that the participants have trouble measuring even after the fact (e.g., how good the obstetrical care really was for a low-birthweight baby left with disabilities). It would be easy to cut spending on Medicare and Medicaid in a number of ways (set global budget caps, eliminate services, deny eligibility), but there isn't sufficient public consensus or political willpower to do so. Managed care and new regulations may bring some relief, but cost pressures will eventually force the public to face these hard choices, and force politicians to deal with the fallout.

SELF-CHECK

- **How did the creation of Medicare and Medicaid in 1965 contribute to increasing hospital costs?**
- **List three ways the government has tried to contain hospital costs through regulation.**
- **What was the purpose of certificate-of-need (CON) legislation?**

SUMMARY

The primary way managers control hospital costs is through the budget process. Often extra capacity and flexibility is built in so that uncertainty and changes are not so difficult to deal with.

Hospitals appear to show economies of scale up to a size of about 120 beds and diseconomies of scale after reaching a size of about 500 beds. For simple services, small hospitals appear to be relatively efficient, but only a large hospital has enough patients of a particular type (e.g., brain cancer) to run a specialized service at an efficient volume. Thus, a hospital may be both too big to deliver some services efficiently and too small to deliver others efficiently.

Cost per day in the hospital varies for many reasons: differences in quality and type of services offered, cost shifting to pay for research and teaching, billing practices, severity of patient illness, prices of labor and other inputs, and differences in production efficiency. Hospitals are multiproduct organizations, providing many types of care; thus, comparisons of cost per day or per case may not be very meaningful indicators of how efficiently a hospital is producing care.

Technology has tended to increase total spending in health care because generous insurance payments and cost reimbursement have given little incentive to develop cost-reducing techniques or to give up a little quality for a large reduction in cost. An increase in capability to improve health often makes more spending worthwhile.

Hospitals compete for physicians, because physicians control the flow of patients (and hence, revenues). Unlike most businesses, hospitals don't compete directly for "customers" because their customers (a) don't pay their own bills and (b) don't make their own choices, but are directed by physicians who act as their agents. Only for some patient-initiated or relatively uninsured services is direct competition important for patients (plastic surgery, childbirth). Larger scale and cost pressures are causing hospitals to compete for contracts, trying to attract employees, HMOs, or insurance companies directly. To do so, they must compete more and more on the basis of price rather than quality.

While able to switch cost from one part of health care to another, regulation hasn't succeeded in controlling the overall cost of health care.

KEY TERMS

Certificate-of-need (CON) legislation	Legislation that required approval of any increase in the number of hospital beds.
Diseconomies of scale	The average cost per unit rises as the quantity produced increases.
Fixed budget	A budget that doesn't change with volume.
Flexible budget	A budget that changes with volume.
Operating budget	A budget that projects all anticipated expenses for the next year.
Pro forma **financial statements**	Projections of incomes, assets, and fund balances for a set period of years in summary format.
Strategic budget	A budget that focuses on long-run changes and plans.

ASSESS YOUR UNDERSTANDING

Go to www.wiley.com/college/getzen to evaluate your knowledge of how hospitals manage and regulate costs.
Measure your learning by comparing pre-test and post-test results.

Summary Questions

1. For which of the following hospital services would one expect to find the most price-based competition?
   (a) Obstetrics
   (b) Emergency care
   (c) Gallbladder surgery
   (d) Nuclear medicine treatments for cancer
2. A _____ budget focuses on long-run changes and plans.
   (a) fixed
   (b) flexible
   (c) operating
   (d) strategic
3. Which of the following factors account for variations in the cost of hospital care?
   (a) Severity of patient's illness and quality of care
   (b) Quality of care and intensity of services
   (c) Intensity of services and cost shifting
   (d) Cost shifting, severity of patient's illness, quality of care, and intensity of services
4. The larger a hospital is, the more it benefits from economies of scale. True or False?
5. The competition for physicians usually results in lower hospital costs for patients. True or False?

Review Questions

1. Why do university teaching hospitals cost so much more per day of care than local community hospitals?
2. Costs per day are usually lower in community hospitals than in university hospitals. Does this mean that transferring patients from university hospitals to community hospitals would increase efficiency?

3. Why do people spend so long waiting to be treated in an emergency room? Would it be more efficient if there were sufficient doctors available so that people could be treated right away?

4. Why have quality improvements in health care caused costs to rise while quality improvements in computers have caused costs to fall?

5. Describe the factors you would expect to be most important in competition for patients for each of the following services. For which services is price more important? Location? Quality? Would hospitals compete for patients or for doctors?

   (a) Heart transplants

   (b) Maternity

   (c) Immunization

   (d) Depression

   (e) Chemotherapy

   (f) Plastic surgery

   (g) AIDS

6. Automation has vastly increased the efficiency and accuracy of laboratory testing. The cost per test has fallen by more than 75 percent in many cases. Do you think that the total cost of laboratory testing has fallen by more or less than 75 percent? Why?

7. CON regulations effectively limited the number of new hospital beds constructed in a region. Who would favor CON? Who would be against CON? When hospitals in a state with CON regulation renovate old buildings, would you expect the cost per bed to be more or less than in a state without CON regulation?

8. How do hospitals compete with each other? For what?

Applying This Chapter

1. Misericordia Hospital had a 20 percent increase in admissions from 1995 to 2000. Total patient care costs went from $50 million to $61 million. Does Misericordia show evidence of economies of scale or diseconomies of scale? Could other factors besides the number of admissions affect the costs of care?

2. The number of patients at Harbordale Hospital increased from 120 to 144 from Monday to Tuesday. The hospital's costs increased $720,000 to $722,000 as temporary nurses were called in to deal with the heavy patient load. Does Harbordale Hospital show economies or diseconomies of scale? Which hospital is better managed for cost control, Harbordale or Misericordia (in problem 1)? Which is more costly, short-run adjustment

between Monday and Tuesday or long-run adjustment between 1995 and 2000?

3. Wills Eye Hospital in Philadelphia is a 114-bed hospital specializing in ophthalmologic surgery. Who do you think competes with Wills Eye?

4. What would you expect to be the effect of a set of regulations limiting hospital revenues to an increase of 1 percent a year on the following?

(a) Number of nurses hired

(b) Number of doctors

(c) Quality of care

(d) Advertising budgets

(e) Emergency room staffing

(f) New construction

Would there be a difference if the regulation applied to just one hospital rather than to all hospitals? Would there be a difference between short-run and long-run effects?

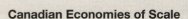

YOU TRY IT

Canadian Economies of Scale

As compared to the U.S., would you expect that economies of scale in hospital services exist differently in a national health system such as that in Canada? Why or why not? Write an essay explaining your answer.

Measing Costs

"Cost is always measured from a point of view." In a brief essay, explain how this statement might be relevant to the determination of (a) economies of scale in nursing homes and (b) optimal staffing in the emergency department.

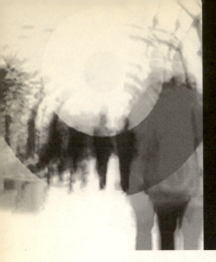

10

MANAGED CARE
The HMO Revolution

Starting Point

Go to www.wiley.com/college/getzen to assess your knowledge of managed care.
Determine where you need to concentrate your effort.

What You'll Learn in This Chapter

▲ The reasons for the development of managed care
▲ How HMOs reduce costs
▲ The difference between HMOs and less restrictive MCOs
▲ Who wins and loses in managed care

After Studying This Chapter, You'll Be Able To

▲ Weigh the pros and cons of managed care for various types of patients
▲ Analyze the sources and uses of HMO funds
▲ Evaluate HMOs from the perspectives of patients, hospitals, and physicians
▲ Assess the future of HMOs

INTRODUCTION

Managed care is a diverse set of contractual and management methods used to arrange the financing and delivery of medical services. Its distinctive feature is that a manager intervenes to monitor and control the transaction between doctor and patient. The primary drive behind managed care has been the rise in health care costs, particularly the rise in the cost of employee health benefits. In an attempt to contain spiraling costs, employers joined health maintenance organizations (HMOs) in record numbers, with contracts and membership rising from 3 million in 1970 to 9 million in 1980, 36 million in 1990, and 104.6 million in 1999. However, total HMO enrollment fell by nearly one-quarter between 1999 and 2004 (78.6 million).[1]

This chapter takes a closer look at the managed care phenomenon, beginning with a discussion of how managed care works to reduce costs. Sources and uses of managed care funds are then examined, as are the different types of managed care plans available. Finally, the chapter concludes with a consideration of whether managed care is indeed a long-term solution to the problem of rising health care costs.

10.1 Why Managed Care?

The primary impetus behind managed care has been the rise in health care costs, and in particular, the rise in the cost of employee health benefits. Traditional corporate health insurance for employees, Medicare, and Medicaid were open-ended entitlement systems. Patients had no reason to worry about costs. Hospitals, doctors, and insurers, being recipients of funds, actually benefited from increased spending. From 1970 to 1980, health care expenditures by businesses rose from 3.1 percent of employee compensation to 4.9 percent. Then, costs grew even more rapidly, and by 1990 these expenditures reached 7.1 percent of employee compensation.[2] Indemnity insurance premiums for BlueCross and BlueShield coverage rose as much as 30 percent a year in many markets during the early 1980s.

In the face of these large increases, prudence and survival demanded that something be done to reduce the cost of health care to businesses. The problems of businesses had actually been made worse by government cost-containment efforts in the 1980s, because reductions in Medicaid and Medicare rates forced hospitals to shift costs by charging more to insured patients (see section 8.3 for a discussion of cost shifting). Businesses became increasingly willing to turn to an outside contractor that could stabilize benefit costs, even if it meant having to accept some constraints and employee complaints.

In a system characterized by a lack of financial restraints, it's not surprising that the United States was spending far more on health care than any other country in the world; the surprise was how little health care the nation was able to buy with all the extra money spent. Despite years of insistence by politicians and physicians that the United States had the best medical care in the world, there is scant evidence that the additional expenditures led to improvements in longevity, infant mortality, morbidity, or days lost from work, relative to other countries spending less than half as much per person.[3] What has become apparent is that the real inflation-adjusted hourly wages of workers have stagnated, and even declined, while the cost per hour of employer-provided health benefits has soared. At the same time, the federal government has been burdened by billions of dollars in deficits attributable to the soaring cost of Medicare benefits. The nation has searched for an organizational structure to control health care delivery to improve efficiency and limit total expenditures. Managed care is one such structure.

10.1.1 Management: The Distinctive Feature of Managed Care

The fundamental difference between traditional medical practice under fee-for-service indemnity insurance and managed care is that with managed care, a manager monitors and controls the transaction between doctor and patient (see Figure 10-1).[4] An outside party, such as the plan medical director, a trained utilization review nurse, or a software program, identifies care that is potentially at variance with accepted clinical practice. This may be done through a statistical profile of each physician's practice, assessment of laboratory testing, a review of individual cases, or a combination of techniques. The manager examines the process of care and controls the flow of funds, facilitating payments in some circumstances and holding back in others. Because the managed care organization (MCO) takes financial responsibility for medical care, it has an incentive to provide care efficiently. To remain viable, it must compete on the basis of both quality and cost.

Figure 10-1

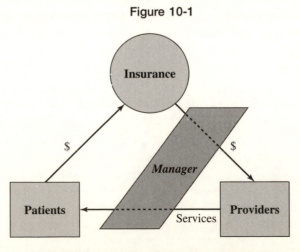

The flow of funds with managed care.

10.1.2 Contractual Reforms to Reduce Costs

Indemnity insurance is a contract to pay for care. The premium must be sufficient to pay for all medical care provided and administrative overhead.

$$\text{Total premiums} = (\text{Price} \times \text{Quantity}) + \text{Overhead}$$

Total costs can be reduced only by reducing one or more of these three elements (see Table 10-1). Because a MCO adds management, overhead increases. This leaves price and quantity as factors that can be adjusted. Of these two, prices are the easiest to cut. Most of the early successes of managed care plans came from the ability to cut the amounts paid to doctors and hospitals. Sometimes these prices were reduced because of excess supply; sometimes the MCO became a big buyer and could exercise market power; sometimes the mere threat of taking patients away, or sending more patients, was sufficient to obtain discounts; and sometimes it was just because no buyer had ever before haggled aggressively in a system that had grown fat and soft.

Cutting prices doesn't change the amount of actual resources used (e.g., physician hours, x-ray machines, hospital beds). It simply means one group (i.e., buyers) is paying less, and thus another group (i.e., sellers) receives less. Presumably, buyers are happy to pay less, but sellers are not happy to receive less. Indeed, faced with an onslaught of discounts, hospitals and physicians finally revolted—blaming managed care for all sorts of evil in the service of greed. Thus, while price cuts are the most readily used method to reduce costs and the source of most savings that MCOs have achieved,[5] there are clear limitations to this strategy.

The second method for reducing costs—cutting the quantity of medical services—has proven to be much more difficult for MCOs. Despite the rhetoric of "restrictive" managed care plans, the reality is that the total volume of services is rarely reduced enough to make a substantial difference in total spending. To reduce quantity of services, both the patient and the physician must agree. The initial idea was that medical services that don't have much of an impact on health could be removed without conflict (i.e., "cutting out the fat"). Yet whether a service is medically useful has nothing to do with its effect on physician income; both vital and merely marginal services bring in the same fee.

Table 10-1: How Managed Care Can Reduce Total Costs

Contractual: Reduce total costs by . . .

Reducing prices.

Reducing quantities.

Substituting cheaper types.

Organizational: Reduce total costs by . . .

Integrating insurance and production in a comprehensive CPGP.

Thus, physicians are harmed by reducing unnecessary medical services even if patients are not.

What actually happened with managed care is that the use of services was bent to follow the contract more closely. For example, because many contracts with hospitals specified a set payment per day, the number of days a patient could stay in the hospital was reduced. However, patients still needed the same amount of surgery, continuing care, drugs, and so on, so the intensity of services was increased—more hours of nursing care and more procedures performed each day. The net result was that the total cost of hospital care wasn't reduced. As long as more nurses are hired, more drugs are used, and more tests are performed, total expenses cannot fall, even though the number of patient days is falling.

The third method many MCOs turned to for reducing cost was to substitute cheaper forms of care—prescribe generic rather than brand-name drugs, have patients see a nurse practitioner rather than a doctor, treat patients with medicine rather than surgery, and so on. The idea was that a manager could identify an alternative form of care that was just as (or almost as) effective but significantly less expensive. Substitution has been practiced effectively for pharmaceuticals, but it has been less successful for other categories of medical care. Even with pharmaceuticals, the savings from use of cheaper generic substitutes has been more than offset by the rise in the total number of prescriptions and increased use of expensive new compounds so that total drug costs per patient have continued to rise.

10.1.3 Reforming the Organization to Reduce Cost

The equation of Cost = (Price × Quantity) + Overhead holds as long as one considers managed care only as a contractual entity that leaves the underlying organization of medical practice the same. An alternative, more radical, reform is to change the structure of medical practice. Instead of having an insurance company/MCO that pays bills and having a set of hospitals and physicians that provide care, a single unified organization could integrate both functions. Kaiser Permanente, Group Health Cooperative, and others had been using closed-panel group practice (CPGP) to do so since the 1940s. In a CPGP, the physicians work

FOR EXAMPLE

The Potential Benefits of Organizational Reform

Changing organizational structure offers great potential for savings but is difficult to bring about, and most CPGPs have rather timidly tried to stay close to "regular" medical practice. The potential for organizational change to reconfigure consumption can perhaps most easily be grasped through a familiar example—music. For 200 years, people have listened to string quar-

(continued)

tets performing Brahms compositions. To perform a 20-minute piece, it takes four musicians playing 20 minutes each (and practicing for years) to bring music to the audience. Whether the year is 1702 or 2002, it still takes four musicians and 20 minutes. There is little room to cut price (musicians have never been all that well paid), and playing the entire prelude in 15 minutes isn't a satisfactory way to achieve efficiency.

However, focusing on the needs of the consumers rather than the producers reveals a new way of listening to music, and it gives rise to a new organization—a recording company. With recording, the performance can be played around the world (although it's not quite as good as being there) for a per person cost that is a fraction of the four musicians' hourly wages. Indeed, when the music is digitized and placed on a compact disc or into an MP3 file, a person can listen to it at home, in the car, or at a picnic dinner on the beach rather inexpensively. If the revolution in musical consumption seems exceedingly far-fetched as an analogy, consider the health effects of smallpox vaccination, better sanitation, heart pacemakers, and the Internet on the practice of medicine between 1900 and 2007.

on salary for the organization, the hospitals are owned by the organization, and the drugs are purchased by the organization. A single entity combines all the complex functions of providing and paying for medical care, which keeps costs low.

SELF-CHECK

- Explain the primary difference between MCOs and traditional fee-for-service indemnity insurance.
- List two options MCOs have for reducing costs.
- How do CPGPs reduce costs?

10.2 Sources and Uses of Funds

Almost 100 million people, 57 percent of those with private insurance, were in either contractual or organizational HMOs in the year 2000, a tenfold (1,000 percent) increase in just 20 years.[6] Another 12.3 million Medicaid enrollees (49 percent of the total) were in HMOs, as were 6.7 million Medicare enrollees (21 percent). Except for Medicare, the old-style indemnity insurance that paid bills automatically without managerial intervention now accounts for less than 10 percent of private insurance.

Table 10-2: HMO Expenses as a Percentage of Premiums[8]

Type of Expense	Percentage of Premium
Physician and outpatient	41%
Inpatient	31%
Administrative	13%
Outside referrals	7%
Emergency	3%
Profit	5%

Most contractual HMOs take 13 to 20 percent of the premiums they receive for administration, marketing, and profit,[7] with the bulk of the funds used to pay medical expenses (see Table 10-2). The largest expense category is physician services. Although hospitals are the largest expenditure item in the health care system in general, HMOs' tight controls over hospitals and coverage of a generally younger and healthier population means that fewer than one-third of HMO premium dollars are used to pay for inpatient hospital services. Some of the HMOs' other expenses are reinsurance (to keep the plan solvent and ensure that patients' bills are paid even if the plan should have a catastrophic loss), taxes, emergency out-of-area services, and certain highly specialized treatments that must be paid for on a fee-for-service basis to noncontracted providers. Over time, the HMO business has become much more price competitive. Administrative expenses and profit margins have been cut as plans have become more efficient; therefore, the percentage of total dollars going to treatment has risen. Competitive standards have been set so that most HMOs offer a similar price (perhaps ±10 percent) for most benefits packages.

FOR EXAMPLE

The Negative Effects of Capping Drug Benefits

One way that MCOs try to save money is by putting limits on the prescription drug benefits for patients. A study published in the *New England Journal of Medicine* found that capping drug benefits actually results in higher overall health care costs.[9] Patients whose prescription drug benefits were capped were more likely than others to visit emergency departments, to undergo non-elective hospitalizations, and to die. The results were even worse for patients with chronic medical conditions such as high blood pressure and diabetes. The study concluded that any savings in drug costs were offset by increases in the costs of hospitalization and emergency department care.

10.3 The Range of Managed Care Plans

MCOs range from unmanaged to tightly managed, as illustrated in Figure 10-2. At one end, under fee-for-service indemnity insurance, the health plan takes all the financial risk but exercises no medical management. Whatever hospitalization, surgery, or drugs any physician decides to order are paid for by the insurance company, without question. There's no haggling over prices. Any difference between premiums and expenses becomes a gain or loss to the insurance company but has no effect on the hospital or physician. The only "control" comes from making the patient pay for some deductibles, coinsurance, or excess over the plan maximums. At the other end of the spectrum is the closed HMO, in which a single organization combines the functions of medical provider and insurance company. It enrolls members; builds hospitals; employs physicians, nurses, and therapists on salary; purchases drugs, beds, cardiac pacemakers, and so on; and controls all finances. Any difference between premiums and expenses is a gain or loss to be shared with the physician group.[10] In between these two ends are a range of contracts that link medicine and insurance but stop short of combining them into a single organization.

10.3.1 Provider Networks

Under pure indemnity insurance, the contract is solely between the patient and the insurance company. Upon submission of a bill, the insurance company sends a check to the patient, who is responsible for all relationships with the providers. In an MCO, the insurance company makes contracts with physicians and hospitals, forming a network of providers. Such a **preferred provider organization (PPO)** limits the patient's choice of physicians and hospitals by paying in full (or a larger percentage) only for care received from approved providers within the network. Patients can choose to see a physician outside the plan or to stay in a hospital that's not part of the preferred group if they are willing to pay a larger portion of the bill (see Table 10-3).

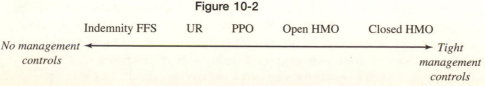

Figure 10-2

| Indemnity FFS | UR | PPO | Open HMO | Closed HMO |

No management controls ← ——————————————————————— → *Tight management controls*

The range of managed care plans.

Table 10-3: Hypothetical PPO Payment

	Within Network	Outside Provider
Hospital	100%	80%
Physician	90%	75%
Therapist	90%	50%
Pharmacies	No copay	$10 copay
Drugs		
In formulary	Covered	50%
Not in formulary	Not covered	Not covered

A PPO is a corporate entity created by a group of doctors, an entrepreneur, a hospital chain, a union, an employer coalition, or the insurer.[11] It has procedures to certify providers (e.g., providers must have valid licenses and meet certain standards) and specifications for reimbursement (e.g., per diems, discounted fees). Contracts may be open or exclusive: A physician may belong to one or many PPOs, an MCO may have one PPO or many, a PPO may contract with one hospital or many, a PPO may contract with one MCO or many. The overlapping contracts and gaps can make the relationships and flow of funds rather complex. Usually, the term *HMO* is applied to a plan that offers care through a single, fairly limited network. A type of HMO called HMO-POS (point of service) allows patients to obtain care inexpensively within the HMO network but also to opt out "at the point of service" and see any other provider by paying extra. The differences between a PPO, an HMO, and an HMO/POS can be subtle, so much so that patients may not even know exactly what type of plan they are covered by unless they examine the contract closely.

10.3.2 Gatekeeping

Two restrictions distinguish partially managed PPO and POS plans from more tightly regulated HMOs:

1. Mandatory authorization for hospitalization
2. Primary physicians acting as gatekeepers

Mandatory authorization means that the physician must contact the health plan, explain why the patient needs hospitalization, and document the severity of illness to obtain approval before admitting the patient. In addition, under a **gatekeeper system,** patients must receive all their primary care from a single physician, and any specialist referrals, surgery, prescriptions, and hospitalizations must be approved in advance by the gatekeeper primary physician. In this way, the plan is able to delegate responsibility for cost control and appropriateness to the primary care physician (PCP).

10.3.3 Capitation

Gatekeeper physicians are sometimes paid a capitation rate, or a fixed amount per member per month (PMPM) for each person enrolled with them.[12] They must provide all primary care for each person and act as managers by coordinating and approving all other services. Paying for the number of people enrolled rather than the number of services rendered changes the economic incentives from "doing more" (fee-for-service) to "doing less" (capitation). With fixed payments per member made in advance, profits are greater when fewer services are used.

What, then, keeps the HMO from doing less and less under capitation, until it maximizes profits by providing no services at all? Quite simply, the need to attract new members and keep the old ones. Competition and the potential loss of enrollment makes HMOs strive to maintain quality and patient satisfaction. Under fee-for-service arrangements, profits increase as more is done. What keeps a surgeon from performing an unnecessary operation in order to make more money? Control over excessive procedures under fee-for-service is largely a matter of professional ethics and disapproval by peers because there is no external reporting and no manager who intervenes to question the appropriateness of treatment.

10.3.4 Withholds

All HMOs must use fee-for-service payment for some types of care, especially for specialty services in which use by enrollees is rare and unpredictable. Using **withholds** is a way of incorporating cost-control incentives into fee-for-service payment. An HMO specialty withhold plan might work as follows: Each specialist receives 80 percent of the agreed amount at the time the patient is treated. The other 20 percent goes into the withhold pool. The HMO projects a total dollar expenditure for specialty referral services for the year. If the total of bills from all specialists is at or below that amount at the end of the year, the withhold pool is distributed in accordance with the amounts billed. In this case, the specialist receives 100 percent of the amount billed but has to wait until the end of the year to receive the last 20 percent. However, if the total billings are more than 20 percent above the projected total, the HMO keeps the withhold pool to help pay for the unanticipated extra volume. In this way, part of the risk is shared with the specialists.

10.3.5 Other Cost Control Methods

HMOs use other management methods to control cost and utilization, including the following:

▲ **Second opinion:** A second doctor must review the record and concur with the initial doctor's recommendation before treatment is rendered.

▲ **Precertification:** Approval must be obtained in advance from the insurance company before elective procedures are performed.

▲ **Pre-admission testing:** Many tests are performed in advance on the patient on an outpatient basis so that he or she spends fewer days in the hospital.

▲ **Concurrent review:** Regular evaluations are made by a case control nurse to authorize a continued stay in the hospital or additional procedures.

▲ **Database profiling:** Graphs and charts indicating the number of services used per 1,000 patients by each doctor or hospital are maintained to identify abnormally high or low patterns of utilization.

▲ **Intensive case management:** A nurse in the insurance company follows and manages any case expected to cost more than $10,000.

▲ **Generic substitution:** A prescription for a brand-name drug is filled with a less expensive generic version if the FDA deems the two equivalent.

▲ **Discharge planning:** A social worker meets with the patient and family early to facilitate rapid transfer home or to a nursing home.

▲ **Retrospective review:** An evaluation is conducted after the patient is discharged from the hospital to deny payment for any medically unnecessary services.

▲ **Audits:** An insurance company representative ensures that all services billed for were actually performed.

FOR EXAMPLE

HMOs Go Corporate

The rapid expansion of HMOs from 9 million enrollees in 1980 to 100 million in 2002 occurred mostly within the corporate for-profit structure. Many HMOs that started as not-for-profits switched to for-profit status to take better advantage of their market opportunities. Why have for-profit firms been more successful than not-for-profits, and why didn't they emerge earlier? Sydney Garfield, founder of the closed-panel HMO Kaiser Permanente, dreamed of "one organized integrality" that encompassed all of medicine—including hospitals, laboratories, physicians, financing, and marketing—as a business under one roof. He was able to maintain unified control by force of personality during Kaiser's formative years but lost control when confronted by these vital questions: Who can borrow enough money to build a hospital? How are wages to be set once profits start rolling in? How can one physician single-handedly manage a group of doctors too large for all of them to be personal friends? The common answer to all these questions lay in the "corporatization" of health care organizations.[13]

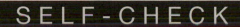

SELF-CHECK

- How does a PPO differ from a traditional HMO?
- Explain what it means for an HMO to use a **gatekeeper system**.
- List at least four specific methods that MCOs use to contain costs.

10.4 Is Managed Care the Solution to Rising Costs?

A large number of studies in many markets over many years have consistently shown that medical care managed and financed through an HMO costs 10 to 20 percent less than under indemnity insurance.[14] Most of the savings are due to two factors:

1. The ability to obtain lower prices by contracting for large volumes of hospital, physician, laboratory, and pharmacy services
2. A substantial reduction in the number of hospital days per 1,000 enrollees

The reduction in hospital days is somewhat offset by a greater use of ambulatory physician services and outpatient surgery among HMOs, but because these substitutes are less expensive than inpatient services, overall dollar savings are realized even when the quantity of services used stays the same or increases.

The following questions have arisen regarding this record of HMO cost reductions, however:

▲ Are some of the apparent savings overstated because HMOs enroll people who are at lower risk to begin with?

▲ Is the quality of care as good when costs are lowered?

▲ Can newer forms of managed care (e.g., independent practice association HMOs, PPOs) reduce costs as much as closed HMOs can?

▲ Will cost reductions be offset by higher administrative costs and profits?

▲ Does the switch to managed care give just a one-time 20 percent reduction in health care costs, or can it slow the rate of price increases?

▲ If most patients and payers are winners, are there also some people who stand to lose from the spread of managed care?

The following sections take a closer look at these questions.

10.4.1 Risk Selection

Most companies that have added HMO options have found that the older and sicker employees have stayed with the indemnity plans. Healthy couples are attracted to the free or low-cost preventive, prenatal, and baby visits offered by HMOs. Older and sicker employees are more likely to have become attached to a particular physician and are thus unwilling to accept an HMO that limits their choice of doctors. Older patients are also more likely to want "the best" care at famous (and expensive) academic research hospitals rather than be limited to the providers within the HMO network.[15] However, there are also some reasons that sicker people might prefer HMOs, such as better coverage of pharmaceuticals, lower copayments, and lack of a deductible. Overall, however, HMOs tend to have a more favorable risk selection.

10.4.2 Quality of Care

Prepaid medical plans have been attacked for providing incentives to reduce services and hence to reduce quality. However, decades of research show that on average, the quality of care in HMOs is comparable to or better than that provided under indemnity insurance.[16] In particular, HMO patients are more likely to receive preventive services, see physicians more often, receive coordinated care from a variety of providers, use primary physicians rather than emergency rooms for acute illnesses, and be subjected to less unnecessary surgery. On the other hand, HMO patients are less likely to receive treatment for some disorders, such as depression and back pain. Also, HMOs use less aggressive therapy and thus more frequently err on the side of doing too little surgery rather than too much. Surveys of consumer satisfaction show mixed results. Patients are usually more satisfied with the financial aspects of an HMO than with an indemnity insurance plan (e.g., no paperwork and billing hassles, no deductibles). However, patients may be less satisfied with service and amenities, particularly when they feel forced to accept an HMO option.[17] The net effect is that quality is roughly comparable in the two sectors—a little better in the HMO for some things, a little better under fee-for-service for others.[18]

10.4.3 Cost Reductions in IPA HMOs, PPOs, and POS Plans

The more open and less restrictive a managed care plan is, the more acceptable it is to new enrollees who are accustomed to fee-for-service care. That's why the great expansion of HMO membership in the 1980s and 1990s occurred in less tightly managed plans. These plans are able to obtain volume discounts but are able to change provider behavior only when they adopt stringent utilization review procedures, carefully assess each day of hospitalization, aggressively substitute less costly drugs and therapies, and, in general, tighten up the management of care.[19] When HMO enrollment accounts for less than one-quarter of a physician's practice, his or her behavior shows little change. When most of a physician's patients are in a single HMO, he or she begins to act much more like a physician in a closed HMO, with lower rates of hospitalization, more careful attention to administrative procedures, awareness of drug and laboratory reimbursement limits, and so on. In short, to get something (cost control), something must be given up (freedom of choice and clinical autonomy).

10.4.4 Administrative Costs and Profits

Some critics worry that reductions in the cost of medical care don't benefit consumers but are taken up by the higher administrative costs required to manage care and by the profits that for-profit HMO companies pay to shareholders as dividends. Because 20 percent of the premiums HMOs receive go toward administrative costs and profit, the concern is justified.

Some well-managed HMOs do a better job of quality control and negotiation with 11 percent of premiums than others do with 15 or 20 percent. As HMOs became more able to control where patients received care, they improved efficiency and, more significantly, were able to take some of the profits that previously had been received by hospitals and physicians.

10.4.5 One-Time Savings?

Will the search by HMOs for market share and greater profits revolutionize U.S. health care or just enrich a few owners and shareholders? In most evaluations so far, only one-time savings have been demonstrated.[20] Managed care may prove to have started a revolution that brought price sensitivity and continuous quality improvement to health care, or it might prove to be just another management fad that has held the attention of politicians and health care administrators for a few decades.

10.4.6 Backlash: Are There Losers As Well As Winners?

There has been a tremendous backlash against managed care, with HMOs attacked as villains in Hollywood movies such as *As Good As It Gets* and *John Q*. Despite Hollywood's spin, managed care has affected hospitals and doctors more than patients—it's just harder to sell a story about how HMOs cut surgical fees or prevent psychiatric hospitals from holding troubled adolescents a few more days to collect additional revenue. The MCO emphasis on preventive services and case management has been notably successful in achieving better outcomes for children with asthma and in reducing expenses while maintaining equivalent survival rates for cardiac care.

Most of the opposition to managed care has come from the traditional powers on the supply side of medicine, licensed professionals, and not-for-profit hospitals, which clearly stand to lose money as costs are cut.[21] Yet it's on the demand side that the weakness of managed care as a strategy for controlling cost is revealed. The problem is that the rather small groups of people who need a lot of care (e.g., the chronically ill, children with HIV/AIDS, the frail elderly) are quite separate from those who can afford to pay for care (the employed). Managed care seeks lower costs for the group of patients being managed and roots out costs that belong to others. Managers are constantly searching for an extra 0.5 percent in savings. Avoiding enrollment of the seriously ill, or even reducing the number slightly, usually reduces costs by more than that. Managed care gives an incentive for efficiency, but it gives an even bigger incentive for exclusion of expensive cases. In this way, it may act to further separate those who are well off from those who are needy.[22]

FOR EXAMPLE

The Enthoven "Managed Competition" Plan

Economist Alain Enthoven published a provocative proposal for a Consumer Choice Health Plan in the *New England Journal of Medicine* in 1978, envisioning a future in which managed care was the norm and fee-for-service was the secondary alternative.[23] It was based on a recognition that consumers, confronted with thousands of possible illnesses, millions of possible prices, and indemnity coverage that was (a) difficult to understand and (b) comprehensive enough to make the effort of comparing costs not worthwhile, actually made decisions that were very remote from the market in which suppliers operated. Consumers looked for plans with low copayments, or coverage of eyeglasses and orthodontics, or benefit maximums set at reassuringly astronomical amounts—factors that had nothing to do with the average total cost of most medical care or the rising premiums that employers had to pay each year, which were reducing profits and wages. In contrast, "consumer choice," as presented by Enthoven, was based on making a choice between two or three competing plans, each with a price that was known in advance and for which the consumer would have to pay the full difference between the low-cost plan and the high-cost plan if he or she preferred to obtain greater choice, more coverage, or higher quality.

Far from being an intellectual abstraction, Enthoven's proposal was based on successful experiences of the Federal Employees Health Benefits Plan, which had worked well for 25 years, offering federal employees a choice from a menu of HMO and indemnity plans in each area.[24] Although by 2000 it was evident that managed care would indeed push indemnity fee-for-service into a small corner, few of the specifics of the Enthoven proposal came to pass. Today, no universal guarantee of basic care for all Americans has been made, employer tax subsidies still favor more expensive plans, and most HMOs don't compete on the basis of care (because they have overlapping lists of hospitals and physicians) but rather on minor contractual stipulations regarding copayments, dental benefits, referral procedures, and the extent of coinsurance.

SELF-CHECK

- What does it mean for an HMO to have favorable risk selection?
- What kind of services are HMO patients more likely to receive than patients with traditional insurance? What kind of services are they less likely to receive?

SUMMARY

The escalation in costs under Medicare, Medicaid, and employer-provided health insurance has been the primary force driving the development of managed care. HMOs reduce costs by saving money on both the demand side and the supply side. They obtain discounts by contracting in volume with physicians and hospitals, substitute less expensive services (e.g., home care instead of hospital stays), and control utilization through the approval process. Managed care has made many doctors bitter because these savings reduce the income and professional autonomy of physicians.

Although managed care has been shown to reduce costs, it is probably not the answer to all of America's health care problems. Some HMOs have made money through risk selection, accepting mostly healthier patients. Other HMOs may find it difficult to maintain quality of care once the easy savings from discounting and substitution have been taken and thus may be tempted to reduce services in precisely those areas where patients, hampered by information asymmetry, depend most on professionals for monitoring quality. Extending coverage to the homeless, those with birth defects, the disenfranchised, and the chronically ill will provide the true test of managed care as a strategy for universal cost control.

KEY TERMS

Gatekeeper system	A system in which a primary physician manages and approves all services for a patient who enrolls in his or her practice.
Preferred provider organization (PPO)	A health insurance plan that offers enrollees a discount for using hospitals and physicians within an approved network of contracted providers.
Withhold	A pool of money for providers that is held back and distributed by an HMO only if total expenses for the year end up at or below acceptable levels.

ASSESS YOUR UNDERSTANDING

Go to www.wiley.com/college/getzen to evaluate your knowledge of managed care. *Measure your learning by comparing pre-test and post-test results.*

Summary Questions

1. The principal incentive for a physician to participate in managed care plans is:

   (a) protecting patient volume and market share.

   (b) higher prices than with traditional fee-for-service payments.

   (c) avoidance of utilization controls and peer review.

   (d) immunity from malpractice suits because the MCO is liable.

2. A managed health plan that allows patients to choose any physician but pays for care more generously if patients choose from a panel of participating physicians is called:

   (a) a health maintenance organization.

   (b) a preferred provider organization.

   (c) an exclusive provider organization.

   (d) a Canadian-style plan.

3. Capitation as a payment method for physicians is most likely to create patient concern about:

   (a) waste of resources.

   (b) overutilization of services.

   (c) underutilization of services.

   (d) unnecessary surgeries.

4. HMOs are more restrictive than PPOs. True or False?

5. Risk selection in HMOs has:

   (a) tended to be adverse for HMOs, which often have more comprehensive benefits and thus attract sicker patients looking for more coverage.

   (b) tended to be adverse for HMOs because sicker persons were attracted by the lower premiums than they would pay in traditional insurance.

   (c) meant that HMOs appear to save cost, but after adjusting for differences in risk, HMOs are actually more expensive.

   (d) tended to result in positive selection of younger, healthier enrollees.

6. Which of the following is most true, historically, of HMOs?

   (a) The major legal barrier to growth has been concern over malpractice issues in a system that rewards limiting care.

(b) The most rapid growth has been in rural areas, where citizens are happy to have organized systems of care.

(c) The major cost savings in HMOs relative to traditional indemnity insurance has been in administrative cost.

(d) Most of the rapid growth of HMOs in the 1990s was in less restrictive HMO types.

Review Questions

1. Which surgeons are more subject to financial incentives when deciding between alternative courses of therapy—fee-for-service physicians who own their own practices or salaried physicians working for an HMO?

2. If an HMO reduces a patient's marginal cost of surgery, hospitalization, chemotherapy, and other expensive items to zero, how can it provide incentives for reduced utilization?

3. In contracting for hip replacements, who would have an incentive to contract on a line-item basis and who would have more incentive to contract on a bundled basis—an insurance company serving as a third-party administrator for a self-insured employer or an HMO offering community-rated plans to employers?

4. Is an HMO able to obtain the biggest discounts where it has a large market share or where it has a smaller market share?

5. Because managed care firms must hire managers to review all hospitalizations and surgeries, isn't managed care necessarily more expensive than unmanaged fee-for-service care due to this extra administrative cost?

6. If ABC corporation shifts from an indemnity plan to an HMO plan that lowers its cost of employee benefits by 35 percent over three years, who benefits? Who loses?

7. Does a surplus of hospital beds in an area make it easier or harder to start an HMO? Does a surplus of doctors? Does a surplus of insurance companies?

8. If a company offers both an HMO and an indemnity plan, which employees will choose which?

9. What are the three main ways HMOs act to reduce the cost of care?

10. Why do "star" surgeons rarely work for HMOs, even the largest and wealthiest ones?

11. What is the purpose of a withhold fund? Do HMOs have substitutes for financial incentives in controlling physician behavior? What factors make these substitutes more or less effective?

12. Is a person who is chronically ill and has a long-term relationship with a physician more likely to choose an HMO, a PPO, or an indemnity plan? How will this affect HMO capitation rates?

Applying This Chapter

1. Mr. Jones is a cranky old man who smokes and drinks so much that his liver and other organs are going downhill. Which payment system—fee-for-service or capitation—provides more incentive to keep Mr. Jones satisfied? Which provides the most incentive to render extra care? Which provides the most incentive to make sure that the level of care is optimized?

2. Systematic differences in risk and cost may be both the biggest threat to an HMO and the ordinary way an HMO or another MCO plans to make its money. Explain.

3. Suppose a family physician has HMO patients who are capitated for primary care, HMO patients who are capitated with a withhold for hospital care, and fee-for-service patients. For which patients is the marginal cost of doing additional laboratory services highest? For which patients is the marginal cost of admitting patients to the hospital the highest?

4. There is some evidence that cost savings from HMOs have tended to be "one-time" reductions. What might produce a one-time saving? What would be necessary in order for savings to be continuous?

5. Why would a patient who belongs to a PPO elect to go to a hospital or clinic that is not on the PPO's coverage list?

Are HMOs Mutually Beneficial?

Newspaper accounts of managed care are filled with gripes from patients and gripes from providers. It has been argued that private contracts, such as insurance, must reflect mutual benefit. Prepare a brief essay that considers whether managed care is the exception to this rule.

"Managed Care Is Neither"

A popular bumper sticker says, "Managed care is neither." Write a brief essay that considers the beliefs that underlie such an assertion. What arguments could be offered to counter this assertion?

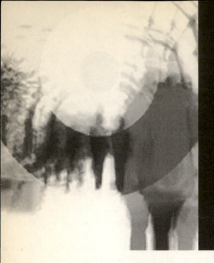

11

LONG TERM CARE
Nursing Homes and Other Elderly Care

Starting Point

Go to www.wiley.com/college/getzen to assess your knowledge of long term care.

Determine where you need to concentrate your effort.

What You'll Learn in This Chapter

▲ The history of long term care (LTC)
▲ The types of LTC
▲ The impact of certificate-of-need (CON) legislation on the LTC market
▲ Medicaid's role in the LTC boom
▲ How LTC differs from most other health care

After Studying This Chapter, You'll Be Able To

▲ Judge whether the government should pay for LTC for middle-class and wealthy Americans
▲ Assess the advantages and disadvantages of LTC insurance
▲ Evaluate attempts to regulate LTC costs
▲ Estimate the future costs of LTC

INTRODUCTION

Of the billions of dollars paid for long term care (LTC), most is spent for institutional services in nursing homes. Yet for every person in a nursing home, there are two equally disabled people living in the community who are cared for by family members and friends. Hence, more care comes from unpaid labor and acts of obligation and love than from patient fees or third-party payments.[1] Although doctors, hospitals, nurses, drugs, and all the other elements of modern medicine are employed in LTC, they are actively involved in only a small portion of the care that patients receive. LTC isn't "medical" in the same way that most acute care is.

The introduction of Medicaid in 1965 fueled the LTC market, and policy makers have been trying to deal with the spiraling LTC costs since then. Certain attempts, such as legislation limiting the construction of new nursing homes, have only served to increase demand and costs. The challenge of meeting both medical and social needs has left legislators uncertain about which aspects of care should be funded through social welfare programs and which should be funded as part of the health care system.

This chapter presents a few aspects of the many and multifaceted economic entities that make up the fragmented LTC sector. It begins with an examination of the development of the LTC market as well as the different types of LTC available. The effects of Medicare and certificates of need on the LTC market are then discussed, as is the concept of case-mix reimbursement. The chapter concludes with a look at the effects of aging on the cost and use of LTC.

11.1 Development of the LTC Market

The number of elderly people in the United States rose rapidly in the years following World War II, from 10 million in 1940 to 17 million in 1965 and 35 million in 2002. This burgeoning group of elderly Americans is relatively healthy, thanks to years of good nutrition and sanitation, and it is relatively wealthy, thanks to pensions and years of saving. After the 1960s, a sizable portion of the population began to be able to look forward to living for many years after working, with no need to depend on their children for financial support. This emerging group of retirees constituted a distinct market. They wanted to enjoy their "golden years" and often looked to each other for social activity. Retirement communities sprang up in Florida, California, and Arizona that catered to this growing group of middle-class elderly people. Retirement communities were specially designed to appeal to the elderly, featuring single-story dwellings without steps, limited traffic, and social centers. This market response to the special needs of the elderly occurred without any reference to medicine or LTC.

Nursing home patients constituted another small group within the elderly population that was destined to grow rapidly during the postwar era. The fraction of total health expenditures devoted to nursing homes, which was less than

Table 11-1: Changes in the LTC Market

	1940	1950	1960	1970	1980	1990	2000
People aged 65+(millions)	9.54	12.40	16.60	20.10	25.71	30.39	34.78
% of population	7.2%	8.1%	9.2%	9.8%	11.3%	12.2%	12.6%
Nursing home $ (millions)	$28	$178	$980	$4,687	$19,989	$54,810	$92,947
% of total health $	0.7%	1.5%	3.6%	6.5%	8.0%	7.9%	7.1%
Home health $ (millions)	–	–	$37	$143	$1,347	$11,056	$32,426
% of total health $	–	–	0.1%	0.2%	0.5%	1.2%	2.4%

1 percent in 1940, more than doubled by 1950, doubled again by 1960, and nearly doubled again by 1970 (see Table 11-1). The fraction of total health spending devoted to nursing homes peaked at 8 percent around 1980 and has held steady since then, and the number of active retirees living in segregated housing with special amenities continues to soar.

Distinguishing active senior citizens from institutionalized patients is easy at the extremes, but there is a range of people in between for whom neat separation is impossible. The simple distinction between "at home" and "in a nursing home" has been replaced by a range of organizational settings, from high-intensity facilities that are almost like hospitals to a variety of intermediate care and assisted-living facilities. The picture is further clouded by the provision of visiting nurse services, Meals on Wheels, home intravenous (IV) and physical therapy, and other supplemental services that make it possible to provide a wide range of care where people live before they become disabled.

Although some disabled younger people receive LTC, the majority of people who receive this care are over age 65, and the rate of institutionalization increases with advancing age (see Table 11-2). Residents in nursing homes are disproportionately female (74 percent) and poor. Older males who are disabled are more likely to be married and hence receive assistance from a spouse or an adult child. Traditionally, care of disabled elders has been provided by adult daughters who were expected to take on the task of caring for one or more parents or parents-in-law after their own children were raised. This informal system was adequate in the 1950s, when most women married and had children early, and didn't have careers. With the majority of women now in the workforce and childbearing frequently delayed so that children don't leave home until the mother is in her 50s, finding time to care for a 78-year-old parent is much more difficult. The "shadow price" (i.e., forgone wage opportunity) of unpaid middle-aged females has become much greater. At the same time, demand has risen. In the 1950s, fewer parents lived past age 70. In addition, families were larger; therefore, middle-aged women were likely to have several sisters to help share the burden. As family size has shrunk and longevity has increased, there have become more elderly disabled parents per potential caregiver daughter. The stress and family complications of providing care have increased. As the supply of unpaid labor has fallen and demand has risen, what was formerly care provided within the household has become care purchased in the marketplace.[2]

Table 11-2: Percentage of Population in Nursing Homes, by Age[3]

Age	Percentage of Population
Under 65	0.1%
65–74	1.1%
75–84	4.3%
85+	18.3%

The care services provided by family members are invisible in national income accounts: No one is billed, no one is paid, and from one point of view, no transaction has taken place. Yet from another point of view, one that predates the existence of money, the obligations of parents to care for children, of neighbors to care for the sick, and of any person present to ease the pain of the dying are fundamental transactions that define society. In LTC, the boundary between market and nonmarket activities is blurred. The fact that nursing home admissions or expenditures double doesn't mean that twice as many disabled people are getting care or that they are getting more or better services. Some of that increase simply reflects the movement of care from the realm of household production and family obligation into monetarized commerce.

FOR EXAMPLE

Nursing Home Costs

The average daily cost of a private room in a nursing home in the United States in 2005 was $203, which amounted to $74,095 per person annually, according to MetLife's annual Market Survey of Nursing Home and Home Care Costs. In 2005, the average stay in a nursing home was 2.4 years, bringing the total average cost to $177,828. The cost represented a 5.7 percent increase over the previous year. The highest rates were reported in Alaska, where the cost was $531 per day. The lowest were in the Shreveport area of Louisiana, at $115.[4]

11.2 Defining LTC: Types of Care

LTC can be provided either at home or in an institutional setting. Institutional settings can be ranked by the intensity of medical intervention they provide, beginning with the most intense:

1. Acute hospitals
2. LTC hospitals that provide rehabilitation and psychiatric treatment
3. Nursing homes (skilled, intermediate care)
4. Assisted living or board-and-care homes

Placement depends on the combined medical, social, economic, and functional needs of the patient. For instance, a postoperative patient who only needs regular bathing and hourly medication could be cared for at home, if he or she has sufficient support from the family. But if that patient doesn't have actively involved family members, he or she may be a candidate for nursing home placement, and if there are no available nursing home beds, the patient might continue to stay in the hospital for many days.[5]

More and more people are also opting for forms of LTC within their homes rather than in institutionalized settings. In fact, home health care is growing rapidly in two different directions[6]:

▲ Medical treatments that used to be performed in the hospital are now being performed in the patient's home, paralleling the trend away from the hospital evidenced by shorter lengths of stay, the growth of ambulatory surgery, and the development of outpatient rehabilitation. For home medical care to be effective, the physician and nurse must be able to count on a high degree of family support to assist in monitoring the patient, administering medication, and performing basic nursing functions, such as feeding, bathing, and changing clothes.

▲ Personal home care is increasingly being provided to otherwise healthy but homebound individuals whose lack of relatives at home is compensated for by having unskilled aides do ordinary cleaning, cooking, and other household tasks. Meals on Wheels, a publicly funded program that delivers hot meals to the homebound, is a good example.

A single provider may offer both kinds of services. For example, a visiting nurse could stop at one house to change an IV antibiotic and proceed to the next house, where the only service she provides is to help someone into a wheelchair.

As elderly people begin to need more care and protection, their likelihood of being placed in a nursing home or another institutional setting depends mostly on the presence of social support. For example, most married people with Alzheimer's disease can continue to live at home and be cared for by their spouses, at least through the early phases of the disease. Those who have children but no spouse are less likely to be able to remain at home, and those with no family nearby are likely to be institutionalized. The extent of disability is the second most important factor. Eventually, almost every family that cares for a person with Alzheimer's becomes overwhelmed by the necessity to provide constant attention, as well as by the pain and alienation of caring for someone who may not know or appreciate any of the things being done. Mental dysfunction is a significant cause in more than half of all LTC institutionalization. Medical needs, while often critical in precipitating a crisis, are relatively less important than social, housing, and functional needs in determining the use of LTC.

The goal of acute care is to increase the patient's level of functioning and reduce the risk of dying. In contrast, most LTC is supportive. Attempts are made to slow the patient's decline and stabilize functioning, but only rarely is an attempt made to achieve a definitive cure, and it's expected that the person will remain dependent. Because acute medical care is focused on cure, the quality of the meals, the room, and social functions are incidentals and contribute little to the total cost of a hospital stay. Most of the cost of LTC, on the other hand, is for helping people with their daily lives, not treatment. Drugs are supposed to help the patient get through the day, not to get better, and curative procedures account for a relatively minor fraction of total expenditures. A physician may show up at a nursing home only once a month. In studies of nursing home costs, physician services account for only 1 percent of costs, as do

FOR EXAMPLE

The Cost of Assisted Living

According to Genworth Financial's annual Cost of Care survey, a private one-bedroom unit in an assisted living facility has an average annual cost of $32,294. Assisted living facilities in Connecticut (Bridgeport area) were the most expensive, at an annual cost of $57,566, while those in North Dakota and Arkansas were the least expensive, charging only $21,000 per year.[7]

Table 11-3: Breakdown of Nursing Home Costs[8]

Category	Percentage
Physician services	1%
RNs (estimated)	9%
Other wages and salaries	53%
Employee benefits	7%
Food	10%
Fuel	4%
Drugs	1%
Other supplies	3%
Insurance	2%
Taxes	2%
Rent, debt, services, profit, etc.	8%

drugs, while wages, salaries, and benefits, mostly for unskilled labor, account for 69 percent (see Table 11-3).

SELF-CHECK

- List three factors that determine the type of LTC a patient receives.
- Distinguish between the goals of acute care and LTC.
- Describe two ways in which home health care is expanding.

11.3 How Medicaid Fueled the Nursing Home Market

The nursing home market was radically transformed, almost created anew, by the creation of Medicaid in 1965. When Medicare was drafted to provide health insurance for the elderly, Medicaid was somewhat of an afterthought. Medicare explicitly didn't pay for the kind of supportive care provided by most nursing homes.[9] It was presumed that housing, nutrition, and personal assistance were individual or family responsibilities. Inability to provide for oneself indicated a need for charity or welfare assistance, not medical insurance.[10] Medicaid was originally intended mostly to expand and consolidate insurance coverage of medical services for indigent women and children. Because it was directed toward a dependent indigent population, Medicaid did pay for social support such as that provided in nursing homes. Therefore, elderly people who were poor, or who could become poor after **spending down** or giving away their savings, could obtain government insurance payments for institutional LTC. Soon Medicaid was funneling billions of dollars each year into nursing homes.

Medicaid now accounts for 52 percent of total nursing home funding, with Medicare paying 8 percent (mostly for skilled medical nursing care and therapy), as illustrated in Figure 11-1. Medicaid is a joint state/federal program, with poor states getting as much as 80 percent of their total Medicaid funding from the federal government and wealthy states getting 50 percent. States are required to cover basic medical services for people who are on public assistance and/or who meet federal poverty definitions, but they have discretion to increase benefits and eligibility above these limits.[11]

Figure 11-1

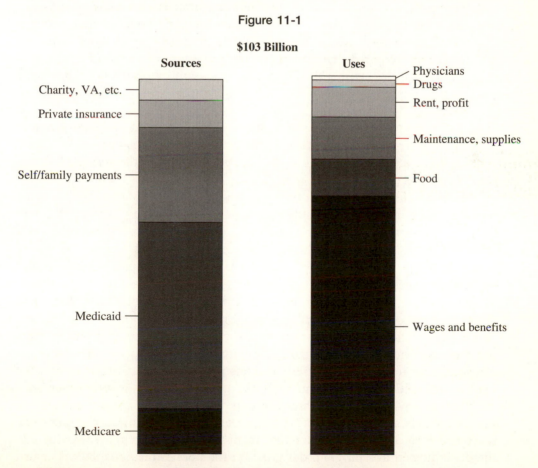

Nursing home sources and uses of funds.

Although nursing homes were only a minor consideration in the creation of the Medicaid program, LTC payments soared out of control, more than doubling every five years. Governors and state budget officials discovered that Medicaid, even with federal matching funds, was an onerous financial burden. In most years since 1965, Medicaid has been the most rapidly growing category of state spending. The surge of Medicaid money into what had been a tiny market caused a rapid increase in prices and a shortage of space for millions of new patients. As prices rose, state financial burdens increased. Any new nursing homes that were built were quickly filled with more of the waiting Medicaid-eligible people, adding millions to state budget outlays. States responded to this financial drain in two ways:

1. **Capping the price they would pay for each day of nursing home care:** The methods of price control varied, but usually regulations were based on costs incurred or on a set percentage increase over prior years.

2. **Halting the construction of new nursing homes:** Control over construction was established by requiring that nursing home owners obtain a certificate of need (CON) before building or expanding facilities. This legislation required that a planning body conduct a study and approve any capital project that would increase the number of nursing home beds in a region.

With these two moves—price controls and capacity constraints—the government created a unique market for nursing home beds. This market's distinctive feature is a constant excess demand but an excess of below-market-price Medicaid patients only.

Many nursing homes admit only private-pay patients. Many patients come into a nursing home with considerable assets, but over the years spend down all their savings by paying for care, and only then do they become poor enough to be eligible for Medicaid.[12] There are stories of couples becoming divorced solely to allow the spouse who is disabled to qualify for Medicaid so that the one who is still living at home can keep the savings accounts. Elderly couples are protected to some extent by federal guidelines that allow the spouse at home to keep the house, car, and some additional assets. Elderly single people may give their assets to their children in anticipation of entering a nursing home. This must be planned with care, however, because most states include recently transferred assets as part of personal funds to be used before Medicaid reimbursement is allowed. Families that would never consider "going on welfare" use asset transfers to make aging parents dependent on state funds as indigents. With 50 percent of all nursing home bills paid for by Medicaid, the conclusion that many middle-class and wealthy people are benefiting from a program designed for the poor is inescapable.[13] The fact that a certain amount of subterfuge is required (e.g., "convenience" divorces,

---

FOR EXAMPLE

Making It Harder to Qualify for Medicaid LTC Benefits

The Deficit Reduction Act of 2005 made it more difficult for individuals to qualify for Medicaid nursing home benefits. It did this by increasing penalties on individuals who have transferred assets for less than fair market value during the past five years and by making individuals with home equity above $500,000 ineligible for nursing home benefits.

---

paper-only transfer of ownership of cars and land, "giving" of money to children that the parent still controls) only makes this process more distasteful and morally undermining.[14] Medicaid is an entrenched part of the nursing home market, but it is not well liked by taxpayers or beneficiaries, and it is difficult to justify Medicaid as being either equitable or ethical when such practices are allowed.

SELF-CHECK

- What was the cause of the major change in the nursing home market in 1965?
- Why do some elderly people **spend down** their savings?

11.4 The Effects of CONs

It's important to understand the implications of regulatory constraints on the LTC market and to examine whose interests are served by creating a situation of chronic excess demand in which frail and sick patients must wait months for beds. For example, the surge of Medicaid money into nursing home care after 1965 meant that there would be a shortage of beds for the years it would take for the market to catch up. In addition, imposing a construction moratorium through the CON process increased the shortage and made it permanent.

It would seem that pushing more money into nursing homes during the late 1960s would have improved the quality of care provided. However, for perfectly sensible economic reasons, conditions actually became worse in most nursing homes. For instance, a nursing home owner does not choose furniture or service based on what can be afforded, but on what will maximize profits. With a long line of Medicaid patients waiting to get in, it was not necessary to keep up

---

FOR EXAMPLE

CONs' Effects on Competition

It has often been assumed that nursing homes with a high percentage of Medicaid patients are less successful than others in attracting private-pay patients and are thus of lower-than-average quality. Studies comparing states with and without CON programs showed that higher percentages of Medicaid reimbursement were indeed associated with lower quality in states where CONs caused a chronic shortage of beds.[15] However, this wasn't the case in the states without CONs. As free entry made more beds available, nursing homes had to compete for Medicaid patients by providing better quality.

---

the appearance of the nursing home to attract new patients, nor was it necessary to provide good nursing service or good food to keep patients there. Because every bed was always filled from the waiting list, profits were maximized by reducing costs (e.g., providing fewer hours of nursing, employing less-skilled nurses, providing less maintenance, purchasing no new furniture). The flood of Medicaid money washed away any incentive to provide high-quality care to attract more patients.

From the beginning, the primary purpose of CONs has been to limit the growth of states' Medicaid expenditures. The crisis atmosphere generated after Medicaid suddenly flooded the market eased over time, and the reflexive need to use regulations to impose order on an out-of-control market faded. Instead, the shortage of beds created by restricting supply became more of an issue. Long waiting lists and the protests of families whose lives were disrupted by having to provide unpaid caregiving put pressure on states to relax or eliminate their CON rules. The length of time a patient has to wait for a bed has fallen in states where CONs have been repealed. Also, the large disparity in waiting time between private-pay and Medicaid patients has been reduced or eliminated as shortages have disappeared. Since 1990, the supply situation has continued to ease, and more and more states are showing declines in occupancy. With empty beds, competition for all types of patients has intensified.

SELF-CHECK

- List two reasons for the shortage of nursing home beds prior to 1990.
- Did CONs give nursing homes incentives to improve quality of care?

11.5 Case-Mix Reimbursement

Even with an adequate supply of beds, the fact that the state pays only a single fixed rate per day for nursing home care means that some patients may be denied care. A patient who is very sick or whose disruptive mental condition requires frequent attention costs more than a patient who is healthy and lucid. With revenue per day fixed, a nursing home can increase profits by accepting only less costly patients who need very little care. To give nursing homes incentives to admit more severely ill patients, some states have developed **case-mix reimbursement** systems that increase payments based on an index of need.

The starting point for determining the reimbursement amount is the patient's level of functioning. Most frequently, this is measured in terms of the number of activities of daily living (ADLs) for which the individual needs assistance (e.g., dressing, grooming, bathing, eating, mobility, transferring, walking, toileting; see Figure 11-2) as well as the level of assistance required. The U.S. General Accounting Office issued a report in 1990, showing that the problem that "heavy care" patients have in obtaining a nursing home bed is substantially reduced in states with systems that adjust reimbursement according to case mix.[16]

FOR EXAMPLE

The Impact of Alzheimer's Disease on LTC

According to the Alzheimer's Association, approximately 4.5 million people in the United States have Alzheimer's disease, and nearly half of all nursing home patients have the disease or a related form of dementia. Medicare costs for beneficiaries receiving residential dementia care is expected to increase 14 percent, from $21 billion in 2005 to $24 billion in 2010. Overall Medicare spending on Alzheimer's care is expected to increase 75 percent, from $91 billion in 2005 to $160 billion in 2010.[17]

SELF-CHECK

- Explain the difference between **case-mix reimbursement** systems and a system of reimbursement based on a fixed rate per day.
- List three ADLs that are factored into a case-mix reimbursement.

Figure 11-2

For each area of functioning listed below, check the description that applies. (The word *assistance* means supervision, direction, or personal assistance.)

Bathing: Either sponge bath, tub bath, or shower

☐

☐

☐

Receives no assistance (gets in and out of tub by self if tub is usual means of bathing)

Receives assistance in bathing only one part of the body (such as the back or a leg)

Receives assistance in bathing more than one part of the body (or not bathed)

Dressing: Gets clothes from closets and drawers, including underclothes, and outer garments, and uses fasteners (including braces, if worn)

☐

☐

☐

Gets clothes and gets completely dressed without assistance

Gets clothes and gets dressed without assistance except for assistance in tying shoes

Receives assistance in getting clothes or in getting dressed, or stays partly or completely undressed

Toileting: Going to the "toilet room" for bowel and urine elimination; cleaning self after elimination and arranging clothes

☐

☐

☐

Goes to "toilet room," cleans self, and arranges clothes without assistance (may use object for support such as cane, walker, or wheelchair)

Receives assistance in going to "toilet room," in cleansing self or in arranging clothes after elimination, or in use of night bed pan or commode

Doesn't go to room termed "toilet" for the elimination process

Transfer:

☐

☐

☐

Moves in and out of bed as well as in and out of chair without assistance

Moves in and out of bed or chair with assistance

Doesn't get out of bed

Continence:

☐

☐

☐

Controls urination and bowel movement completely by self

Has occasional "accidents"

Supervision helps keep urine or bowel control; catheter is used or is incontinent

Feeding:

☐

☐

☐

Feeds self without assistance

Feeds self except for getting assistance in cutting meat or buttering bread

Receives assistance in feeding or is fed partly or completely by using tubes or intravenous fluids

---

ADL evaluation form.

Source: Adapted from Katz et al., "Studies of Illness in the Aged. The Index of ADL: A Standardized Measure of Biological and Psychosocial Function," *Journal of the American Medical Association* 185:94ff, 1963.

11.6 The Effects of Aging on Cost and Use

The Medicare program is immensely popular (and immensely expensive) because it serves every elderly person, regardless of need, and, therefore, it provides an upper-middle-class standard of care to all, using taxpayers' money. Attempts to forge an equally popular LTC program have failed. A major reason is that most of the features that characterize medical care (e.g., randomly occurring illness, reliance on physicians when quality can be a life-and-death issue, rapid technological innovation) are missing in LTC. Instead, much of the cost of LTC is for housing, food, and social amenities—things normally identified as personal responsibilities or lifestyle choices rather than medical care. The boundaries between medical care, social services, and living expenses often become unclear. Distinctions between professional services and unpaid family help are often similarly unclear. The differences between medical care and LTC suggest that the types of health insurance financing developed for medical care may not be appropriate for financing the costs of assisted daily living that is characteristic of most LTC.

What difference does it make if LTC is called medical care or not? In a word, money. Distinguishing services as medical makes it more likely that those services will be covered by insurance, more likely that the people providing the services will be licensed, and more likely that quality will be regulated and that choices by consumers in the marketplace will be supplanted by professional standards. LTC has more in common with social insurance programs such as disability, workers' compensation, pensions, and Social Security than with medical insurance programs. Yet the tremendous cost of expanding entitlements and the lack of taxpayer support have caused many advocates to try to find ways to "medicalize" LTC to increase the flow of funds to professionals and institutions.

11.6.1 LTC Insurance

Most medical care is paid for through third-party insurance, which has been around for quite some time. On the other hand, private LTC insurance didn't even come into existence until the 1980s, and it still pays for less than 3 percent of nursing home and home health care bills. There are several major reasons LTC insurance isn't as attractive to consumers as insurance for acute medical care.

For one, the incidence of disability requiring LTC isn't so much random as delayed. If we live long enough, almost all of us will need some form of LTC. Yet if we wait until age 70 to purchase LTC insurance, the premiums will be very high because the likelihood of loss is so great. A more prudent course would be to plan in advance. However, people who purchase LTC insurance at age 40 will have to wait many years to obtain benefits. Financially, they may do almost as well if they put aside savings to be used for LTC if the need arises, letting interest accrue over the intervening years. In addition, people may die without entering a nursing home, and hence the money used for LTC premiums could instead be passed on

> ## FOR EXAMPLE
>
> ### The Cost of LTC Insurance
>
> A typical LTC policy might offer a $150 daily benefit with four years of coverage and inflation protection of 5 percent. In 2002, such a policy cost approximately $1,474 if purchased at age 50; rising sharply with age, to $2,862 at age 65 and $8,991 at age 79. The increase in price with age is due to the increased likelihood of developing conditions that result in the need for LTC. Just under one-fifth of all seniors experience some degree of chronic physical impairment, increasing to more than half of all seniors age 85 and older.[18]

to their heirs. If one did end up needing a lot of LTC and ran out of savings, there would always be Medicaid to fall back on. Why should people pay premiums for 30 years when the government would pay if they really needed help?

A final barrier to LTC insurance is the nature of the benefit: payment for a nursing home stay. Unlike payment for acute medical treatment, which is expected to improve health or reduce the risk of premature death, payment for nursing home care just makes it easier to be taken from home and be placed in an institution. It's difficult to get excited about paying thousands of dollars to merely slow the rate of decline and extend the number of years spent living with disability. Upon reflection, it becomes clear that the greatest beneficiaries of LTC insurance are not the patients but their children and the Medicaid program. Children benefit because they may find it easier to send a disabled parent to a nursing home if the charges are paid for by insurance. In addition, children protect their inheritance by having the risk of caring for a disabled parent insured. Medicaid also benefits because nursing home charges are paid through premiums rather than state and federal tax monies.

11.6.2 Aging and LTC

It is widely assumed that aging increases the need for and the use of medical services. This assumption, at least in its simplest form, isn't well supported. Treating disease in a patient who is expected to die of other causes within 5 years is less valuable than treating a young patient likely to live another 50 years. When scarce medical resources have to be allocated, most people, even the elderly, support favoring the young. With the advent of Medicare, older people spent about twice as much money on medical care as the middle aged in 1970, four times as much in 1987, and nearly five times as much in 1998 (see Table 11-4 and Figure 11-3).[19] The reason so much more money is spent on medical care for the elderly today than 50 years ago is because the system has made more money available, not

Table 11-4: Health Care Spending of Young and Old, 1953–1995

	1953	1963	1966	1970	1977	1987	1995
All people	$88	$141	$182	$292	$658	$1,776	$2,884
People under age 65	$85	$135	$155	$236	$512	$1,287	$1,946
People age 65 and older	$108	$191	$445	$799	$1,856	$5,360	$8,953
Ratio: Over 65/ under 65	1.28	1.41	2.87	3.39	3.63	4.16	4.60

because today's elderly are sicker. Comparisons made with other countries confirm that income and insurance, not aging, have caused expenditures to rise.[20]

Compared to those in years past, today's elderly are healthier and less likely to be disabled. Much of the growth in spending has been for the oldest old and for LTC rather than for curative medicine or surgery.[21] The data suggest that the

Figure 11-3

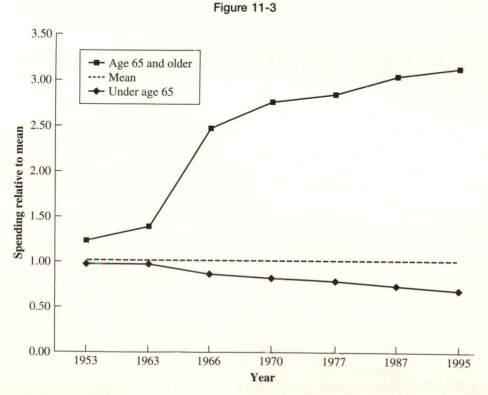

Health care spending of the old and young, 1953–1995.

number of elderly is growing and cumulative disability is increasing but that health status at age 65, at age 75, and even at age 85 is markedly improving. Spending on medical care is significantly higher for the last year of life than for other years—but that final year, by definition, only occurs once in each lifetime. Furthermore, heroic efforts to save life that seem necessary at age 30, and perhaps justified at age 70, look intrusive and wasteful at age 90. Thus, the actual pattern of spending for medical intervention peaks at about age 75 and begins to decline after that, as family and physicians become more willing to accept the dictates of nature. Total health spending continues to rise with advancing age only because more is spent for nursing home, hospice, home health, and related supportive care.

The market for supportive services among the elderly is affected not only by demand but also by supply. In this regard, it's important to remember that most care is actually provided by unpaid family members and friends. Recent estimates suggest that the increase in the number of healthy older people able to care for others, and particularly the increase in the percentage of the elderly who are male (and thus likely to be married to the more numerous females), will reduce the number of elderly people placed in institutions.[22] The lack of someone at home to care for a person—not just disability—drives up the rate of nursing home admissions.

SELF-CHECK

- What are the pros and cons of "medicalizing" LTC?
- List three reasons people don't buy LTC insurance.
- Briefly explain why Americans spend more money on care for older people today than they did 50 years ago.

SUMMARY

Although most LTC expenditures are for nursing home care, most care of the disabled elderly is provided by unpaid family members and friends. As the number of elderly has risen, more and more LTC has shifted from unpaid household production to commercial market purchases of care.

Nursing home economics is dominated by a two-part market. Private-pay patients tend to pay more and sometimes receive better care. Medicaid patients must demonstrate to the state that they qualify by being poor. The state pays their bills but won't pay as much as a private-pay patient would pay; this leads to a chronic excess of Medicaid patients trying to get into beds that nursing home owners preferred to fill with private-pay patients. CON regulations led to an increase in the shortage of nursing homes, causing patients to wait months for a bed. In a shortage situation, patients most in need of nursing home care are most likely to be denied a bed because their care tends to be more costly than that for patients with fewer needs. To alleviate this problem, some states have replaced the flat-rate per diem with a rate that is case-mix adjusted for differences in need. Such systems help match reimbursement with cost but can never be perfect.

LTC primarily provides assistance to people with disabilities to help them perform activities of daily living, and financing is appropriately done through social insurance. "Medicalizing" LTC enables providers to tap new sources of funding, allows workers to justify licensure, probably increases quality, and clearly increases total costs.

People in the United States are living longer. Although this means that there will be more and more elderly people, the average person age 75 will be healthier, more likely to live at home, and more likely to be able to care for a spouse or friend so that he or she, too, can live at home rather than being admitted to a nursing home.

KEY TERMS

Case-mix reimbursement	Adjustment of reimbursement provided by a state to a nursing home to account for differences in patient diagnoses and sometimes for the severity of illness as well.
Spending down	The process of spending or giving away assets by elderly persons so as to qualify for Medicaid reimbursement of LTC expenses.

ASSESS YOUR UNDERSTANDING

Go to www.wiley.com/college/getzen to evaluate your knowledge of the market for LTC.

Measure your learning by comparing pre-test and post-test results.

Summary Questions

1. LTC spending has remained constant since 1965. True or False?
2. Which of the following are types of LTC?
    (a) Hospitals providing rehabilitation and psychiatric treatment
    (b) Nursing homes
    (c) Assisted living or board-and-care homes
    (d) All of the above
3. A possible effect of the CON process for nursing homes is:
    (a) increased price due to restrictions on entry.
    (b) increased price discrimination.
    (c) reduction of barriers to entry because firms can agree to share services.
    (d) increased elasticity of demand as substitutes are diminished.
4. Which of the following statements best describes the relationship of Medicaid to nursing homes?
    (a) Medicaid is important for nursing homes, but it covers only posthospital stays for skilled care and thus pays for less than 10 percent of nursing home care.
    (b) Because most nursing home patients are elderly, Medicaid pays for significantly less nursing home care than Medicare.
    (c) Most Medicaid recipients are in young families, but the largest Medicaid expenditure is for the elderly in nursing homes.
    (d) Although Medicaid is the most important third-party payer for hospitals, most nursing home care is still paid for out-of-pocket by patients or their families.
5. The ADLs used in some nursing home payment systems:
    (a) reflect specific diagnostic categories similar to diagnosis-related groups (DRGs) but targeted to the elderly.
    (b) are an attempt to keep patients from being able to switch from private-pay to Medicaid without clear justification.
    (c) are measures of cognitive awareness from the Alzheimer's Disease League scales.
    (d) are measures of functional ability to perform certain tasks.

6. Which of the following is *not* a reason for the lack of popularity of LTC insurance?

   (a) Benefits help mostly heirs and Medicaid, not those who pay the premium.

   (b) In order to be affordable, insurance must be purchased so far in advance that savings are a good alternative.

   (c) Medicaid protects persons without private insurance against catastrophic large expenditures.

   (d) The incidence of need for LTC is much more sporadic and random than the incidence of acute illness.

Review Questions

1. Who provides most of the care for elderly people who need assistance with the daily tasks of living? How do these helpers get paid?

2. Does the federal-/state-funded Medicaid program expand or contract the market for private LTC insurance? Who would benefit from a federal subsidy of private LTC insurance plans?

3. What characteristics of LTC make it unlike other health care? Are these the most important characteristics limiting the market for LTC insurance?

4. Do the elderly pay to be cured or to be cared for?

5. As people live longer, does that mean that they are healthier and thus spend less on medical care, or more disabled and thus spend more?

Applying This Chapter

1. Does the administrator of a hospital want to admit patients who are sicker than average or healthier than average? Does the administrator of an LTC facility want to admit patients who are sicker than average or healthier than average? Why do LTC administrators face financial incentives that are different from those that hospital administrators face?

2. Draw a set of supply and demand diagrams illustrating how CON legislation could cause waiting lists and increase the price of care.

3. Hospitals compete for doctors and the newest technology. How do nursing homes compete? Does price play more or less of a role? What about technology?

4. Would a shortage of beds created by regulation make it easier or more difficult for a nursing home administrator to racially discriminate among patients for admission?

5. To measure the productivity of medical care, economists attempt to measure outcomes of treatment, such as increases in longevity, fewer sick

days, and increased earnings. Which measures would you use to compare the productivity of two nursing homes?

6. In hospitals, payment for care is frequently on a per-case basis, adjusted for the patient's diagnosis (e.g., by DRG). Case-mix-adjusted payment has also been used in nursing homes but is quite different in its operation. Discuss the differences between the hospital and nursing home settings that must be accommodated in a case-mix-adjusted payment system. What would happen if nursing homes were paid by DRGs in the same way as hospitals?

The Market for LTC Services

Several major trends have characterized labor markets in the United States over the past 80 years: Wages have increased, life expectancy has increased, and female workforce participation has increased. Write a brief essay discussing how each of these factors has affected the market for LTC services. Which has been more important in determining the shape of LTC markets: changes in labor market factors or changes in medical technology?

Put Yourself in Their Shoes

Answer the following questions in a brief essay: If you were elderly, would you be in favor of or against a proposal to increase the amount paid per day under Medicaid? Which factors would your response depend on?

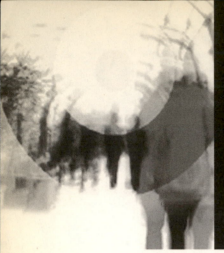

12

PHARMACEUTICALS[1]
The Prescription Drug Marketplace

Starting Point

Go to www.wiley.com/college/getzen to assess your knowledge of the pharmaceuticals market.
Determine where you need to concentrate your effort.

What You'll Learn in This Chapter

▲ How funds flow through the pharmaceutical industry
▲ The importance of research and development of new drugs
▲ How regulation has changed the industry
▲ The major markets for prescription drugs
▲ The role of marketing

After Studying This Chapter, You'll Be Able To

▲ Argue whether high drug prices are justified
▲ Evaluate the role of marketing to physicians and patients
▲ Assess the reasons the pharmaceutical industry is so profitable
▲ Predict the future of the industry, based on current research and development payoffs

INTRODUCTION

In any given week, more than 80 percent of U.S. adults use some form of medication, with 50 percent taking a drug prescribed by a doctor.[2] The average American fills 11 prescriptions per year, spending approximately $771 annually. This chapter examines the "ethical" prescription pharmaceutical market.

Sales of creams, ointments, vitamins, herbal supplements, headache pills, digestive aids, and other over-the-counter (OTC) medications, which can be obtained without a prescription, amount to around $30 billion—a large sum, but only a fraction of the $188.5 billion spent on prescription drugs in 2004.[3] Drugs account for 10 percent of national health expenditures but are a much larger part of the cash flow in health care because the pharmaceutical industry is so concentrated and profitable. With many prices far above marginal cost, drug companies are vulnerable to criticism, and repeated calls have been made for price controls. However, it's evident even to critics that pharmaceuticals have been one of the major technological success stories of the twentieth century, with new drugs extending life span and productivity at much lower cost than surgery and hospitalization. The gains in health directly attributable to profit-driven pharmaceutical innovation are collectively worth far more than all sunk costs and shareholder profits.

This chapter unravels some of the intricacies of the pharmaceutical market and its role in health care economics. It begins by examining the flow of funds into the market as well as how these funds are used. The special role of research and development (R&D) in the pharmaceutical industry is then discussed. Finally, the chapter concludes with a look at the structure of the pharmaceutical industry and the different types of competitive practices drug companies employ in an attempt to obtain a larger share of sales.

12.1 How Funds Flow In

As with all other health care services, funding for pharmaceutical products comes from a variety of sources, including patients, employer and private insurance, and federal and state governments (see Table 12-1). The process of obtaining a prescription drug begins with the patient visiting a physician. After making a diagnosis, the physician may give the patient a prescription for a specific drug and directions for its use. In the United States, all drugs are approved for sale by the **Food and Drug Administration (FDA),** the federal agency that has jurisdiction over the labeling, manufacture, and sale of food and drugs for human consumption. Although all drugs are approved by the FDA based on specific indications, physicians can prescribe drugs as they think appropriate. The actual prescription may be written using the scientific name of the drug or a brand name made up by the manufacturer that first patented the drug.

Table 12-1: Sources of Funds for Pharmaceutical Products[4]

Source	Percentage of Funds
Private insurance	39%
Medicare	27%
Out-of-pocket	16%
Medicaid	12%
Other public programs	6%

Usually, the patient takes the prescription to the local pharmacy, where a licensed pharmacist fills the prescription. Pharmacists provide additional information about how to take the drug and its potential side effects. If the drug has been in use for a time, the original patent period may have expired, and there is apt to be a **generic drug** available. The generic version is an FDA-approved drug that is identical in chemical composition to the brand-name drug but that is produced by a competitor and usually sold for a much lower price. The pharmacist usually substitutes the less expensive generic version unless the prescription explicitly requires the brand name. (In 2001, 47 percent of all prescriptions were filled with generics.) The average prescription has a retail cost of about $50 to $70 for brand names and $23 for generics (see Table 12-2).[5]

Most patients have insurance and pay only the copayment, which currently averages $10 for generics and $22 for preferred brand names (those on the second tier of insurance company formularies).[6] Some insurance plans require the patient to pay a percentage of the price (coinsurance) rather than a specified amount, and other insurance plans require the patient to pay in full when the prescription is filled and send a copy of the bill for full or partial reimbursement later. These alternatives are more confusing and more cumbersome, which is one reason the market has shifted over time to the copayment system run by a new form of contractual intermediary—**pharmacy benefit managers (PBMs)**. PBMs are subcontractors chosen by insurance companies to develop benefit plans, administer claims, and manage relationships with pharmaceutical companies (i.e., manufacturers) and retail pharmacies. PBMs don't have any direct control over physicians' prescribing behavior. However, by creating a formulary (i.e., a list of preferred drugs) and setting copayments, PBMs indirectly influence physicians' choices through patients' pocketbooks. In addition, PBMs have become sophisticated about calling physicians and suggesting product substitutions.

In 1970, 82 percent of all drug costs were paid by patients out of pocket. The little bit of drug insurance that was available operated retroactively through "major medical" benefits, requiring the patient to submit bills and wait for payment, or through government programs for the indigent. This situation was

Table 12-2: Pharmaceutical Sales, R&D, and Profits (in Millions)[7]

Major Brand Pharmaceutical Manufacturers

	Total 2001 Revenues	U.S.	R&D	Profit	A Major Drug	U.S. Sales of This Drug
Pfizer	$ 32,084	$ 17,631	$ 4,847	$ 7,752	Lipitor	$ 4,423
GlaxoSmithKline	29,847	15,474	5,496	4,498	Flonase	N/A
Merck	47,716	12,519	2,456	7,282	Zocor	$ 4,690
Johnson & Johnson	33,004	10,922	3,591	5,668	Procrit	$ 2,335
Bristol-Myers Squibb	19,423	10,505	2,259	2,570	Glucophage	$ 2,655
Lilly	11,543	7,627	2,235	2,809	Prozac	$ 1,659
Wyeth	14,129	6,983	1,869	2,285	Effexor	$ 1,098
Pharmacia	19,302	6,512	2,949	1,291	Celebrex	$ 2,447
Schering-Plough	9,802	5,059	1,312	1,943	Claritin	$ 2,716
Abbott	16,285	3,770	1,578	1,550	Depakote	$ 869

Generic Manufacturers

	Total 2001 Revenues	U.S.	R&D	Profit	A Major Drug	U.S. Sales of This Drug
Teva	$ 2,077			$ 278	Fluoxetine (Prozac)	
Ivax Corp	1,215			236	Onxol (Taxol)	
Watson Phamaceuticals	1,161			116	Diliatizem (Cardizem)	
Andrx	740			73	Loratadine (Claritin)	
Barr Laboaratories	510			63	Oral contraceptives	

Biotechnology Firms

	Total 2001 Revenues	U.S.	R&D	Profit	A Major Drug	U.S. Sales of This Drug
Amgen	$ 4,016		967	$ 1,120	Epogen	$ 2,109
Biogen	1,043		366	273	Avonex	$ 972
Genentech	2,082		613	404	Humulin	$ 1,061
Incyte	219		183	(188)		
Millenium	246		510	(192)		

reversed by 2004, when only 25 percent of prescription costs were paid out of pocket.[8] Shifting payments to insurance and providing a "drug card" that could be used at the local pharmacy required the development of PBMs, which took care of all claims and rebates that had to be processed. PBMs expanded rapidly and were responsible for more than half of all prescriptions filled in 2002.

12.1.1 Medicare and Medicaid Funds

Until the introduction of prescription drug coverage in Medicare (through Medicare Part D), Medicare was a minor source of funds in pharmaceuticals, accounting for less than 2 percent of all spending. With Part D, Medicare has become a major player, accounting for 26.6 percent of total pharmaceutical spending. The Medicare prescription drug plan had a dramatic impact on the flow of funds in the pharmaceutical market, significantly increasing the growth of public spending on prescription drugs while slowing spending growth by the private sector. Medicare payments for prescription drugs jumped from $3.4 billion in 2005 to $56.3 billion in 2006, a whopping 1,576 percent change.[9]

Medicaid's share of national spending on drugs dropped after Part D was introduced, going from 19.1 percent of expenditures overall in 2005 to 10.7 percent in 2006.[10] In most Medicaid plans, patients pay nothing or a small copayment (perhaps $2) after they obtain a drug card. The pharmacy bills the Medicaid

FOR EXAMPLE

Negotiating for Drug Prices: The VA vs. Medicare Part D

One of the success stories of the Department of Veterans Affairs (VA) hospitals and clinics is that they can offer their patients high-quality care at a much lower cost than the national average. This is due in part to the fact that the VA negotiates directly with drug manufacturers to get lower drug prices. The VA is able to achieve lower prices because of its huge buying power. When Medicare Part D was enacted, Congress explicitly prohibited Medicare from directly bargaining for lower drug prices. Instead, it left it up to the private insurers handling the prescription drug benefits to negotiate with manufacturers. In a 2006 report comparing Part D plan prices with prices negotiated by the VA, VA drug prices were a median of 46 percent lower than Part D prices, and for some common drugs, the differences were extreme. For instance, the lowest annual VA price for cholesterol-lowering drug Zocor (20mg) was $127.44, while the lowest Part D plan price was $1,275.36, a 901 percent difference. For Fosamax (70mg), a drug used to treat osteoporosis, the lowest annual VA price was $265.32, while the lowest Part D plan price was $727.92, a 174 percent difference.[11]

program (or its PBM) directly for the cost of the drug, plus a dispensing charge (about $5). State Medicaid agencies keep track of the drugs purchased through their programs and obtain rebates from manufacturers of single-source drugs (i.e., drugs that can be obtained from only one manufacturer).

12.1.2 Inpatient Pharmaceuticals

The process of receiving a drug as an inpatient in a hospital differs significantly from the process used for outpatients. Again, it begins with a physician writing a prescription, but in this case, the prescription goes directly to the hospital pharmacy. The prescription is filled by the staff pharmacist and administered to the patient by the nursing staff. All medications are carefully noted on the patient's hospital chart.

Payment for an inpatient's drug depends on how the hospital is reimbursed for its services. Under Medicare, the hospital receives a flat, fixed payment based on patient diagnosis and the average cost of treating a patient with that diagnosis (through a diagnosis-related group [DRG]; see Chapter 8). A component of this payment is based on average drug usage, but the hospital doesn't receive payment linked directly to drug usage. A number of states have adopted all-payer DRG reimbursements that extend this form of payment to all patients. If the hospital is being paid on a per diem rate, average drug usage is generally incorporated into the daily rate. Again, the hospital doesn't receive any payment directly associated with drug utilization. Only in cases in which the hospital is paid on a "charges" basis is drug utilization itemized and billed directly to the patient or third-party payer. Thus, in many cases, the hospital bears the full marginal cost of the drug.

Because hospitals often bear the marginal cost of the drugs they administer to patients, they have a strong financial incentive to minimize the overall pharmaceutical budget. In pursuit of this objective, a hospital may establish its own formulary of drugs it keeps in stock and from which physicians may prescribe. By negotiating with pharmaceutical companies over the inclusion of particular drugs on the formulary, the hospital is able to utilize its market power to obtain discounts on drugs. However, a hospital must balance these economic decisions against antagonizing the physicians on the hospital medical staff, on whom the hospital must rely for admissions.

SELF-CHECK

- What role does the **FDA** play in the pharmaceutical drug market?
- Describe the function of **PBMs**.
- Explain the difference between **generic drugs** and brand-name drugs.

12.2 Uses of Funds

When a person goes to a local pharmacy to fill a prescription, the money that pays for the prescription is usually distributed as follows:

▲ 20 to 25 percent of the total goes to the retailer to cover the costs of labor, overhead, and profit.

▲ 70 to 80 percent goes to the pharmaceutical company that manufactured the drug.

▲ 2 to 3 percent goes to a wholesaler that obtains drugs from many manufacturers and warehouses and delivers them to a variety of retail pharmacies.[12]

The flow of funds is complicated because most payments come from insurance companies (which must be compensated for bearing the risk) and go through PBMs (which must be compensated for processing claims and negotiating). The flow of funds also depends, in part, on the negotiating power of each party. A simplified diagram of this flow is presented in Figure 12-1. Patients

Figure 12-1

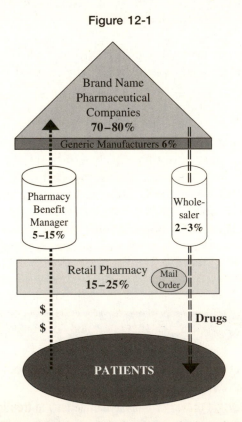

Flow of funds in the pharmaceutical market.

using their own money are not involved in this complex set of transfers—and they lose! Patients without insurance pay list rather than discounted prices, which are 5 percent to 45 percent higher than what health maintenance organizations (HMOs), insurance companies, and Medicaid plans pay for filling identical prescriptions at the same pharmacy.[13]

12.2. Retail Pharmacies

There are approximately 52,000 local pharmacies in the United States, with more than one-third of them in five large chains (i.e., CVS, Walgreens, Rite-Aid, Eckerd, Wal-Mart).[14] Increased competitive pressure and the need for sophisticated information systems for billing insurance, ordering, marketing to consumers, and preventing drug interactions have caused the number of pharmacies to fall and an increasing number of them to be in chains. Patients with chronic illnesses who take large quantities of medicines on a continuing basis have increasingly turned to mail-order and Internet pharmacies, which have even lower prices and distribution costs. Mail-order pharmacies now account for about 15 percent of retail drug sales. Most retail pharmacies purchase inventories from wholesalers that buy both generic and brand-name drugs from the manufacturers. Because of the many drugs available, most local pharmacies don't carry a large inventory of each drug but rely on computerized inventory systems to get deliveries from the wholesaler daily. Wholesalers and pharmacists usually can't switch patients from one product to another (except for generic products). As a result, they are unable to exert market power against the manufacturer but instead must pay the full list price of the drug—often called the average wholesale price (AWP). Hospitals purchasing drugs for inpatient use may buy directly from the manufacturers, but they usually purchase from wholesalers.

PHARMACOECONOMICS

Are new drugs worth the high prices drug companies charge to cover their R&D and marketing costs? Should we really pay $2 per pill (or $250 or $1,500 per prescription) for a particular drug? Could the company get by with charging only $1.50 per pill? Conversely, from the company's point of view, because blockbuster drugs are rare and must cover the cost of many failed R&D efforts, could the company reasonably charge $2.50 per pill? An entire discipline with its own scientific journals, conferences, and university professorships has developed to answer these questions. Known variously as **"pharmacoeconomics,"** "disease management," and "outcomes research," this discipline attempts to determine the following:

✔ How much of a gain in health (outcome) will a certain drug provide?

✔ How much will people value that gain?

✔ Do other drugs provide similar effectiveness in treating this disease?

(continued)

✔ How many people will benefit from this drug?
✔ Will some people benefit more than others?
✔ Will some people value the drug more than others?

These questions have become increasingly pressing as the cost of pharmaceuticals has soared. Australia, Canada, Sweden, and other countries with national health systems have created expert panels of health economists to advise governments on whether a new drug should be added to the national health insurance plan and on the maximum amount that should be paid per treatment. Even in the United States, where administrative price controls don't exist, drug companies have found it useful to employ health economists to estimate the potential size of the market for a new drug and to create an economic justification to help sell the drug to price-conscious buyers with limited budgets (e.g., Medicaid, hospital pharmacies, PBMs). Indeed, so many economists are looking at the value of drugs that many doctors and pharmacists think that this is all there is to health economics, and they use the term "health economics" as a synonym for pharmacy value studies, without considering all the other issues covered in the chapters of this textbook.

12.2.2 Wholesalers

Pharmaceutical wholesalers are limited to warehousing and distribution; they play no role in the acquisition of patients or insurance financing. Thus, the physical movement of drugs—buying and selling on the wholesale side—is totally separate from the complex flow of funds on the patient/retail side. Moving drugs is fairly cheap and accounts for only a fraction of total costs, despite the large volume of items being shipped.

12.2.3 Insurance Companies and PBMs

The financial side of the pharmaceutical business is made up of insurance companies and PBMs. Some large insurers (e.g., Aetna, CIGNA, WellPoint) have their own PBMs. Managed care has had a major impact on the way the pharmaceutical industry conducts business. PBMs consolidate the purchasing power of multiple insurance companies and employer health benefits plans covering millions of people and thus can force manufacturers to give sizable discounts. More than half of the total pharmaceutical dollars now flow through PBMs, leaving perhaps one-quarter to one-sixth still flowing through unmanaged insurance payment systems.

The PBM gets fees from the insurance company for handling claims but gets most of its funding from pharmaceutical manufacturer discounts. Although the prescription passes through the wholesaler at list (i.e., AWP) price with a retail markup, the PBM negotiates with the manufacturer, and a rebate of 5 to 15 percent is paid directly to the PBM. Medicaid gets a special superdiscount of 15.1 percent, based on the best available price given to any nongovernment buyer.

12.2.4 Pharmaceutical Firms

In 2002, about $120 billion went to the pharmaceutical manufacturing companies, accounting for the bulk (70 to 80 percent) of all drug costs. The top brand-name blockbuster drugs (e.g., Celebrex, Claritin, Lipitor, Zocor) have more than $2 billion in annual sales, and a single drug can make or break a company. The largest pharmaceutical companies (i.e., Merck, Johnson & Johnson, Pfizer) each had more than $30 billion in sales in 2002, and the top 10 pharmaceutical companies accounted for 68 percent of all prescription dollars.[15] Conversely, while generics accounted for 47 percent of all prescription volume and represented 4 of the 10 most frequently prescribed drugs in terms of units, they accounted for only 18 percent of total sales in dollars. Only one generic firm, Teva, had prescription sales of $2 billion or more.

The industry has been shaken up by a series of scandals in the past few years. According to *Forbes,* the 10 largest drug makers lost $130 billion in combined market value in 2005 and 2006, at a time when many companies were experiencing market gains.[16]

Funds that flow into pharmaceutical firms are used in a variety of ways. For example, they are used to support R&D efforts as firms seek to develop newer and better drugs before their competitors. These funds are also used to support the marketing and promotional efforts needed to get physicians to prescribe their drugs rather than competitors' drugs. In addition, some of these funds are used to cover the costs of manufacturing, distribution, and administration that go along with any production process, and a portion of these funds are profits, which are either given to stockholders in the form of dividends or reinvested in the company in the form of retained earnings. A breakout of the uses of funds is shown in Table 12-3.

Manufacturing the drugs takes about one-quarter of pharmaceutical companies' resources. As a result of the need to maintain high quality standards, most drugs are manufactured in small batches rather than in a continual process. Although large batches are generally more economical to manufacture, there is a greater variance in the quality of the product and a greater chance that some of the units will have either too much or too little of the

Table 12-3: Uses of Funds for Pharmaceutical Products

Uses of Funds	Percentage
Sales, marketing, and administration	31%
Cost of goods	30%
Net income	20%
R&D	13%
Taxes	6%

active ingredients. With pharmaceutical products, such deviations could be deadly; hence, small manufacturing batches are the norm. The initial development of the sophisticated extraction and production process is very costly and constitutes a large fixed cost.

Advertising and promotional activities account for 20 to 35 percent of the pharmaceutical dollar. These activities primarily consist of detailing, sampling, and journal advertising. Of these, detailing and sampling are the most important. With detailing, a representative of the pharmaceutical firm calls on individual physicians. During these meetings, the representative discusses one or two products. The representative may give the physicians literature on the drug, as well as free samples to pass on to patients. In addition, the detailer answers questions the physicians have about the drug or its use. The information presented and literature given to the physician must meet with strict FDA guidelines. Studies have shown that detailing can have a large impact on a physician's prescribing behavior.

R&D accounts for 10 to 25 percent of the total pharmaceutical dollars. Viewing R&D in this manner, however, is somewhat inappropriate because it gives the impression that R&D activities are funded by current sales, a notion perpetuated by the drug industry itself. It's more appropriate to view R&D expenditures as investments rather than as current-period expenses. The primary incentive for current R&D efforts is the future cash flows expected from these investments.

Profits account for 10 to 25 percent of the pharmaceutical dollars. The pharmaceutical industry is consistently ranked as one of the most profitable industries by *Fortune* magazine, and this has been the case for many years. In 2005, the pharmaceutical industry's profitability was reported as 15.7 percent of sales, making it the fifth most profitable industry.[17]

FOR EXAMPLE

Pitching Pills

Pharmaceutical manufacturers spend vast amounts of money marketing their products. According to *Forbes* magazine, the top 10 drug firms direct twice as much money toward marketing as they do toward research. And of the $42 billion spent on research, $9 billion of that is spent on clinical trials for drugs that have already been approved or will be soon, often in an attempt to provide new ad slogans for their drugs (e.g., "In a trial comparing Drug A to Drug B, Drug A was more effective, with fewer side effects"). The industry is constantly pumping more money into marketing to physicians, having tripled the number of drug representatives calling on physicians in the past 10 years. There are now about 100,000 representatives, which means there's one seller for every nine doctors.[18]

12.2.5 Cost Structure

The economics of the pharmaceutical industry are dominated by fixed costs. Discovery, R&D, regulatory approval, and market introduction all are sunk costs when the first pill is sold. The cost of manufacturing an additional unit is a fraction of the price, usually less than 20 percent, and sometimes amounts to mere pennies on the dollar. After fixed costs are recovered, each additional unit sold is almost pure profit. This makes it worthwhile to put millions, even billions, of dollars into marketing. Other industries where most costs are fixed, such as information technology (e.g., software, Web sites), media (e.g., movies, CDs, books), and luxury goods (e.g., clothes, perfume) tend to use mega-marketing techniques for the same reason: The gross margins (i.e., revenue-variable cost) are very attractive.[19]

In other parts of the pharmacy industry—retail drug stores, wholesalers, insurance companies, and PBMs—costs rise almost proportionately (perhaps 80 percent) with volume. Because there are substantial incremental variable costs per unit, it's not worth pushing so hard for more sales or putting so much money into marketing. Hence, behavior in these parts of the industry resembles that of more traditional firms.

SELF-CHECK

- Indicate who gets the majority of revenue from the sale of a prescription drug. Who else gets revenue?
- List three of the most profitable pharmaceutical manufacturers.
- What percentage of the pharmaceutical dollar goes to R&D? What percentage goes to advertising and marketing? What percentage is profit?

12.3 Research and Development

The pharmaceutical industry consists of many small companies, each producing only one or two products, and about 25 global corporations that have broader product lines. Even in the largest corporations, however, one or two blockbuster drugs are responsible for most revenues. Competition for the development of these key products, through R&D activities, is fierce. The success or failure of even a single product could mean the success or failure of the corporation. As a result, R&D activities drive competition in the pharmaceutical industry. The cost of developing a new drug ranges from $150 million to $1.5

billion, and the process can take up to 10 years. Once a new product is developed, patents protect it from competition. Patents give the innovator the exclusive right to manufacture and sell that product, once the drug is approved, for up to 22 years from the time of discovery. Pharmaceutical firms spent an amount equal to 17.7 percent of sales on R&D in 2001, more than four times the 4 percent of sales spent by the average nonpharmaceutical firm.[20]

On average, only one out of five drugs for which an application is filed with the FDA ultimately obtains FDA approval for use. As a result of the lengthy testing and approval process, a total of more than 10 years generally elapses from the time the firm first begins spending money on researching a new product until a successful drug is introduced to the market. Thus, each individual marketed drug represents a substantial investment of resources for the firm. These investments are made in the anticipation of obtaining future profits on the manufacture and sale of the drug. The estimated average cost of a drug development project in 2002 was approximately $800 million. A portfolio of patents, and the creativity and expertise of the scientists who generated them, are major assets to the pharmaceutical firm. Mergers are often carried out to obtain a set of patents, to fill out a product line, or to create synergies in research. While marketing benefits from increased company size, it appears that economies of scale and scope are quite limited in research.[21] Indeed, some of the most innovative work is performed in small boutique biotechnology firms composed of a few scientists moonlighting from a university laboratory, suggesting diseconomies of scale.

FOR EXAMPLE

Global R&D Spending: The 10-90 Gap

Analysts refer to the under-funding of R&D on diseases that predominantly afflict people in poor countries as the 10-90 gap—meaning that just 10 percent of global health R&D funding is devoted to diseases and conditions associated with 90 percent of the world's health problems. Consider malaria, which kills more than one million people each year, most of them children, and most of them in low- and middle-income countries. In sub-Saharan Africa, where almost 90 percent of all malaria deaths occur, the estimated economic toll of the disease is $12 billion a year in lost gross domestic product. A report by the Malaria R&D Alliance found that Malaria is responsible for 3 percent of all the lost years of productive life caused by all diseases worldwide, but it receives only 0.3 percent of all funding. In comparison, diabetes gets about 1.6 percent of the total money spent on medical research, while it accounts for 1.1 percent of all the productive years of life lost to disease. In other words, the burden to society of diabetes is about one-third that of malaria, but it gets almost six times more R&D funding.[22]

SELF-CHECK

- Explain the importance of patents for pharmaceutical R&D.
- How long does it typically take for a drug to be approved by the FDA?
- Do pharmaceutical manufacturers spend, on average, more or less on R&D than nonpharmaceutical firms?

12.4 Industry Structure and Competition

The market for pharmaceutical products can be divided into three segments, based on the type of buyer:

1. Individual patients
2. Group purchasers (e.g., hospitals, PBMs)
3. Government

In the traditional retail market, physicians prescribe drugs, and consumers and/or insurers pay for them. Because these actions are separate, individual patients have little influence over what the physician prescribes, and, as a result, this market segment isn't very price sensitive. The second market segment, which has been growing in importance, is the group purchasers. In this market, drugs are purchased directly by PBMs and hospitals, and a physician's choice of which drug to use is constrained by the use of a formulary and ordering directives. Because PBMs and hospitals can shift a large number of patients from one product to another, they have some market power, and are more sensitive to prices. Exercising this market power enables discounts to be obtained from drug manufacturers. The third market segment consists of the largest purchasers of pharmaceutical products: state and federal government. Governments make and interpret the rules, potentially giving them absolute control over the market.

12.4.1 Market Segmentation: Types of Buyers

Competition for sales differs significantly across the three segments discussed in the preceding section. In the traditional retail market for individual patients, where consumers (patients) are price insensitive, competition takes place among products on the basis of product quality and physician detailing. Studies have consistently shown that detailing greatly influences a physician's choice of drugs. Moreover, when a physician becomes familiar with a particular product, its method of action, and its potential side effects, he or she may be reluctant to try a new product unless it offers either a substantial advantage in efficacy or a decrease in side effects. Price tends not to be an important criterion for consumers.[23] Thus, competition in this market is usually based on product quality, effectiveness, and detailing; hence, generics haven't been able to make significant inroads in this market.

To date, government purchasers have chosen not to fully exercise their market power on a drug-by-drug basis but instead have adopted a standardized discount policy that pharmaceutical firms can either accept or reject. Under this policy, the government is rebated an amount equal to 15.1 percent of the average wholesale price for Medicaid purchases, or equal to the best deal given by the drug company on a particular product.

The growth, and most of the change, has come in the "managed" segment: HMOs, PBMs, and hospitals paying directly for drugs can influence physicians' prescribing patterns through a formulary. These group purchasers are the ones most interested in, and able to assess, price and cost-effectiveness. This is the segment in which generics have had the most impact because they are chemically identical to brand-name products and sold at a much lower price (up to 60 percent less). For example, when the patent expired on Eli Lilly's blockbuster drug Prozac, 70 percent of prescriptions were switched to generic substitutes within a single month.[24] Unless a drug has demonstrated clear superiority through health economics outcomes research studies, price-sensitive managers choose the less costly product.

12.4.2 Contractual Responses to Pharmacy Benefits Management

Managed care greatly increases the elasticity of demand. Organized payers with sophisticated information and outcome assessment methods are able to switch large numbers of patients from one drug to another in response to small changes in relative prices. Pharmaceutical firms can respond in several ways to this shift in market power.

The first response is by reducing prices. Pharmaceutical firms can compete with one another through successive reductions in the prices of their competing products. During the past few years, there has been increased price competition, particularly in pharmaceutical categories in which several branded products exist, such as antihypertensives and cholesterol reducers. Price reductions reduce profitability and thus are not popular with pharmaceutical firms. These firms argue that continued reductions would reduce funding for research and eventually lead to fewer new drugs.

A second response to the increased elasticity of demand is the development of new ways to differentiate among products. Pharmaceutical firms try to differentiate their products from those of their competitors and develop "value" messages about their products. For example, rather than simply showing that a cholesterol drug can reduce low-density lipoprotein (LDL) cholesterol by x percent, pharmaceutical firms have undertaken studies to show what that percentage reduction means in terms of reduced coronary events (e.g., heart attacks, strokes) and to show that reducing these events reduces future health care expenditures and improves the quality of patients' lives.

A third response involves developing contractual relationships that serve to "lock in" customers to a specific product line. These are often called "disease management programs."

12.4.3 Value and Cost: The Role of Marketing

The structure of the pharmaceutical industry is dictated by a single fact: The large and important costs are all sunk costs. The value of a drug depends on how useful it is in treating disease, not how many years it took to conduct clinical trials or perfect the production process, nor on the number of failed projects the company had to fund in order to get a winner. Research and testing to bring a pill to market costs so much more than manufacturing that there is essentially no rational connection between price and cost, however measured. Instead, value and price depend on therapeutic effectiveness.[25]

Medical "value" is worthless economically unless potential buyers know how effective a drug is. This means marketing. It's inevitable that marketing will be much more important and expensive than physical distribution—as it is for other products with a similar cost structure, such as software, movies, CDs, and perfume. Most of the pharmaceutical marketing is directed toward doctors because they are the ones who write prescriptions. For each practicing physician, pharmaceutical companies spend more than $2,500 on meals, events, and scientific meetings (some conducted in very nice resorts).[26] Spending on personal visits by industry representatives and free samples runs more than $10,000 per doctor. The size of the expenditure on marketing indicates how valuable the power to influence doctors is in terms of company profits.

While clinical value may not depend on marketing, economic value does. Once a drug is launched in the market, any distinction between the value added from increased therapeutic effectiveness and the value added from increased marketing isn't meaningful. Perfectly good drugs have languished almost unused for years because they weren't being advertised and detailed to doctors.

When marketing launches a drug, the brand name is worth something, even if the drug has been superceded by superior competitors; this is kind of like old sports stars still being used to sell athletic shoes. The brand-name version often continues to sell at the old high price even after the patent has expired in order to capture the consumer surplus of customers who are not price sensitive. Also, competition from generic manufacturers has created incentives for research-based brand-name companies to introduce and subsequently patent minor changes in their most important products. These changes might include introducing a sustained-release or once-a-day formulation or changing the route of administration from injection to inhaler or pill. AstraZeneca made such an effort to shift users of Prilosec, its blockbuster anti-ulcer drug, to a new, improved version, Nexium, which retained the distinctive purple coloration of the original and incorporated minor modifications protected by new patents to limit the impact from generic competitors.

The Prilosec/Nexium example illustrates an important aspect of the pharmaceutical market: Competition is between treatments for a specific disease (in this case, ulcers). Most drugs don't compete with one another because they are used for different illnesses. The real market is "treatments for disease X" and thus is much narrower than "all prescription drugs." Firms focus their research and marketing efforts on a particular set of diseases (e.g., cardiovascular, neurological, gastric), making the effective market share (and market power) of the top firm, or top three firms, more significant than it appears to be when reviewing industrywide statistics.

12.4.4 Control of Distribution and Marketing

Wholesalers distribute drugs. They buy in bulk from pharmaceutical manufacturers and distribute on demand to retail pharmacies and hospitals. The customer isn't involved in this back-office physical distribution network, and it's a commodity business with low margins. Conversely, the PBM never touches the physical product but controls the flow of customers and money, and for performing this market aggregating function, it is paid handsomely. The essential element here is control. Assume that a drug cures a horrible disease and thus is worth more than $1,000 to the patient, but production cost is only $1. This difference is up for grabs. If there is lots of competition, prices may get forced down toward $1.50, providing just enough for the costs of manufacture, distribution, and small profits. If patents or market power keep competition out, then profits of $100 or $500 or even $999 per customer are possible. It's that possibility which makes marketing so valuable.

The essential question is control—who "owns" the business. To a large extent, the business of patients is controlled (owned) by the doctors, who write the prescriptions for them. However, doctors are prohibited by law and ethics from taking any of that $999 in surplus value of a drug. If there's only one treatment for an illness, and it is protected by a patent, the company with the patent in effect "owns" the business. The main question becomes how much business (i.e., total sales) there will be. In this case, the company may detail doctors to push them to prescribe more, but it doesn't have to worry about competing drugs. If there are two or more treatments for an illness, however, the situation becomes more complex. In theory, the choice should be made by the patient, balancing therapeutic effectiveness, cost, and side effects. In this case, marketing focuses directly on the patient in the form of DTC advertising.

FOR EXAMPLE

Claritin: Direct-to-Consumer Advertising, Over-the-Counter Medication, and Pricing

Claritin had a tortuous transition from laboratory to market. Schering-Plough submitted a new drug application (NDA) for the compound (scientific name, loratadine) in 1980 but didn't obtain approval until 1993, by which time there were only five years left on the basic patent.[27] The FDA felt little pressure to approve what was classified as a "me-too" drug promising little clinical advance over existing prescription and OTC antihistamine remedies for allergy and hay fever. However, when FDA rules regarding direct-to-consumers (DTC) advertising were relaxed in 1997, Schering-Plough spent $322 million on promoting Claritin to the public. Ads featuring clear skies and happy faces (with pollen-carrying flowers in the background) were seen on TV shows, billboards, bus stops, and leaflets handed out on street corners. Sales of Claritin ballooned to more than $2.6 billion in 2000.

In clinical trials, 46 percent of allergy sufferers showed improvement with Claritin, compared with 35 percent who showed improvement when given a placebo. Tests indicated that Schering-Plough's old drug, Chlor-Trimeton, now sold inexpensively OTC, was equally or perhaps more effective in relieving symptoms—and may not have been much more sleep inducing when used in a low dose. Was it really worth paying six times as much for the new version? The question rarely arose because prescriptions were covered by insurance. WellPoint, a large health insurance company, sued in 1998 to force Claritin and similar allergy drugs to be sold OTC without prescription, claiming that they clearly were safer than the existing OTC medications such as Chlor-Trimeton. If Claritin were declared safe enough to be used without a prescription, then it would no longer qualify for insurance reimbursement, consumers would have to pay out-of-pocket, and demand would become much more price sensitive. Despite concerted efforts by Schering-Plough and other pharmaceutical firms, the insurance companies made a persuasive case. In November 2002, the FDA approved Claritin for OTC use. Schering-Plough's stock dropped precipitously as the price of Claritin had to be cut, and cut again, to compete in the more wide-open OTC market and as Johnson & Johnson and Wyeth geared up production of generic versions of loratadine to sell at less than $20.

Pharmaceutical companies have ramped up their DTC advertising in recent years; DTC advertising accounted for 12 percent of prescription drug growth in 2000.[28] However, most of pharmaceutical companies' marketing efforts (e.g., detailing, scientific meetings at nice resorts) are still directed at doctors.

Notice how little market power and how little excess profit the pharmacy is able to get. Even though pharmacies are the point of contact where the patient obtains the drug, they have to fill the prescription as written by the doctor or as modified by the insurer (e.g., generic substitution, tiered copayments) and are not allowed to try to shift patients from A to B. Pharmacies are almost as neutral and powerless as wholesalers: They simply distribute pills from manufacturer to patient. There isn't a lot of excess profit to be obtained here. Actually, one of the most lucrative parts of the retail pharmacy business is all the other stuff (e.g., candy, bandages) that pharmacies sell at above-average markups to people who come in to fill their prescriptions. That is, the pharmacy doesn't "own" the prescription business (because there are so many retail pharmacy competitors and because wholesale prices are fixed), but it does own the idle shopping time of the patient who is waiting to have his or her prescription filled—and can exploit that to sell high-markup magazines, mints, and other items.

12.4.5 Research and Innovation

Research is a sunk cost for drugs already on the market. These drugs would still be manufactured even if prices were reduced to the level of marginal cost, but then no new research would be undertaken. The high prices are the incentives for investing millions of dollars in the hope of making a discovery. Almost every economist and politician accepts this simple premise connecting research expenditures and innovation to the promise of future profits. However, some issues remain. How much profit is necessary to provide an incentive? It's not clear whether more R&D spending leads to the development of more innovative new drugs. Much of the expenditure goes for imitative "me-too" drugs to fight off the competitive threat from generics and chemically related drugs that other companies have made sufficiently different (by adding some side molecules or by using a new production process) to engineer around existing patents and claim their own brand names. Whereas 46 percent of all new drug approvals in 1991 were for new molecular entities (NMEs), by 2001, only 35 percent of approvals were for new molecules. Furthermore, only 7 of these 24 NMEs were ranked by the FDA as priority drugs promising important advances entitled to expedited review, compared with 19 in 1999.[29] During the 1990s, research spending grew from $10 billion to $30 billion, yet the number of important new drugs brought to market fell, and the number of applications for approval submitted by pharmaceutical companies to the FDA declined from 2,116 to 1,872. Most reputable analysts agree that the major financial problem facing the industry is a lack of important new drugs in the pipeline. More than 10 years of increased R&D spending haven't provided impressive results, making it difficult to argue that having a bit more profit to pour into laboratories would make a big difference in the rate of therapeutic advances or drug discovery.

It may be that research productivity is in a stage of decline. Some analysts suggest that "discovery" methods have been played out, with most significant compounds already investigated and under patent, so that any surge of new drugs will have to come from new areas of research.

SELF-CHECK

- List the three major types of buyers in the pharmaceutical market.
- Explain the difference between a drug's clinical value and its economic value.
- Compare the pharmaceutical market power of pharmacists to that of physicians.

SUMMARY

The average American fills 11 prescriptions per year. Pharmaceuticals were a $188.5 billion industry in 2004, for which government and private insurance paid two-thirds of the bill. Of all the funds flowing in, about 70 percent go to pharmaceutical companies, 20 percent to retail pharmacies, and 10 percent to PBMs and insurers—much of that in the form of rebates from manufacturers.

Pharmaceutical manufacturing is among the most successful of industries, having greatly improved human welfare and generated enormous profits. A single successful drug can earn more than $5 billion in a year and can make or break the company. However, R&D of new products is a risky, lengthy, and costly process. Only 1 in 1,000 compounds initially studied eventually makes it to the market. On average, the time from discovery to successful market introduction is more than 10 years, at a total cost of $800 million. The hope of making large profits from discovering the next blockbuster product keeps pharmaceutical firms investing in R&D and fuels progress in the pharmaceutical industry.

The dominant economic feature of the pharmaceutical industry is the large sunk costs, first for R&D and then for the marketing blitz required to launch sales. The marginal cost of producing additional pills is small; therefore, most of the price is pure profit once the large fixed costs are covered. The ability to control the flow of funds determines who will hold on to most of these profits: the brand-name manufacturer with the patent, the generic competitor, the government, the physician, the PBM, the insurance company, or the patient.

Pharmaceutical manufacturers have begun to respond to changes in their markets brought about by managed care and generic competition. These changes include the use of discounts, disease management programs, and the development of various forms of risk-sharing contracts.

KEY TERMS

Food and Drug Administration (FDA)	The U.S. federal agency that has jurisdiction over the labeling, manufacture, and sale of food and drugs for human consumption.
Generic drug	A drug that is identical in chemical composition to a brand-name pharmaceutical preparation but is produced by competitors after the firm's patent expires and is usually sold for much less than the brand-name drug.
Pharmacoeconomics	Cost–benefit analysis of drugs; assessment of the market for a drug.
Pharmacy benefit managers (PBMs)	Subcontractors chosen by insurance companies to develop prescription drug benefit plans, administer claims, and manage relationships with pharmaceutical companies (i.e., manufacturers) and retail pharmacies.

ASSESS YOUR UNDERSTANDING

Go to www.wiley.com/college/getzen to assess your knowledge of the pharmaceuticals market.

Measure your learning by comparing pre-test and post-test results.

Summary Questions

1. PBMs offer prescription drug coverage directly to consumers at much lower rates than traditional insurance companies. True or False?

2. Today, the vast majority of prescription drug costs are paid out of pocket. True or False?

3. Medicare Part D makes prescription drug coverage available to everyone enrolled in Medicare. True or False?

4. The introduction of Medicare prescription drug coverage resulted in:

    (a) a decrease in the growth of Medicaid spending on prescription drugs.

    (b) a decrease in the growth of private-sector spending on prescription drugs.

    (c) an increase in the growth of public-sector spending on prescription drugs.

    (d) All of the above

5. Because of the reimbursement structure for inpatient pharmaceutical use, most hospitals have a strong incentive to maximize the amount they spend on prescription drugs. True or False?

6. The majority of the money spent on prescription drugs goes to:

    (a) the retailer.

    (b) the government, in the form of taxes.

    (c) the manufacturer.

    (d) the wholesaler.

7. "Detailing" in pharmaceuticals refers to:

    (a) the extensive information concerning product contents and effects that must be published on the container.

    (b) the emphasis on absolute purity in manufacturing because of the importance of reputation in a product that can be lethal if contaminated.

    (c) the precise listing of drugs that can be paid for under a managed care plan.

    (d) personal contact with physicians by representatives of pharmaceutical firms for marketing.

8. Competition in pharmaceutical products:

   (a) is similar in all market segments because a drug is a homogeneous product rather than a personal service.

   (b) in the hospital market is largely on the basis of efficacy because the patient is not very price sensitive while in an inpatient setting.

   (c) isn't very price sensitive in the retail pharmacy market even though patients are more likely to be paying out-of-pocket.

   (d) in the government market is mostly over cost-effectiveness, in order to be included in formularies. - List of pharmacedicals a pharmacy carries

9. Which of the following are considered to be sunk costs of a drug when the first pill is sold?

   (a) Discovery and regulatory approval

   (b) R&D

   (c) Regulatory approval and market introduction

   (d) Market introduction, discovery, regulatory approval, and R&D

10. Due to the intense demands of research, only large pharmaceutical companies are capable of producing innovative new drugs. True or False?

11. The public sector is the largest purchaser of pharmaceuticals. True or False?

12. Managed care has which of the following effects on the demand for pharmaceuticals?

    (a) It increases demand.

    (b) It increases elasticity of demand.

    (c) It increases prices.

    (d) It has no effect on demand.

13. Marketing increases the clinical value of drugs. True or False?

Review Questions

1. What is the function of a prescription for a drug? Who benefits when drugs are restricted to prescription status?

2. Who benefits and who would loses now that outpatient drugs are covered by Medicare?

3. What is the function of a patent granted on a pharmaceutical product? Does it benefit only the firm that holds the patent?

4. What determines the price of a drug?

5. Why are fixed costs more important for pharmaceuticals than physical therapy? How does this affect marketing expenditures?

6. Do patents raise or lower the productivity of research?

7. How are prescription costs "managed" by insurance companies?

8. What fraction of the total cost of pharmaceuticals is paid for directly by patients? Does this mean that price is more or less important for drugs than for other types of medical care?

9. How is most pharmaceutical research paid for? What is the most costly aspect of pharmaceutical research?

10. How many distinct market segments exist in the pharmaceutical industry? How do these segments differ?

11. On what basis do pharmaceutical firms compete in each market segment? Is price a more important factor for the choice of which doctor to see or for which drug is prescribed?

12. Do hospitals have more of an incentive to control the costs of surgical implants, anesthesiologists' fees, or pharmaceuticals? In which case do they bear the highest fraction of marginal cost? In which case do they receive the highest fraction of marginal revenue?

13. How would a change in the length of the patent period affect the structure of the pharmaceutical industry?

14. Marketing accounts for a much larger portion of the cost of pharmaceuticals than the cost of other forms of care. Why? To whom are most pharmaceutical marketing efforts targeted?

Applying This Chapter

1. When a brand-name drug loses patent protection and competing generic products enter the market, does the price of the brand-name drug increase or decrease?

2. Why is so much more spent on marketing drugs than on marketing surgery or psychotherapy?

3. Because FDA regulations limit the entry of new drugs into the market, do they constitute an "unfair restraint of trade" that reduces competition and raises prices to consumers?

4. The FDA lifted restrictions on TV ads for prescription drugs in 1997, allowing manufacturers to advertise drugs without including lengthy disclaimers explaining the often numerous side effects. How has this regulatory change affected the market for pharmaceuticals?

YOU TRY IT

Off-Label Drug Use

Physicians and researchers often discover new uses for drugs that have aleady received FDA approval. The FDA consider these to be "off-label" uses because rigorous trials to test the safety and effectiveness of the drugs for these uses haven't been presented to the FDA for approval. However, it's perfectly legal for physicians to prescribe drugs for off-label uses, and it's a fairly common practice. For instance, Viagra was originally approved for treating chest pain; when researchers recognized its usefulness for treating erectile dysfunction, it was prescribed for off-label treatment of this condition (and was eventually approved by the FDA for this use). In 1997, the Food and Drug Admininistration Modernization Act made it legal for pharmaceutical companies to provide physicians with certain kinds of information about off-label uses for drugs. Write a brief essay considering the possible implications of prescribing drugs for off-label use. Who benefits? Who loses?

Canadian Prescription Drugs

There has been a lot of news coverage about the fact that prescription drugs in Canada are often a lot less expensive than those in the United States. Given what you have learned about the distribution and pricing of pharmaceuticals, who do you think is responsible for the lower prices in Canada: pharmacies, wholesalers, or pharmaceutical manufacturers? Explain your answer in a brief essay, being sure also to address the following questions: Do you think it should be legal for residents of the United States to order their drugs from Canadian pharmacies in order to save money? If the majority of people did this, what would be the effect on the U.S. drug market?

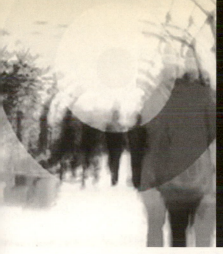

13

INTERNATIONAL COMPARISONS OF HEALTH AND HEALTH EXPENDITURES
A Global Perspective

Starting Point

Go to www.wiley.com/college/getzen to assess your knowledge of international health care.
Determine where you need to concentrate your effort.

What You'll Learn in This Chapter

▲ Global disparities in health care spending and health
▲ Health care as a luxury good
▲ Health care spending in low-, middle-, and high-income countries
▲ The relationship between spending and a nation's health
▲ The international trade in health care

After Studying This Chapter, You'll Be Able To

▲ Assess the relationship between a nation's gross domestic product and its citizens' health
▲ Critique the concept of health care as a national luxury good
▲ Evaluate the value of increased spending on health care for low-income countries, middle-income countries, and high-income countries
▲ Evaluate the impact of the international trade of knowledge and health professionals

INTRODUCTION

Any assessment of health economy around the world must take into account the world's tremendous diversity in population, economic growth, and health status. Health care spending, education, and status vary considerable among high-, middle-, and low-income countries.

This chapter takes a look at variations in health care among nations in different income classes. One very important point raised in this chapter is that nations spend more money on health care because they have more money to spend, not because they have greater medical needs. In addition, just because wealthier countries are healthier and spend more on medical care doesn't necessarily mean that higher spending levels buy better health.

This chapter concludes with a brief section on international trade in health care. It's interesting to note that even though health care is among the world's largest industries, it accounts for only a tiny fraction of world trade.

13.1 Health Care Differences Among Nations

There were more than 6 billion people in the world in 2002, distributed across some 200 countries. Health care expenditures for these 6 billion people totaled $3.5 trillion that year.[1] The 285 million people living in the United States at the time represented 5 percent of the worldwide population total, but U.S. health care expenditures, $1.5 trillion, accounted for more than 40 percent of total health spending. Although China was the world's largest country, with 1.3 billion people, it accounted for less than $0.3 trillion in health care spending. Health expenditures per person in the United States were 10 times the worldwide average in 2002, twice as much as the $2,009 per person spent in Japan, and 20 times the per person average of $45 (approximately $205 in international purchasing power parity [PPP] exchange rates) in China (see Table 13-1).[2]

The extra $1.2 trillion spent in the United States purchased a lot more hospitals, physicians, drugs, and technologically sophisticated equipment for U.S. citizens. But how many additional years of life, how much reduction in morbidity and mortality, did all these extra medical inputs yield? Could the United States have done as well, or become even healthier, while spending less? Many factors other than hospitals and doctors are responsible for differences in health among China, the United States, and other countries, but $1.2 trillion is a significant amount to spend on health care.

When comparing health care among nations, it's important to recognize the economic status of the countries being studied. For instance, Mozambique, Tanzania, and Ethiopia are among the world's poorest countries. These predominantly rural countries depend on subsistence agriculture and have limited government, little accumulation of savings or investment, per capita incomes of less than $500, and rapidly expanding populations facing repeated threats from

Table 13-1: Comparision of Health and Expenditures Across Nations[3]

	Population (millions)	Growth % Rate	Life Expectancy	% Age 60+	Mortality Under 5	Mortality 15–59	GDP (per capita)	GDP (PPP)	% Urban	% Agr.	Health % of GDP	Expenditures (International $)	% Govt.	% Private	% Out-of-Pocket	% Prepaid Plans
World	6,122	1.6	65.1	9.8	.064	.247	$ 4,890	$ 6,490	46	4	5.7	$ 573	.62	.38	.32	.08
Sudan	32	2.3	55.9	5.5	N/A	N/A	330	1,298	N/A	N/A	4.7	51	.21	.79	.79	.00
Kenya	31	2.5	48.9	4.2	.114	.537	360	975	32	27	8.3	115	.22	.78	.56	.05
Pakistan	145	2.6	61.3	5.8	.110	.216	470	1,757	36	26	4.1	76	.23	.77	.77	.00
India	1,025	1.8	60.8	7.7	.094	.257	450	2,149	28	28	4.9	71	.18	.82	.82	.00
China	1,292	0.9	71.2	10.0	.037	.132	780	3,291	32	17	5.3	205	.37	.63	.60	.00
Turkey	68	1.7	69.0	8.5	.043	.162	2,900	6,126	74	18	5.0	323	.71	.29	.29	.00
Mexico	100	1.7	74.2	7.1	.030	.140	4,400	7,719	74	5	5.4	483	.46	.54	.50	.04
Poland	39	0.1	74.0	16.6	.009	.150	3,960	7,894	65	4	6.0	578	.70	.30	.26	.00
U.K.	60	0.3	77.5	20.7	.007	.089	22,640	20,883	89	1	7.3	1,774	.81	.19	.11	.17
Canada	31	1.0	79.3	16.9	.006	.079	19,320	23,725	77	2	9.1	2,534	.72	.28	.16	.71
Japan	127	0.3	81.4	23.8	.005	.072	32,230	24,041	79	2	7.8	2,009	.77	.23	.19	.01
Germany	82	0.3	78.2	23.7	.005	.091	25,350	22,404	87	1	10.6	2,754	.75	.25	.11	.50
U.S.A.	285	1.1	77.0	16.2	.008	.114	30,600	30,600	77	2	13.0	4,499	.44	.56	.15	.63

starvation. One out of 10 children die before age 5, and life expectancy is less than 60 years. At the other extreme are Sweden and Switzerland, whose urbane citizens enjoy average incomes of more than $30,000, where most deaths occur after age 75, and where average life expectancy exceeds 78 years. Development economists categorize countries as low, middle, or high income, broken down as follows:

▲ **Low-income countries (less than $1,500 per capita income):** More than half the world's population still lives in low-income, rural agricultural countries. Most countries in Africa are toward the bottom of the distribution. The two developing giants in this category, China and India, have 1.292 and 1.025 billion people, respectively. China's recent rapid development could transform the economy within 20 years.

▲ **Middle-income countries ($1,500 to $7,500 per capita income):** Middle-income countries are home to 1.5 billion people. Such countries include many Latin American countries; most of the formerly socialist countries of the former Soviet Union and Eastern Europe; South Africa; Saudi Arabia and other oil-rich states of the Middle East; and Asian countries with emerging economies, such as Korea.

▲ **High-income countries ($10,000 or higher per capita income):** 850 million people live in high-income countries, which include the Western European countries and the United States, Canada, Japan, Australia, and New Zealand.

A nation's health resources generally increase with income, while the extent of illness and need for medical care are reduced. The high-income countries had 2.5 doctors and 8.3 hospital beds per 1,000 people in 1990. (This chapter uses 1990 statistics to enable greater range of international comparisons.[4]) The average life expectancy was 78 years, with more than half of all deaths occurring after that age. In contrast, the low-income countries of sub-Saharan Africa could afford to spend only $12 per person on health care and had just 0.1 doctors and 1.4 hospital beds per 1,000 people. Life expectancy averaged 52 years, and half of all deaths occurred in children under age 6.

13.1.1 Size of the Market

The United States is by far the largest health care market in the world, with a 42 percent share of total global health care spending. In contrast, the world's most populous country, China, has only a 7 percent share, and the second most populous, India, has only a 2 percent share. In dollar terms, China's market is roughly the same size as the state of Ohio. All the very-low-income countries together, with a total of 2.5 billion people, account for less than 2 percent of the world's health care spending (about one-third as much as the state of California) (see Figure 13-1).

The disparity in health resources isn't as great as the disparity in health spending because wages are lower in low-income countries; therefore, 75 percent less health care spending usually translates into a somewhat less severe reduction in the

Figure 13-1

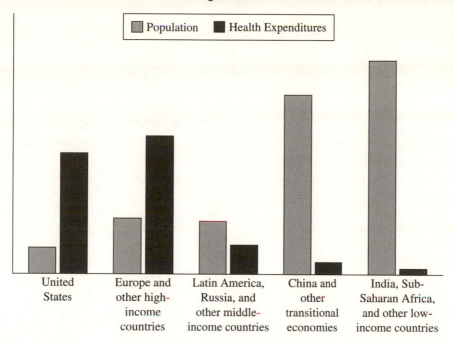

International comparison of market size.

number of doctors or nurses.[5] Still, the gap between high-income and low-income countries is substantial (see Table 13-1). Some goods, such as pharmaceuticals, are traded internationally, and their prices are somewhat consistent across countries; thus, any decline in spending causes an equivalent decline in usage. Such internationally traded items take a much larger portion of health care budgets in low-income countries (25 to 50 percent) than in high-income countries (5 to 15 percent). There are vast disparities between rich and poor. Haves and have-nots face such different choices that they almost seem like inhabitants of different planets or different centuries. What is common and readily accessible to most citizens of high-income countries are the favored privileges of a few government officials, industrialists, and celebrities in low-income countries. Medical care as practiced in the developed world is but a dream as distant as Hollywood for most of the world's population.

SELF-CHECK

- Indicate life expectancy for low- and high-income countries.
- What was total worldwide health spending in 2002?
- What was the United States's share of global health spending in 2002?

FOR EXAMPLE

The World Trade Organization and World Health

Cheap access to prescription drugs is crucial for the health of people living in low-income countries, many of whom could never afford to pay the rates pharmaceutical companies charge for drugs in the United States and Europe. Until recently, companies based in poor countries such as India produced cheaper, generic versions of brand-name drugs, undercutting the price of the drug sold by the patent holder, sometimes by thousands of dollars. Such practices made medicine far more affordable for the people in the poorest countries, who might otherwise have had to go without lifesaving drugs. However, recent global patent rules established by the World Trade Organization (WTO) are requiring member countries to provide exclusive marketing rights to holders of pharmaceutical patents for at least 20 years. Critics of these new rules worry that when such laws are implemented in India and elsewhere, it will be very difficult for companies to produce and distribute low-cost generic versions of patented brand-name drugs to developing countries. They argue that the U.S. and European-based pharmaceutical companies will profit, at the expense of sick people in poor countries.

13.2 Health as a National Luxury Good

Nations spend more money on health care because they have more money to spend, not because they have greater medical needs. This statement isn't very surprising when considering whether Bangladesh (gross domestic product [GDP] $400 per capita) will spend more or less than Belgium (GDP $24,000 per capita) on health (see Figure 13-2). Yet the fact that health care spending is unrelated to medical needs contradicts most people's personal experiences. On an individual level, people spend more on health care if they become sick. However, on a national level, spending decisions are made through a political process in which leaders decide how much of a country's resources should be spent on health care. Thus, just because more people have AIDS in Kenya than in the United States doesn't necessarily mean that Kenya spends more money on AIDS than the United States.

As the focus shifts from the individual to the nation as a whole, the significant determinant of spending shifts from "medical need" to "available income" (see Figure 13-3). For example, most countries spend two to five times as much on elderly people as they do on young and middle-aged people. However, this doesn't mean that if a country's population is older than average, it will spend more on health care than a country with a younger population.[6]

Figure 13-2

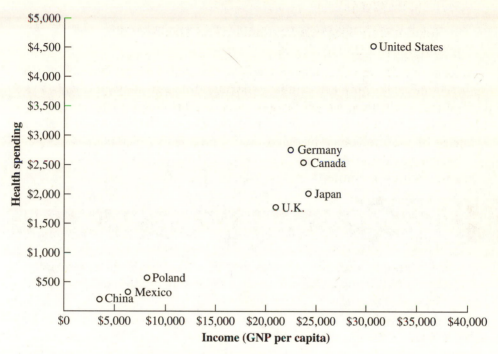

Health expenditures related to income.

Source: World Health Report 2002.

Figure 13-3

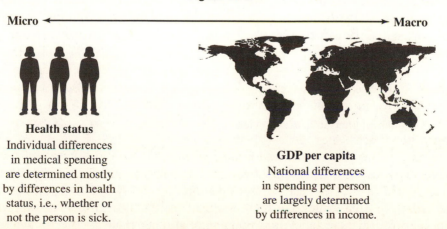

Micro and macro determinants of health spending.

FOR EXAMPLE

The Relationship Between Population Age and Spending: England vs. the United States

England has an older population than the United States and health statistics that are roughly equivalent on many measures (life expectancy 77.5 years vs. 77.0 years, infant mortality 7 percent vs. 8 percent), but England spends significantly less on health care on average ($1,774 per person versus $4,499), largely because per capita income is lower ($22,640 vs. $30,600).[7]

SELF-CHECK

- On a national level, which is a more important factor in determining the amount of money spent on health care: medical need or available income?
- Why is medical care considered a luxury good?

13.3 Does More Spending Improve Health?

Compared to other countries, wealthier countries are healthier, and they spend more on medical care. Can one then conclude that more spending buys better health? Not necessarily. Many factors associated with higher incomes, such as education, nutrition, and sanitation, are also known to improve health. Furthermore, life expectancy has increased greatly in many poor countries over the past 20 years, even when the availability of doctors and GDP per capita has declined. On the whole, three factors influence a nation's health:

1. Economic growth
2. Advances in public health and medical research
3. The use of medical care services

Thus, if a country has no knowledge of what to do to improve health, money is worthless, and medical knowledge alone is useless in the face of extreme poverty, which leads to death from starvation.

Figure 13-4 illustrates that there is a relationship between per capita income and average life expectancy and that the relationship has changed over time. A likely explanation is that movements along the curve reflect the combined

Figure 13-4

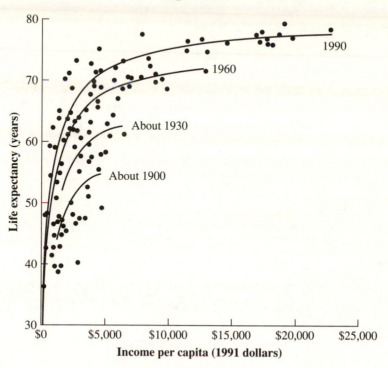

Life expectancy and income per capita.

effects of more income and more medical care, while the shifting of the curve reflects the universal effect of increased knowledge, which is a public good. In poor countries today, sanitation, basic nutrition supplements for infants, and control of preventable disease are still of primary importance. In these situations, studies have indicated that maternal education and literacy are often more important than income in preventing childhood disease and death.

Separate assessment of the effects of living standards and use of medical care is difficult because both generally rise or fall together. Japan, for example, has achieved a phenomenal 25-year increase in life expectancy since World War II, but there's no easy way to determine how much is due to the rapid economic growth and how much is due to the deployment of modern medical care. The achievement of relatively high life expectancies in some low- or middle-income countries with relatively low use of sophisticated medical treatments (e.g., 72 years in Malaysia, 75 years in the Czech Republic, 76 years in Costa Rica) suggests that the incremental effect of medical care alone is probably modest. Analysis across many countries reveals that where there is greater equality of income, the average level of health is higher. The greater the degree of inequality, the more likely it is that some families will be so lacking in food and amenities that

> ## FOR EXAMPLE
>
> ### Knowledge Is Healthy
>
> A piece of evidence related to the effect of knowledge on health is provided by studies of childhood mortality in the United States around 1900.[8] In that era, children of well-to-do physicians were just as likely to die before age 5 as children of poor laborers living in tenements because both the wealthy and the poor used the same ineffectual health practices. As the importance of infection prevention and nutrition were revealed, physicians' families were able to take advantage of their better education and resources so that child mortality declined much more rapidly in this group than among low-income laborers.

deaths from infantile diarrhea, tuberculosis, and other preventable or treatable illnesses will occur.

SELF-CHECK

- List three factors that influence a nation's health.
- What impact does income inequality have on a nation's health? Is it more or less important than overall income level?

13.4 Low-Income Countries

Low-income countries face very different health care problems than wealthy, industrialized countries. Their populations are generally rural, with many children and a heavy burden of infectious disease and stunting (i.e., abnormally low height and/or small body size) due to occasional malnutrition. However, government officials living in the capital have incomes, tastes, and health care needs much more like those of people in developed countries. This can lead to a major misallocation of resources, such as building a modern research hospital that provides excellent care in the capital, even though much of the rest of the country lacks access to a doctor or a nurse, and children remain unvaccinated so that preventable disease epidemics remain common. It's not unusual for as much as half the entire health budget of a low-income country to be spent in the capital city, with a large part going to equip and staff the leading hospital. (In contrast, the Johns Hopkins University Hospital takes about 0.6 percent of the U.S. health care budget.)

In low-income countries, ruling politicians and leaders of the medical profession naturally tend to favor maintaining a state-of-the-art facility with modern technology, even when doing so drains funds from the village clinics and nursing care that can do more to reduce infant mortality and raise life expectancy.

Even in very-low-income countries, medical schools train many specialists who want to perform technologically advanced procedures rather than primary care generalists able to treat most common illnesses.

Studies by the World Bank have also found that the status of women is a major determinant of health in low-income countries. Access to knowledge is one factor related to women's status. In countries where most women are illiterate and uneducated, there's no way for them to know about sterilization of water, proper nutrition, or care of children with childhood infections. Women are also more likely than men to make family health a priority, so the more power and knowledge a country's women have, the more likely it is that the country's population will be healthier.

Starvation remains a problem in many of the lowest-income countries. In Nigeria, 43 percent of children aged 2 to 6 are stunted (i.e., low height for age); similarly, 32 percent of children in Kenya and 65 percent of children in India are stunted. Compare these percentages to stunting rates of 22 percent in Mexico, 4 percent in Japan, and 2 percent in the United Kingdom and United States.[9] This situation occurs not because of lack of food but because the food doesn't get to where it is needed most. No simple solution presents itself because the defects in economic organization that cause mismanagement of food are the same as those responsible for a lack of economic development in the first place. National governments that maintain order, handle their budgets and money supply prudently, and support market-oriented policies are usually able to grow out of the low-income category over time.

13.4.1 Health Care in Kenya

Kenya provides a good example of how the health care system works in low-income countries. The economy of Kenya, like that of many poor nations, is dominated by agriculture. Its most significant exports are coffee, tea, cotton, and minerals. Kenya's 34 million people had a per capita income of about $460 in 2005. Total health expenditure per capita is $65. (Note that income is difficult to measure or define in a traditional agricultural economy such as Kenya's; therefore, any figure should be considered approximate.) The population is growing rapidly (2 percent per year), with almost half of the population under the age of 15. Enrollment of children in primary school is 92 percent, and nearly three-fourths of all adults are literate. About 40 percent of the population lives in cities. The government is relatively stable for such a poor country. Average life expectancy, 45 years, has plummeted sharply in the past 15 years due to the high rate of AIDS. Child mortality is 129 per 1,000 for males and 110 per 1,000 for females; adult mortality rates have skyrocketed due to AIDS and are now at 477 per 1,000 for males and 502 per 1,000 for females.[10]

The health system is split almost equally between the public and private sectors (see Table 13-2). The Ministry of Health runs 80 hospitals, 41 district health centers in the provinces, 178 rural health centers, and about 1,200 subcenters and dispensaries. District medical officers are physicians, usually assisted by one or more nurses and a hospital secretary (i.e., administrator).[11] Below the district level, most facilities are operated by paraprofessionals, and at the dispensary level, by community workers or untrained auxiliaries. Despite a stated emphasis on primary care and rural development, more than 35 percent of the entire national budget is spent on the showcase Kenya National Hospital in Nairobi. Some government agencies, such as the Ministry of Transport and the Coffee Board, run health services for their workers, as do the dozen or so corporations that have more than 500 employees.

Religious missions are a very important part of the health care system, running 40 hospitals, 84 health centers, and 173 clinics. Although the origins and management of these facilities are religious, 60 percent of their funding comes from patient fees, about 25 percent from government subsidy, and 15 percent from donations. Thus, they are considered part of the private sector. Overall, about 22 percent of Kenyan health expenditures are derived from foreign aid.

The Kenyan government actively encourages private-sector health care. Private hospitals, supported entirely by fees, are viewed as being of higher quality

Table 13-2: Health Expenditures in Kenya[12]

	$ (Millions)	Percentage
Government		
Ministry of health	204	42%
Municipalities	27	6%
Other government	6	1%
Private Sources		
Voluntary agencies	6	1%
Religious missions	28	6%
Corporate clinics	2	<1%
Household spending		
Hospitals	45	9%
Physicians and healers	36	7%
Drugs	114	24%
Other	16	3%
Total	484	Approximately $20 per person

than public hospitals and are growing rapidly. The government runs the National Hospital Insurance Fund for high-income workers through a mandatory 2-percent wage tax (there is no employer contribution) designed to reimburse people for stays in private and religious hospitals or private rooms of public hospitals. However, this plan covers only 12 percent of the population. The effectiveness of the plan may be further limited by its low payout rate: Only 60 percent of the hospital insurance premiums collected have been used to pay claims or administrative expenses, allowing 40 percent to be held by the central government.

Most physicians (70 percent) in Kenya work full time in private practice. The 30 percent who work for the government or missions also engage in private practice after clinic hours. There are, perhaps, 2,000 physicians actively in practice in Kenya, with almost half of them in Nairobi (although it has only 7 percent of the nation's population). In contrast, there are about 19,000 traditional healers and herbalists practicing in Kenya, most of them in the countryside. A physician earns roughly 30 times as much as a traditional healer. A small fraction of the population, the 2 or 3 percent who belong to upper-income families living in the major cities, accounts for more than half of all private expenditures for medical care. About one-third of expenditures come from the 10 percent who are middle-income city dwellers. The poor who have flocked to the cities account for less than 2 percent of private spending, and the bulk of the population still living in rural areas accounts for just 17 percent of private expenditures. Here, the flow of medical resources clearly follows the flow of funds. The disparity between members of the elite who live in the capital and the vast rural population that subsists by farming is clearly visible in morbidity and mortality statistics and remains a large problem facing health care in Kenya.

FOR EXAMPLE

AIDS in Sub-Saharan Africa

Sub-Saharan Africa has the world's highest rates of HIV infection. At the end of 2005, there were 24.5 million people in sub-Saharan Africa living with HIV. Globally, 64 percent of all people living with HIV live in sub-Saharan Africa. In 2005, the region was home to 2 million children under 15 years of age living with HIV, constituting almost 90 percent of the total number of children living with HIV in the world. Fewer than 1 in 10 of those children were getting basic support services. An estimated 12 million children under the age of 17 living in sub-Saharan Africa (just under 10 percent) have lost one or both parents to AIDS. In 2005, an estimated 2.7 million people in the region became newly infected with HIV, and 2 million adults and children died of AIDS. Around 1 in 6 people in need of treatment in the region were receiving it (i.e., 17 percent, or ??,000 people).[13]

> ## FOR EXAMPLE
>
> ### The Economic Toll of HIV on Kenya
>
> The economic toll of HIV/AIDS on Kenya's economy is very significant, particularly given that 80 percent of HIV infection occurs in the economically active age group of 15 to 49 years. The Kenyan Ministry of Health cites a 1996 study that projected the Kenyan GDP would be 14.5 percent lower in the year 2005 than it would be without the AIDS epidemic, while per capita income would drop by 10 percent. The study also predicted a 15 percent drop in savings and labor productivity.[14]

SELF-CHECK

- Where are the best medical facilities usually located in low-income countries?
- What impact does the education level of women have on health status in low-income countries?
- List some key factors affecting people's health in low-income countries.

13.5 Middle-Income Countries

Turkey, Mexico, Thailand, and South Korea are examples of countries that are in the process of industrialization. Subsistence agriculture and poverty are still the norm in the remote rural regions of these countries, but the bulk of the population has moved into cities and works for wages. The shift from rural agricultural labor to urban wage labor presents a major organizational problem: how to develop a comprehensive health insurance system able to fund a higher level of health care. Rapid economic growth allows some countries to expand government services; thus, a predominantly public system is created. In other countries, such as Korea, a strong tradition of industrial paternalism leads to private insurance based on employment benefits. Some countries began with a public system and switched to reliance on the private sector, while others are moving in the opposite direction.

In almost every middle-income developing country, the health insurance system is in transition. Even when coverage is universal by law, the reality is that access to medical care is very uneven. The urban ghettos and impoverished rural villages frequently lack sanitation. Restrictions and incompleteness in the health insurance system may prevent poor citizens from using medical facilities even when those facilities are accessible geographically. Thus, the disadvantaged populations disproportionately get sick and die. At the same time, expanding incomes have brought the lifestyle-related illnesses of the wealthy countries, such as heart disease and lung cancer, to prominence. (The growth markets for cigarettes in the twenty-first century are China, India, and Asia, not Europe and North America.) Finally, the middle-income countries are still likely to misallocate resources: Large research hospitals in the cities are accompanied by a lack of village clinics in the countryside and the training of too many specialists and not enough primary care physicians or public health experts.

13.5.1 Health Care in Mexico

With a 2001 per capita GDP of $6,200, an average life expectancy of 73 years for males and 78 years for females, and a young population (34 percent under age 15) of 101 million people that is growing rapidly (1.4 percent per year), Mexico is similar to many other countries that have transitional economies.[15] The bulk of the people have moved off farms into cities to find industrial and service jobs, but agriculture and export of raw commodities still make up a substantial part of the economy, and illiteracy is still a problem in rural areas. The government is politically stable, with a relatively more open, multiparty democracy.

The government enacted a comprehensive social security system, IMSS, in 1943, relatively early for a transitional economy, but it covered only industrial workers and their dependents.[16] A nationwide network of IMSS health centers, polyclinics, and hospitals was built. The Ministry of Health and IMSS-Solidaridad provide services for around 40 million uninsured Mexicans, mainly the rural and urban poor. In 1960, a plan for government employees, ISSSTE, was established, and a modern and technologically sophisticated network of hospitals and clinics was built, with generous funding, to accommodate this favored group of employees. ISSSTE, IMSS, and the medical services for the armed forces and employees of the national oil company (PEMEX) provided the top tier of health insurance and covered about half the population (see Table 13-3).

Table 13-3: Health Insurance Coverage in Mexico[17]

Source	Percentage
Mexican Institute for Social Security (IMSS)	39%
Institute for Government Workers (ISSSTE)	8%
Other federal agency plans	2%
Secretariat of Health and Welfare (SSA)	21%
Marginal families program	13%
Private medical care	5%
Unprotected population	12%

The private market provides services both at the bottom of the income distribution (where public services are inadequate) and at the top (where wealthier people can buy state-of-the-art medical care), with the middle occupied by three separate tiers of public care. The private sector consists of providers working in hospitals, clinics, offices, and folk medicine units on a for-profit basis. Around 25 percent of the people enrolled in social security agencies and 40 percent of the uninsured report a private provider as their usual source of primary care.

Most physicians in Mexico work in salaried positions for ISSSTE, IMSS, or social security agencies and also have private practices as well. Yet even though Mexico has considerably fewer physicians per 100,000 population than in the United States (about one-fourth as many), a large pool of unemployed or underemployed physicians (more than 30 percent of all physicians) can't find a government job or attract enough private patients to make a living from medicine.

The government has identified three main challenges for the Mexican health system: equity, quality, and financial protection. To meet these challenges, three basic initiatives have been implemented: (1) programs to confront the backlog of common infections and reproductive health problems that mostly affect the poor, (2) a major initiative to improve the quality of care both in the public and private sectors, and (3) an ambitious effort to provide universal health insurance. The universal health insurance program will provide regular access to quality care and financial protection to almost 40 million Mexicans who are presently uninsured. Relative to those in other transitional economies, the health care system in Mexico seems to work reasonably well. Yet glaring deficiencies in finance (i.e., the per capita expenditure in Mexico is below the Latin American average) and in organization (i.e., lack of coordination and production efficiency) remain.

SELF-CHECK

- In middle-income countries, are health care systems largely public or private?
- List some factors that affect the health of people living in middle-income countries.
- List one positive and one negative impact of increasing incomes on health in middle-income countries.

13.6 High-Income Countries

Among high-income countries, there is considerable variation in the use of medical care inputs (e.g., doctors per 1,000 population, ranging from 1.4 to 4.3; hospital beds per 1,000, ranging from 3.9 to 16.1), organization of services, reliance on taxpayer financing, and total cost, but there is remarkably little variation in health outcomes. Life expectancy in the 23 high-income countries is between 76 and 81 years, and infant mortality is between 4 and 8 per 1,000 births.

More variation in health statistics exists between regions within any one of these countries than across all 22 countries together. Given the small differences in average health outcomes, it's difficult to say that one country's system is better or worse than another's. What is clear is that many health problems are concentrated in specific, underserved populations, usually ethnic minorities or areas of extreme poverty.[18] Although tremendous resources are available for advanced experimental treatment, electronic scanning for diagnosis, and long-term rehabilitation, there is still a lack of primary care resources to ensure that every child is immunized, that all pregnant women receive adequate prenatal care and nutrition, and that every person has a primary physician to contact when in need of advice or care. In many ways, high-income countries face the same problems of maldistribution and misallocation in the delivery of medical care as low-income countries, but at a different level (see Figure 13-5).

13.6.1 Costs and Cost Control

Rapidly rising health care costs have created fiscal difficulties in all high-income countries. Although attempts at cost control have varied widely, there has been a degree of convergence across nations so that most spend between 6 percent

Figure 13-5

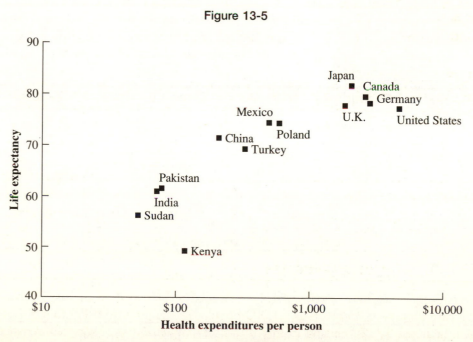

Health expenditures and life expectancy across countries.

and 10 percent of their GDP on health care, with the notable exception of the United States, which spent 16.8 percent in 2007. The United States spends by far the most on health care yet ranks twenty-second out of 23 countries in number of patient bed days per 1,000 population (only Greece is lower), ninth out of 14 in number of physician visits per person, and twelfth out of 18 in number of prescriptions.[19] There is no consistent relationship between costs per capita and the number of services provided, hospital beds, physicians employed, or extent of public or private insurance. Reducing the number of visits, drug prices, hospital days, and other micro-level variables hasn't been successful in controlling health system costs. A comprehensive examination concluded that there appears to be no relationship between success in containing costs and ways of organizing services.[20]

How have Japan and the Western European countries been able to keep health care costs so much lower than the United States while maintaining equal or better health outcomes and patient satisfaction? For one, many attempts to control costs in the United States have been directed at the individual level, using deductibles and copayments to moderate demand, yet the use of pooled financing that protects patients from risks also insulates them from costs. Consumer choice doesn't lead to lower expenditures when consumers are spending someone else's money.

European countries have operated largely on the supply side, constraining the provider system rather than individual demand. The number of health care workers and their wages has been limited and is often subject to nationwide bargaining and controls. Purchasing of expensive new diagnostic and therapeutic technology has been restricted (see Table 13-4).[21] It has been argued that the flaws of governmental control (e.g., lack of innovation, consumer responsiveness) and the flaws of insurance markets (e.g., lack of cost control, gaps in coverage) are leading toward a convergence of public and private in a blended contractual model—what is known

Table 13-4: Medical Technology per Person in Three Countries, 1992–1993

	Canada		Germany		United States	
	Number	Per Million Persons	Number	Per Million Persons	Number	Per Million Persons
Open-heart surgery	36	1.3	61	0.8	945	3.7
Cardiac catheterization	78	2.8	277	3.4	1,631	6.4
Organ transplant	34	1.2	39	0.5	612	2.4
Radiation therapy	132	4.8	373	4.6	2,637	10.3
Lithotripsy	13	0.5	117	1.4	480	1.9
MRI	30	1.1	296	3.7	2,900	11.2

Source: Dale A Rublee, "Medical Technology in Canada, Germany, and the United States: An Update," *Health Affairs*, 13, Vol. 4 (1994): 113–117.

in the United States as managed care (see Chapter 10).[22] Government will be responsible for setting the rules and the overall limits on the amount to be spent and ensuring that everyone receives coverage, while market competition will be used to maintain the quality and amenity of services and provide local control.[23]

13.6.2 Health Care in Japan[24]

Japan is one of the world's highest-income countries. Life expectancy in Japan is the highest in the world: 78 years for men and 85 years for women. However, the level of health care spending is only half that of the United States and 7.4 percent of Japan's GDP. This figure is perceived in Japan as a sharp rise in comparison with 5.5 percent of GDP in 1990, the peak of the country's boom years. Since then, health care spending has risen by 40 percent while the economic system has suffered.

While the technology used in the Japanese health care system is similar to that used in the United States, the organization and flow of funds and, hence, the quantity and intensity of use, are considerably different.[25] In Japan, all citizens are covered by some form of insurance and are able to choose any physician or hospital they wish, with no bills other than modest copayments per visit or per day. Japan's universal health insurance system functions as a financing mechanism as well as the means of health policy implementation. By using a uniform fee schedule, the government is able to macro-manage provider behavior as well as national health care spending.

Physicians are clearly split into two groups. Generalist physicians are private solo practitioners providing primary and secondary care as small businesses, earning a substantial portion of their income from markups on pharmaceuticals and laboratory tests. Specialist physicians work in hospitals on salary and generally earn much less. Unlike in the United States, a patient undergoing surgery at a hospital in Japan receives a single bill that includes both room and board and the surgery fee. Surgeons are employees of hospitals and aren't allowed to charge patients independently. Some argue that this combined bill may be one reason that giving gifts to the doctor is a customary practice in Japan. Private practitioners cannot attend to hospitalized patients, and hospital physicians are not allowed to have a private practice on the side. The average private practice had revenues of 146 million yen and expenses of 122 million yen in 2001, making the average family doctors' income about 24 million yen (i.e., $200,000). This is three times the average annual income of salaried workers and much higher than the annual salary of $100,000 to $150,000 earned by hospital specialist doctors.

Japanese hospitals are also split into two groups. Large public and university hospitals contain medical schools and research facilities, and they may also have large outpatient departments providing primary care. Small facilities owned by private practitioners provide less sophisticated treatments and simple therapeutics. For-profit, investor-owned hospitals are prohibited in Japan. Controls over utilization are not stringent. There is no preauthorization for surgery, there is no requirement for a second opinion, and there is no statistical profiling or concurrent review as there is under managed care in the United States. With no limits imposed, length of stay tends to be very long—30.4 days for general acute hospitals and 377 days for psychiatric hospitals.

Universal health insurance coverage is obtained through myriad funding bodies, all regulated by the Ministry of Health, Labor, and Welfare (MHLW) (see Figure 13-6). Society-managed health insurance (SMHI) covers the employees of the large corporations. Corporations with a minimum of 700 employees may opt to establish their own health insurance societies as distinct legal entities whose assets are shielded from liabilities of the parent corporation. Approximately 1,800 such SMHI societies exist, and virtually all corporations known worldwide, such

Figure 13-6

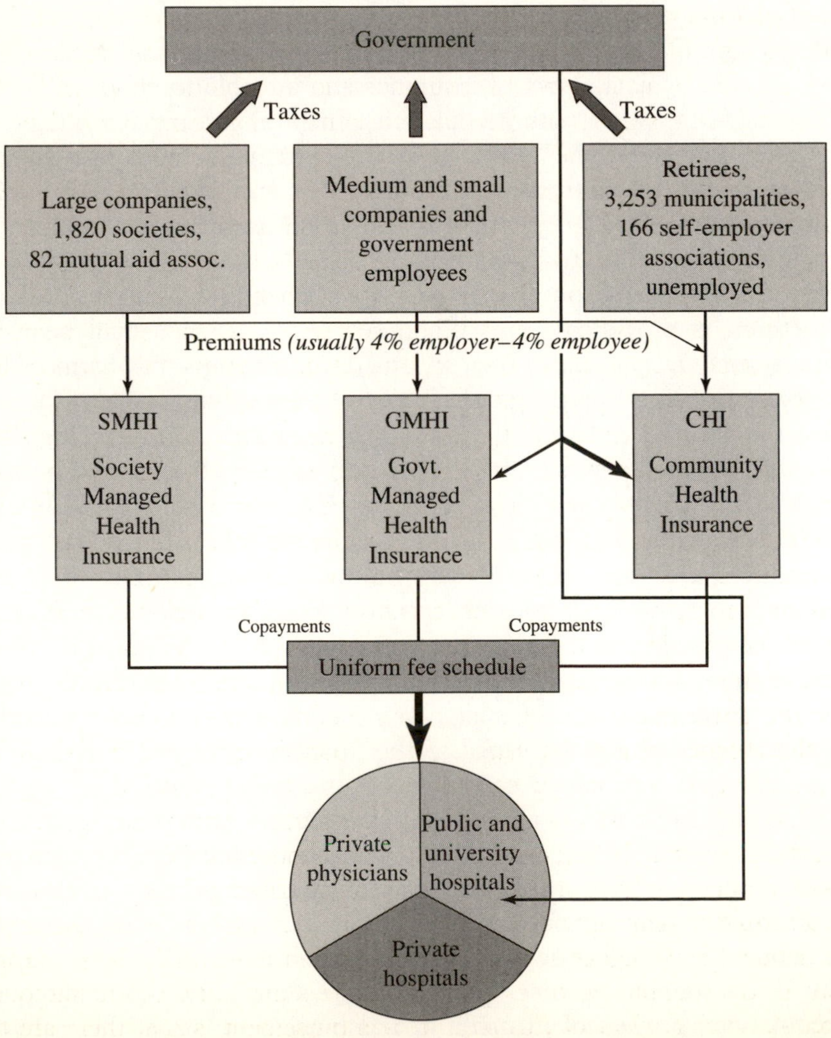

Flow of funds in the Japanese health care system.

as Sony and Toyota, have them. SMHI premiums are 6 to 9 percent of salary, split equally between the employer and the employee. Large-company employees tend to have the best salaries, with young workers (typical retirement age is 60) in good health, making these societies financially viable without subsidy. Small- and medium-sized corporations are covered by government-managed health insurance (GMHI). The premium for GMHI, 8.5 percent of salary, isn't sufficient to cover costs, and subsidies are provided through the MHLW.

The self-employed, the unemployed, retirees, and all others are covered by local community health insurance (CHI) plans administered by the 3,200 municipal governments (i.e., cities, towns, and villages ranging in size from a few hundred to several million people). Premiums for CHI are levied on household income but vary widely by municipality and are subject to a cap of $4,300 per household. Although enrollment in municipal CHI and payment of premiums is compulsory for all people not covered by SMHI or GMHI, about 10 percent of families default on payment, and penalties are rarely enforced because most defaulters have few assets. Most CHI spending is for health care of the elderly, whose incomes are small. Substantial subsidy (almost 50 percent) is required from the central government to maintain solvency of the CHI plans. Hence, although the Japanese health care finance system superficially resembles a large number of independent insurance pools, the extent of transfers and cross-subsidies means that these plans are linked through the MHLW into what is, in effect, a form of social insurance that equalizes medical purchasing power across all people.

In contrast to the fragmentation among insurance plans, reimbursement to providers is standardized, with little concern for differences in the type of facility, severity of illness, or geographic variance. The fee schedule and drug prices are set by the government every two years, after negotiation with the Japan Medical Association and insurance plans. These fees are administratively negotiated provider payments, not "prices," and are adjusted in response to political agreements, not changes in demand. For instance, the fee schedule implemented in 2002 introduced a 30 percent cut for hospitals whose surgical cases don't reach specified minimum numbers in each category, giving an obvious incentive to concentrate surgery in a smaller number of hospitals.

Because all reimbursement is regulated by the uniform fee schedule, it's possible for the government to exert rather rigid control over total expenditures, even in the absence of a global budget. The financial incentives regarding specialization and high technology are almost exactly the opposite of those in the United States, where doctors doing high-tech procedures garner the most prestige and the most income. In Japan, a doctor who chooses to become a specialist gets prestige but must give up the lucrative office-based primary care practice. The fee schedule system can reverse the dynamics of a market (where the services most in demand have higher prices, which in turn brings forth a larger supply). In Japan, if a procedure becomes popular, its fees are often cut to discourage provision. A notable effect of this shift in reimbursement is that there are two-thirds fewer surgical operations in Japan than in the United States.

FOR EXAMPLE

Cultural Attitudes Toward Care: Japan vs. the United States

Can you imagine a group of U.S. executives or lawyers suspecting their own heart failure being willing to wait patiently for hours in a public clinic to be served alongside the unemployed or accepting a situation in which two out of three who currently would be receiving a bypass graft or new pacemaker are sent home with pills instead? This is often the case in Japan. Then, when adversity strikes, can you further imagine that the American patients would not sue? The sources of such differences in attitude between the United States and Japan go beyond language, currency, and government. Although cultural studies lie a bit beyond the scope of this book, one can clearly see that culture profoundly affects the health systems of the two countries just by looking at the differences in physician salaries, relative differences in the uses of drugs versus invasive therapy, and ownership of facilities and equipment.

The structural flaw in Japan's universal health insurance system is that all employees will eventually retire and migrate to the underfunded CHI. Japan's complex and bureaucratic health care system has remained viable because of strong price regulation, constant economic growth, and a relatively young population. The Japanese system is a way of reaching equilibrium through consensus, which is vastly different from the sprawling mixture of regulated and competitive markets in the United States. However, the Japanese economy is stagnant and weakened by a long slump, the population is rapidly aging, and calls for deregulation are increasingly popular. How Japan copes with these daunting challenges will be one of the great social experiments in health economics.

SELF-CHECK

- Is income distribution a problem in high-income countries?
- What percentage of GDP do most high-income countries spend on health care? What percentage of GDP does the United States spend on health care?
- In high-income countries that are able to contain the costs of health care, do the restraints come from the demand side or the supply side?

13.7 International Trade in Health Care

Health care is among the world's largest industries, accounting for 10 percent of gross world product but only a tiny fraction of world trade. Products (e.g., drugs, equipment) are much more likely to be bought and sold across national boundaries than are services. Trade in services is usually limited to a small amount of border crossing, such as when a Canadian citizen disgruntled with a long wait for elective surgery crosses into the United States or an uninsured Hispanic worker from Texas crosses to Mexico for cheaper hospital and physician care. The part of the health care system most subject to international movement—trade in people and skills—doesn't appear in the world economic accounts.

13.7.1 Pharmaceuticals

The pharmaceutical trade is one of the world's truly global businesses (see Chapter 12). Drugs made in England or France cross pharmacy counters in the United States as readily as drugs made in Chicago, and research is as likely to be conducted in Genoa or Geneva as it is in Georgia. Companies cross international boundaries and link major markets. Protectionist legislation still gives local firms an advantage, but it's common for more than 25 percent of a large pharmaceutical company's sales to occur outside the country where it is headquartered, and some companies' sales are mostly international.

There are three major pharmaceutical markets in the world today:

1. Japan
2. The United States
3. The European Union

The ability of Japanese doctors to profit from prescribing gave them the highest rate of prescription drug use in the world. Thus, with only half as many consumers, the Japanese market was larger than the U.S. market in 1990 ($51 billion vs. $48 billion). However, the decade-long recession in Japan has caused a relative decline even though the percentage of health expenditures spent on drugs there still exceeds that in the United States (16.8 percent vs. 10.4 percent). The European Union accounted for about $40 billion, and all the developing low- and middle-income countries together accounted for $44 billion.[26] Only the major market countries have the research infrastructure and a protected domestic market of sufficient size to cover the massive fixed costs of discovering and testing new drugs. Many developing countries allow local companies to make copycat versions of brand-name drugs. Clinical tests constitute a sizable portion of drug companies' costs and provide an interesting opportunity for international trade. By carrying out trials in a foreign country, a firm may be able to significantly reduce the cost per patient of developing a drug and may face lower liability due to any adverse reactions the experimental drug might produce.

13.7.2 Equipment

Medical equipment is less open to international trade than pharmaceuticals because it can't simply be packed in a box and shipped. Skilled technicians are required to maintain and use these sophisticated devices, and the ongoing labor costs are much larger than the manufacturing costs. When a new technology is developed, it is usually produced and supported by a local firm or the local branch of a global firm within a few years.

13.7.3 Services

Health care is limited to national boundaries. The U.S. Medicare program doesn't pay for surgical operations in Mexico, nor does it cover Canadians who come to the United States. Therefore, the border-crossing trade in medical services that does occur is usually paid for privately. Private investment in the small fee-for-service or insured hospitals and clinics that exist alongside national health facilities in the United Kingdom, Sweden, and elsewhere is often international. Yet the true test of international trade in medical care looms in the proposals for full integration of service markets within the European Union. Under such a system, a Belgian patient might opt for heart surgery in one of the major Parisian hospitals, or a Swiss factory worker might decide to seek psychiatric care in Germany. To date, however, every country in the European Union has jealously guarded its health care system, and such freedom of choice is available only to a few employees of international companies.

13.7.4 People and Ideas

There is substantial movement of medical personnel and ideas across national boundaries. Most specialists in developing countries receive some of their training in Europe or the United States, bringing home skills of immense value.

The extraordinary increase in life expectancy that has swept the world is perhaps one of the greatest benefits of international trade. As public goods, information and scientific discoveries cannot be owned or charged for by a particular firm or country. What is somewhat surprising is the extent of trade in the reverse direction—doctors and nurses who come to work in the United States from low-income countries. More than 12 percent of all U.S. physicians are immigrant doctors. Similarly, a large number of licensed nurses were educated overseas. There are more Filipino nurses practicing in the United States and Canada than in the Philippines. This flow of highly trained labor from less-developed to more-developed countries has much to do with the labor supply and with the incentive structure created by the size of the market. Limits on the numbers of physicians and nurses imposed through the U.S. educational system mean that there is room for those who have received training overseas and are willing to work for less. Also, truly outstanding neurosurgeons are able to earn more in the United States than in Mexico and may be tempted to go where their skills command the highest reward—just as Latino baseball players and movie stars do. There's also a niche at the bottom of

FOR EXAMPLE

Telemedicine: Off-Shoring Medical Services

Radiologists are highly specialized physicians who are trained to read x-rays and MRI scans. And according to E. Stephen Amis, Jr., chair of the board of chancellors at the American College of Radiology and chair of radiology at Albert Einstein College of Medicine in the Bronx, there's a severe shortage of radiologists in the United States. "Demand for radiologists is growing at twice the rate that we're turning out the radiologists," Amis reported to the *New York Times*. In particular, hospitals have trouble filling positions for radiologists who are willing to work nights, handling x-rays and scans for middle-of-the-night emergencies. A few entrepreneurs have come up with a unique way to handle the shortage: Send the images via the Internet to radiologists working in countries where it's daytime during America's night, such as Australia and India. Unlike most other physicians, radiologists don't require close patient contact to do their job; all they need is access to the scans. These firms can't just hire anyone off the street, though; the radiologists must be licensed in the state in which the hospital is located, as well as by the hospital itself. And because Medicare doesn't pay for services provided outside the United States, the overseas radiologist does a preliminary reading, which is used to guide treatment during the night, but the final reading must be performed by a local staff radiologist, who then bills Medicare.[27]

the market that attracts foreign labor. Caring for the elderly in nursing homes is so demanding and underpaid that it's difficult to find competent staff willing to work for minimum wage. These positions are attractive to immigrants who are able to obtain steady employment and benefits in jobs that require a lot in the way of patience, endurance, and strength but not in language or education.

SELF-CHECK

- Which aspects of health care are most likely to be traded on the international market? Which are least likely?
- What percentage of the worldwide GDP does health care take up?
- What are some problems associated with selling medical equipment overseas?

SUMMARY

There is a tremendous disparity in health between rich and poor nations. The poor countries of sub-Saharan Africa have very little health care and low life expectancies. Many people there die before the age of 5. The wealthier countries of Europe, North America, and Japan have more health resources to be applied to much less need. People in these countries have a longer life expectancy, with most deaths occurring after age 70.

Average spending on health care is determined primarily by national income per capita, not the health needs of individuals. Increased per capita income is also a major factor explaining increased life expectancy. The United States is the world's largest health care market, accounting for 40 percent of all health expenditures, even though it has only 5 percent of the world's population. Significantly higher medical expenditures don't appear to have made U.S. citizens significantly healthier. U.S. life expectancy ranks about in the middle of developed high-income countries.

Lack of organization, maldistribution, and political instability are perhaps even more important than low income in causing poor health among many low-income countries. Even in middle- and high-income countries, many of the worst health problems result from the uneven distribution of health care and the inability to effectively target care to those most in need.

Cost control in Europe—that is, constraining supply and putting limits on the system as a whole—appears to have been more effective than in the United States. Japan's inexpensive health care system is much less technology-intensive than that of the United States, using only one-third as much surgery but more drugs.

There is very little international trade in health care services. Global trade in health care is dominated by pharmaceuticals. However, the invisible trade in knowledge and health professionals has the largest effect on national health care systems.

ASSESS YOUR UNDERSTANDING

Go to www.wiley.com/college/getzen to evaluate your knowledge of international health care.
Measure your learning by comparing pre-test and post-test results.

Summary Questions

1. Nations that spend more money on health care do so because they have greater health care needs. True or False?

2. One explanation for higher health spending in the United States is the standard of living, measured as GDP. Relative to other industrialized countries, health spending in the United States:

   (a) is approximately what would be predicted from the usual relationship between GDP and health spending.

   (b) is well above what would be predicted from the usual relationship between GDP and health spending.

   (c) is well below what would be predicted from the usual relationship between GDP and health spending.

   (d) seems to have an inverse relationship with GDP rather than the usual positive relationship.

3. In which of the following variables is the U.S. value the lowest relative to other major industrialized countries?

   (a) Health expenditures as a percentage of GDP

   (b) Proportion of the population covered by guaranteed insurance

   (c) Per capita health expenditures

   (d) Specialist physicians as a proportion of all physicians

4. Which statement best expresses the relationship between inequality and health?

   (a) The level of national income (i.e., GDP) determines the average level of health, and income distribution within the country is relatively unimportant.

   (b) The disparity in health spending among countries is smaller than the true disparity in health resources (e.g., doctors, nurses).

   (c) Although there are wide differences in the income levels of nations, there is relatively little variation among nations in per capita health spending after adjusting for local price levels.

   (d) For a given average per capita income, average health levels are higher where there is greater equality of income within a country.

5. Which of the following is *not* a reason why European countries have generally been able to keep per capita health care costs so much lower than has the United States?

   (a) Most European countries have concentrated their controls on the supply side, constraining the system rather than demand for services.

   (b) The number and pay of health care workers are often subject to national or regional bargaining.

   (c) Europeans have been more willing to accept lower health outcome levels, probably because of their experience of war and deprivation.

   (d) Purchase and use of expensive diagnostic and therapeutic technology has been restricted.

6. International trade in the health sector:

   (a) is largest in the area of personal services because people living close to borders routinely cross over to receive care (e.g., Canadians coming to the United States for elective surgery).

   (b) rarely involves pharmaceuticals because the licensing and patent laws in different countries make firms worry about losing their research investment.

   (c) mostly involves public health because governments find it easier to work out the issues than do private contractors.

   (d) often involves movement of professionals (e.g., physicians, nurses) either for training or practice.

Review Questions

1. How many people are there in the world today? What fraction of them live in high-income developed economies? What fraction of total health expenditure is accounted for by high-income countries?

2. How much is spent per person on health care in Kenya? How much is spent per person on health care in the United States? In Mexico? What are the primary factors accounting for these differences?

3. What is the largest global health care market?

4. Is the relative inequality in the distribution of health greater between countries or within countries? What could be used as evidence to support your answer?

5. It's clear that national health expenditures rise with income per capita. Do health outcomes improve in the same way?

6. Why is the status of women particularly important as a determinant of health in low-income countries? Why would this change (or at least not be as detectable) as a country's per capita income rises?

7. In Japan, specialists generally earn much less than generalist physicians, the reverse of the situation in the United States. What accounts for this reversal?

8. Although all the industrialized wealthy economies share some difficulty in controlling health care expenditures, it appears that European countries have done better on average than the United States. What are the principal differences in strategies for controlling expenditures?

9. Which types of health care labor are most likely to be traded between countries? Why?

10. Which types of health care goods are most likely to be traded between countries? Are there more or fewer barriers to trade in health care than in other sectors?

Applying This Chapter

1. As an officer of the World Health Organization with a budgetary allocation of $100 million, which programs would you fund if you wanted to make the greatest impact on health, measured as the increase in life expectancy multiplied by the number of people affected?

2. Patents on pharmaceuticals encourage manufacturers to invest in research and development of new drugs because a patent guarantees the manufacturer exclusive rights to sell the drug for a set number of years. However, patents also restrict competition and artificially inflate prices, sometimes pricing them out of the reach of poor people or forcing people to forgo other basic goods and services in order to purchase life-saving medicines. How should this conflict between economics and ethics be resolved?

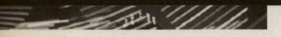

YOU TRY IT

Outsourcing Medical Services

An increasing number of jobs in the medical field are being performed overseas. Jobs being outsourced are frequently "back office" jobs, such as medical transcription, medical coding, and hospital collections. Write a brief essay discussing the potential economic benefits and downsides of such job outsourcing.

Restricting the Sale of Drugs

It's a common practice for pharmaceutical companies to limit the release of new and improved versions of drugs to high-income countries such as the United States and Germany, while delaying the release to low-income countries such as Kenya and Haiti. Yet, it's often the case that patients in less developed countries need the drugs just as much as patients in wealthy countries. Write a paper, explaining why you think pharmaceutical companies would restrict the sale of new drugs to high-income countries.

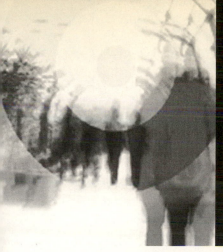

14

DYNAMICS OF HEALTH SPENDING
The Present and Future of Health Care Economics

Starting Point

Go to www.wiley.com/college/getzen to assess your knowledge of the dynamics of health spending.
Determine where you need to concentrate your effort.

What You'll Learn in This Chapter

▲ The difference between individual and national perspectives on health care spending
▲ The dynamics of health system changes
▲ The history of cost-control regulations
▲ The role of labor in health care spending
▲ The economic analysis of decision making
▲ Issues involving the allocation of health care resources
▲ The future of health care

After Studying This Chapter, You'll Be Able To

▲ Assess health care from micro and macro perspectives
▲ Estimate the time it takes various sectors of the health care field to respond to changes in the economy
▲ Evaluate the effectiveness of cost-control regulations
▲ Assess the process of health care decision making
▲ Evaluate the efficiency of the economy in allocating resources
▲ Predict key issues in the future of health care in the United States

INTRODUCTION

This chapter considers one of the most important questions facing health care economists and policy makers in general: How much of a nation's wealth should be devoted to health care? One problem that plagues any attempt to address national health care policy is the time it takes for health care spending to respond to major economic changes, such as a drop in gross domestic product (GDP) or inflation. Policy makers attempt to control costs by imposing regulations on the health care system, but because of the slow pace of economic change, it's difficult to know whether regulations are necessary or even effective. An added problem is that most health care spending is for labor, so cost containment measures often involve cutting wages or laying off personnel, which are always unpopular actions.

In addition to examining perspectives on spending, the dynamics of change within the health system, cost-control regulations, and labor costs, this chapter summarizes the contribution and role of economic analysis in health services, largely by focusing on the types of questions that can be addressed by economics. Finally, the chapter concludes with a brief look at what will likely be trends in health care economics in the years to come.

14.1 Individual and Societal Perspectives on Spending

Looking at health care spending from an individual perspective, or what economists call a micro perspective, and from a community, or macro, perspective can be revealing. Consider hospital expenses:

▲ From the point of view of an individual, there are no hospital expenses unless one is admitted for treatment.

▲ From the point of view of the community, there are expenses regardless of the number of patients receiving treatment on a particular day. The hospital must be maintained, the laundry washed, staff paid, and magnetic resonance imaging (MRI) devices serviced. As a matter of fact, only a small fraction of the total cost of hospital care (e.g., drugs and supplies, food, nursing overtime) varies with the number of patients. Most costs are relatively fixed.

An individual assumes that if he or she becomes sick and needs hospitalization, the care will be provided. However, if all hospital beds are full, the next patient cannot be admitted, and the hospital must displace someone whose need for the bed is less pressing. A **capacity constraint,** or the fact that there aren't enough services to meet demand, limits the total amount of resources available. Similarly, if twice as many people in the United States got sick next winter as this winter, the nation couldn't suddenly substantially increase the number of doctors.

> ### FOR EXAMPLE
>
> #### Capacity Constraints
>
> To get a better grasp of capacity constraints, consider what happens when people try to win a gold medal at the Olympics. While additional training and effort can increase the probability that any individual can win the gold, for the group as a whole, the number of medals is fixed—there is only one gold. If everyone tries harder or trains more, there's no corresponding increase in medals. Similarly, studying harder may increase one student's chances of getting into Harvard medical school, but whether all applicants study harder doesn't affect the number of medical students at Harvard next year. Many resources have capacity constraints, and the factors that determine individual and group consumption are not connected. If there are 10 hearts available for transplant, then only 10 people can get heart transplants. Being young, being a better match with donor tissue, having better insurance, and having political connections can all help an individual increase his or her personal chance of getting a transplant, but for the group as whole, the number of transplants is fixed.

To some extent, each doctor would work harder and see more patients, but the capacity constraint means that for the most part, this surge in demand would be met by doctors giving each patient fewer minutes of attention, keeping some patients who are mildly ill from making return visits, and other adjustments.

Health insurance shows the same disparity between individual and group perspectives. To an individual, medical expenses resulting from an accident are something the insurance plan has to pay; the person's personal insurance premiums are fixed and paid in advance. Yet from the point of view of the group, all expenses must be paid out of premiums. If more accidents than anticipated occur, a premium increase for all group members is required, or the insurance plan becomes insolvent.[1]

For most countries, including the United States, funding is national in scope. Thus, we don't expect to see major differences in health care as we cross the border from Texas into Arizona, or in Mexico as we cross the border from Sonora into Chihuahua. Yet crossing the national border from Arizona into Sonora or Texas into Chihuahua reveals a vast disparity in the use of medical resources, costs, and prices.

Disparities in health care of this sort were once found within a single country. At the end of the nineteenth century, for example, New Yorkers living on Park Avenue and those living in the tenements of lower Manhattan occupied different social and medical worlds. To some extent, disparities still exist within each country today—for instance, between the suburbs and the inner city or between the mainstream medicine provided to most Americans and the care available to residents of isolated Native American reservations in the United States. The crucial determinant of the health care available to a group of people is the amount of resources available to that group, often measured by average income per capita. The essential question then becomes, What is a group? Why are Mexican-Americans living in San Diego getting more medical care than their relatives and friends across the border in Tijuana? Why are some Indian tribes not sharing in the wealth of the average American? Defining who is and who is not part of a group determines who does and who does not have access to health care.

SELF-CHECK

- List two different perspectives on health care spending.
- Is a country's health care spending usually based on an individual or national perspective?

14.2 Dynamics of Health System Change

If per capita income falls, health care spending must also fall. Yet it's impossible to make this economic adjustment all at once. Usually, the country goes into debt during the transitional period. Even for an individual, adjustments to changes in income are not instantaneous. If you were to lose your job today, you wouldn't immediately move into a smaller apartment, drive an older car, or wear less fashionable clothes. In fact, if you lose your job today, you'll probably go out and spend a little extra money to keep up your spirits. Next week, you'll cut back, but not too much, because you probably expect to find another job soon. If you're still out of work six months later, you'll find that your clothes and your house and your car start getting shabby, and you might think about downsizing your lifestyle. After you get a new job, it will take time to build your savings back up.

When college students graduate and begin to earn good wages, they find it easy to live and save part of their salary because their lifestyles are still somewhat geared to being a student. Consumption for the newly employed doesn't usually rise as fast as their incomes rise. During this "I can't figure out how to spend it all" period, savings accumulate. Later on, with a fancy lifestyle suitable for a young stockbroker or lawyer, they find it difficult to see how one could have lived on so little money as a student, or even on what they earned three years before. Consumption is geared to expected income, whether $15,000 or $150,000. The amount of income saved depends not so much on how high the income is but on transitional (i.e., permanent income/life cycle) factors and the extent to which a person is willing to give up current pleasures for retirement or future consumption. If a young lawyer who has just bought a new Mercedes loses his job, he will discover one of the underlying and seemingly unfair truths of human behavior: It's a lot easier and more fun to adjust spending upward than downward.

Economists can study the pace change by looking at the dynamics of health spending. **Dynamics** is the study of how things change over time, so a study of the dynamics of health spending analyzes how changes in health care spending occur over time rather than simply what is true at a single point in time. The focus on dynamics reminds us of the importance of the speed of adjustment when designing policy or forecasting the impact of policy or other shocks to the system.

The dynamics of adjustment for individuals (micro) and for nations (macro) are similar, except that macro adjustments usually take longer because the system as a whole must change. People who still have their jobs must be convinced that it's necessary to cut back, to reduce the provision of public goods, or to change the tax code. Achieving a consensus to alter organizations and revise institutional structures is extremely time-consuming. The health care system, based on professional ethics, institutional obligations, and shared public values and reliant on a complex set of public and private financing mechanisms, is even more difficult to change than most other sectors of the economy. Health care lags behind other sectors in adjusting to economic conditions.

How long does it take for health care to adjust? From one to five years, on average, but some parts of the system take even longer. For example, even if everyone in Congress decided today that we need more health care or less health care, this decision couldn't be carried out for months, and its full effects would take years to work their way through the system.

FOR EXAMPLE

Timing the Expansion of Physician Supply

Suppose that policy makers decide we need to increase the number of physicians practicing in this country. It takes at least a year to enroll more students in medical school, and it takes much longer to build new medical schools. Medical students take four years to graduate and another three or four years to complete residencies and enter practice. Thus, eight years after a decision to expand a medical school has been made, there are still no extra doctors in practice. Something might be done to reduce the rate of retirement, but effectively, the quantity of doctors in practice who graduated in a particular year in the past was fixed once they left school. Thus, it took until 1985, 20 years after the Health Professions Educational Assistance Act of 1963, before the expansion in physician supply was a real force in the market—and by then Congress had changed its mind. Similarly, it takes 40 years, until all graduating physicians have retired, before the full effects of such decisions work through the system.

Some aspects of health care can be adjusted more quickly than others. Whereas it can take several years to increase the number of physicians, the supply of nurses is much more flexible because, typically, there are many licensed nurses who are temporarily not working or working part time; therefore, an increase or a decrease in demand is quickly translated into a change in the numbers employed. Clerical, maintenance, and other less-specialized labor adjusts even more smoothly and rapidly because people can move between health services and other sectors of the economy in response to changing conditions. The average adjustment period for all medical spending is 2.7 years.[2] Here's how quickly some key components of the health care system adjust:

▲ Hospitals, the largest component of health care expenditure, are quite rigidly institutionalized and dependent on public or third-party financing. As one would expect, they take a bit longer to adjust, 3.0 years.

▲ Physician services are somewhat more flexible and adjust a bit more quickly, with a lag of 2.5 years.

▲ Spending on drugs, much of which depends on direct consumer decisions and is paid for out-of-pocket with current income, takes only 1.3 years.

▲ Long term care, a mixture of flexible personal spending and rather inflexible Medicaid spending, adjusts in 2.5 years, on average.

▲ Construction, at 3.5 years, takes the longest to adjust. Capital must be accumulated in advance to fund new construction, and the decision to build depends on long-run future economic considerations, not just revenues and expenses today.

The time required to adjust also depends, in part, on the magnitude of the change. A massive revision of the system, such as that which occurred in 1965 with the introduction of Medicare and Medicaid, may take several decades to complete. In fact, some argue that one reason health spending is so high in the United States is because the country is still using a health care system constructed on the lines of the Great Society envisioned during the 1960s, when economic growth was steady and strong. This system isn't appropriate to the more constrained conditions and budget deficits prevailing in 2007.

What are the consequences of slow adjustment in the health care sector? Importantly, it buffers the economy. During a downturn, Medicare and Medicaid spending usually continue; therefore, health care workers are less likely to lose their jobs than workers in the farming, housing, or financial services sectors.[3]

The delay in adjustment can also have adverse budgetary consequences. Because spending continues to rise in a recession, even though government tax revenues fall, a deficit builds up. In theory, such periods of excess spending average out over time with underspending during periods of rapid growth. However, it's easier to obtain agreement to pour money into the health care sector and save jobs during a recession than it is to hold back and save money during good times.

Politicians want to get elected. They need results that will affect the economy and the voters in the near term. Extra government spending during a recession meets these needs; extra saving when the economy starts to grow again usually doesn't. It's difficult to get politicians to behave in a way that benefits the long-term public interest because it's difficult to get voters to behave that way. One consequence of this is well known: a U.S. deficit of a trillion dollars. Eventually, just like the out-of-work lawyer running up his charge cards, we will have to bring spending back into line and balance the budget. But that is in the long term, and the elections keep coming up quickly.

SELF-CHECK

- Which is faster: adjustment time for health care for nations or that of individuals? Briefly explain why.
- On average, how long does it take the health care system to adjust?
- List one negative and one positive consequence of the slow adjustment time for health care.

14.3 Controlling Health Costs: The Push to Regulate

Analysts have questioned why a cost-control policy that seems so successful in one instance, or so successful among individuals or physicians or hospitals alone, fails to reduce total costs. It's because the consequences of income for spending are established only at the level where the budget constraint is fixed. For some types of health care, this is the individual household, and for others, it's the hospital, region, or the insurance plan, but for much of medicine, the national budget constraint is most relevant.

The lagging response of the health care sector to economic changes makes management easier in one respect: Budget forecasts are usually accurate because the system is slow to change, and much of the movement over the next few years reflects what has already occurred in the broader economic indicators, such as the consumer price index (CPI) and GDP. However, this same inertia also makes it difficult to balance the budget. In a recession, expenditures continue to

---

FOR EXAMPLE

Washington's Recession and Subsequent Cost Controls

In 1965, Washington was a robustly growing state with above-average per capita income, 108 percent of the U.S. average. Growth continued in 1966 and 1967, with per capita income rising above 110 percent of the U.S. average and the state population growing 3 percent per year, as people migrated to the state to look for good jobs, particularly in the aerospace industry. Growth slowed in 1968 and again in 1969, before the recession caused real per capita incomes to fall in 1970 and 1971. Boeing, which accounted for one in four jobs in metropolitan Seattle, eventually laid off half its workforce. Local businesses were devastated, and many retail stores closed. In 1972, the state population declined and per capita income fell to the U.S. average. The state suffered a fiscal crisis as tax revenues fell. In 1973, the legislature passed an act creating the mandatory Hospital Rate Review Commission that was among the toughest in the nation. In 1974, hospital expenditures per capita declined 2.8 percent in real inflation-adjusted terms.

A dynamic model that incorporates lagging income and inflation effects shows that the decline resulted from a delayed response to the severe state recession, not from regulation. Hospital expenditures would have declined anyway because of the recession, even if the legislature had failed to pass any acts. Eventually, the state legislature came to the same conclusion, and the hospital rate commission was disbanded. If the researchers responsible for the initial analysis of the cost commission had been able to wait 10 years for more information, they would have concluded that the controls didn't have much effect because the level of per capita hospital expenditures in Washington was essentially unchanged relative to projected levels or the U.S. average in 1990 compared with 1973.

---

climb, even as revenues fall. The budgetary gaps created by delays in the adjustment of spending to changing economic conditions may force governments to put cost controls on health care. Almost every inflationary spike or sharp recession is followed by a new attempt to regulate hospital rates, ration health care, establish price controls, cap revenues, or use another method to stem rising costs.

Legislatures don't get together to pass cost-control measures for health care because the economy is doing well. Economic crises bring about a call for legislatures to do something, but these crises eventually push spending down, regardless of whether legislatures act. The ability of politicians to dictate spending independent of the rest of the economy is limited, particularly during the next one to four years. Incomplete adjustment to inflation and recession is apt to simultaneously exert pressure on legislatures to do something about excessive health care costs and force future spending downward, thus often creating a questionable correlation between the enactment of regulation and the temporary moderation in costs.

14.3.1 An Example of Price Controls: The "ESP" Program

America's economic growth slowed toward the end of the 1960s, and a recession occurred in 1970. Unlike previous recessions, however, with this one, there was no moderation in prices. This combination of slow or negative GDP growth with high inflation, called *stagflation,* rudely ended the dream of permanent stability and prosperity. President Nixon stepped in to impose shock therapy, in the form of wage and price controls with the Economic Stabilization Program (ESP), on August 15, 1971. In retrospect, the U.S. experience from 1971 to 1975 served mostly to confirm the lessons learned from wage and price controls imposed by other governments around the world over the past two millennia: Controls were routinely evaded, and prices shot up as soon as the controls ended in April 1974.

Yet at the time, the public, government officials, and even many economists thought that price controls on health care had been successful. They thought so because there was a clear moderation during 1971 in both nominal and real health care costs from the 1966–1970 trends, falling from 11.1 percent to 9.3 percent and from 6.1 percent to 3.5 percent, respectively. The dip was even more pronounced for the narrower measure of hospital costs, which grew 8.3 percent in 1970 but only 3.4 percent in 1971.[4] Comparing trends before and after introduction of ESP makes it appear that the controls were effective in reducing spending, yet most of the decline would have occurred anyway due to the slowdown in GDP growth and lagging adjustment to a rapid increase in inflation.

14.3.2 A Second Example: The VE to Control Costs

After the expiration of ESP, health care costs were freed from external economy-wide controls, although they continued to be regulated by cost reimbursement rules (see Chapters 5 and 8). Medicare, in particular, attempted to constrain costs, but without notable success. In April 1977, President Carter made a legislative proposal to regulate hospital revenues. The hospital industry was strongly opposed to the measure and formed the Voluntary Effort (VE) coalition of providers and payers in December 1977. Flyers and buttons were printed to promote voluntary efforts to reduce the rate of cost increases. The VE coalition set a national target for holding cost increases to 2 percent less than the previous rate, or to 3 percent above the rate of inflation. Hospital price increases did moderate in 1978 and 1979, and VE's proponents loudly proclaimed the effectiveness of the plan. In November 1979, Congress cited these claims in debate before soundly defeating Carter's legislation to regulate hospital revenues.

This tale of voluntary regulation would normally have been forgotten and relegated to footnotes, but the story lingered on because claims of effectiveness were uncritically accepted. The claims of VE's success appear plausible until the data are examined more closely. Hospital costs had already begun falling in 1977, before VE. They declined further in 1978 and were below the target. Even VE believers referred to the American Hospital Association's luck because the VE coalition didn't even convene a meeting until December 1977 and, therefore, had no time to directly affect hospital behavior that year. The financial reports on which the 1978 National Health Expenditures (NHE) figures were based came mostly from hospitals whose fiscal years ran from July 1, 1977, to June 30, 1978. For these hospitals, fiscal year 1978 was half over before the VE coalition met.

Luck, however, was only one factor in the "success" of VE. The main reason that nominal health care expenses were lower than expected was that hospital wages and supply prices hadn't yet caught up with the surge of inflation that began in 1977. There was no decline in hospitals' use of real inputs (e.g., labor full-time equivalents, supply items); there was only a delay in price adjustment that made nurses and technicians temporarily inexpensive. In 1979, however, there was a real decline in health care spending. Nominal expenditures per capita rose by only 10.8 percent, 0.5 percent less than the year before. This drop placed spending almost 2 percent below the predicted value. Was this a real VE effect? Probably not. VE was a program promoted by the hospital industry to control *hospital* expenditures. Therefore, the effect of VE should have been greatest in the hospital sector, resulting in a lower rate of increase in hospital spending than nonhospital spending, which wasn't under the purview of VE. In fact, the opposite was the case: Nonhospital expenditures rose more slowly in 1979, at less than half the rate of hospital expenditures.

14.3.3 A Third Example: The Medicare Prospective Payment System with DRGs

In October 1983, Medicare radically changed its method of paying hospitals from cost reimbursement to a new prospective payment system (PPS) based on the expected cost of each admission, categorized into diagnosis-related groups (DRGs). This new cost-control plan did work, in some ways. There was a significant reduction in the rate of increase in Medicare Part A (inpatient) expenses and in hospital expenses generally. However, this was accomplished primarily by hospitals shifting services to outpatient and day surgery categories covered under Medicare Part B. Total health care expenditures per capita continued to rise at historically high rates (see Figure 14-1). In 1985, 16.9 percent of the $407.2 billion spent on health care was paid for by the federal government, and by 1990, the fraction actually increased to 17.7 percent of the $643.4 billion spent that year, even though reduction in the federal deficit was an explicit objective of the Medicare legislation. PPS clearly had a large effect on the health care system. Administrators and doctors panicked, employment was (temporarily) held below trends, and the average length of stay for patients fell sharply. However, there were no long-run reductions in the total costs of health care.[5]

Figure 14-1

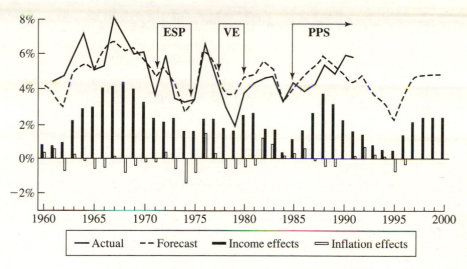

Health spending and price controls, 1960–1990.

14.3.4 Why Do People Believe Cost Controls Work?

The idea that ESP, VE, and PPS regulations were "effective" in reducing expenditures lingers because a superficial before-and-after comparison in each case showed a decline in spending that the public and legislators could understand, and it was quickly reported in the newspapers. People didn't recognize that these declines were delayed effects of the adverse economic conditions that had caused the regulations to be proposed in the first place. Also, the declines in spending in one reimbursement category (e.g., Medicare Part A) due to regulations look like effective cost controls until it's realized that these costs were just shifted to another area (Part B). A more human reason for the persistence of this belief is that many analysts and politicians worked thousands of hours to draft and implement these regulations, becoming so personally committed that it was hard for them to accept that so much well-intentioned effort had so little effect over the long run.[6]

Health care expenditures are never too high or too low in an absolute sense; rather, they are out of line with the spending that can be afforded under current economic conditions. A theory of health care cost regulation must start with the realization that shared costs, and governmental expenditures in particular, are always regulated, even when no external regulatory agency is in operation. Furthermore, costs can be ratcheted up or down within the existing framework by making administrative procedures tighter or looser, even if no legislation is passed. Regulation is always an essential part of health care system management in a modern nation.

SELF-CHECK

- List three ways the government has tried to regulate costs in the past 40 years.
- Explain the effectiveness of these cost-control measures.

14.4 "Spending" Is Mostly Labor

What does it mean to control costs? Because health services are mostly labor, costs are primarily a function of the number of people employed in the health sector and the wages (or professional incomes) they are paid. Cost control must be employment control. Yet it's easier for politicians to say that they will control costs than to say that they will have people laid off or cut wages, which is one reason there is so much more rhetoric than action in health care cost control.

Every occupation within the health services field has its supply and demand most strongly influenced by the particulars of licensure statutes and relations with the dominant medical profession. Yet what is true of each of the parts is not true of the whole. Most of the growth in health employment comes from adding new occupational categories rather than by expanding numbers within an existing occupation.

14.4.1 Employment

Employment in health care has grown more than twice as rapidly as total U.S. employment over the past 100 years: 3.4 percent versus 1.5 percent for the period 1900–2000. Consequently, the share of total employment accounted for by health care has increased from 1.2 percent in 1900 to 7.7 percent (i.e., 1 out of every 13 workers) now. The average annual growth rate of this sector between 1958 and 2002 was 4.8 percent—more than double the annual average growth of total U.S. employment. During this period, health care sector employment never contracted, in contrast to total employment, which experienced four major contractionary episodes. Health care employment shows less fluctuation because it adjusts more slowly and gradually to economic shocks.[7]

Although the enactment of Medicare and Medicaid in 1965 created a fundamental change in reimbursement and flow of money into the system and was ultimately responsible for a rise of more than 10 percent in the number of health care jobs, it had no visible effect on health employment during 1965 or 1966. Not until 1967 did employment begin to soar, leaping 3.7 percent above the trend in that year, 2.4 percent in 1968, 1.2 percent in 1969, 0.6 percent in 1970, and 0.4 percent in 1971. The average lag between the enactment of Medicare and the creation of an additional job was 3.5 years.

FOR EXAMPLE

Hospital Employment Data

The Bureau of Labor Statistics (BLS) records employment within industries by Standard Industrial Classification (SIC) codes and has identified health care services (SIC 808) as a category since 1958, providing annual observations since that year. (SIC 80806 is the subcategory "hospital employment.") The BLS data are based on the SIC code of the employer; therefore, a nurse, medical technician, or doctor employed at a manufacturing firm wouldn't be counted as a health care employee, but a hospital secretary would be.

14.4.2 Wages

From 1980 to 2002, while real wages in the rest of the economy were essentially flat (rising by less than 2 percent), average health care wages rose by 26 percent, and the increases for hospital employees and self-employed physicians were even greater. There does not appear to be any consistent correlation between economic growth (i.e., GDP) and health care wages. Other than the apparent surge due to Medicare, no government policy appears to have significantly altered the health care wage trend. The adjustment of health care wages to changes in the rate of inflation is slow.

Real health expenditures per capita in the United States grew 5 percent per year from 1960 to 2002, outpacing the 2 percent rate of growth in per capita incomes and thus consuming an ever-larger share of GDP. The labor portion of this 5 percent annual increase can be broken down into a 4 percent increase in employment and a 1 percent annual increase in real wages[8]; therefore, increased intensity of medical services and more nurses, perfusionists, occupational therapists, and so on per patient day, is by far the more important cause of increased spending over this time span. However, since 1980, excessive compensation growth in the health care sector relative to the rest of the economy has accounted for a significant proportion of spending increases. With both wages and employment increasing faster than in other occupations, it may well be that health care professionals are getting more than a fair share of the nation's economic growth.

Although the power of licensed health professions to control entry and wages is a major cause of delayed adjustment, it's not the only one. The dominance of not-for-profit firms and third-party financing is also an important factor in creating labor market rigidity. Health services in the United States are currently undergoing significant institutional changes. The pattern of slow and delayed adjustment over the past 40 years indicates that the ultimate outcome of these changes will not be revealed for a considerable period of time.

SELF-CHECK

- What is the largest category of health care spending?
- Have the wages of health care workers grown more slowly or more quickly than those of the average U.S. worker?

14.5 Forcing the Question: Who Gets Healthy and Who Gets Paid?

The most important contribution economists can make to the operation of the health care system is to be relentless in pointing out that every choice involves a trade-off—that certain difficult questions regarding who gets what and who must give up what are inevitable and must be faced, even when politicians, the public, and patients would rather avoid them.

Health economists give economic advice, not patient care. They estimate, evaluate, and explain the decisions to be made, but they don't make the decisions or carry them out. This analysis of decision making can be thought of in terms of three levels:

1. What are the questions?
2. Who makes the decisions?
3. What are the answers?

FOR EXAMPLE

What, How, and for Whom?

In the words of Paul Samuelson, "Every economy must answer a triad of questions: *what, how,* and *for whom.*"[9] In the case of cancer, one could ask what symptoms or diagnoses are to be treated? On an inpatient or outpatient basis? By generalists or specialists? Who is to receive first priority for treatment (e.g., those who plan ahead and show up first, who are most ill, who are most likely to recover, or who are best insured?). Although these questions can be asked independently, the answer to one question influences all the others: *for whom* affects *what* and *how,* and vice versa. Any answer also determines who pays, who gets paid, and how much; that is, it determines the distribution of income as well as the distribution of health care.

14.5.1 The Most Basic Level of Economic Analysis: What Are the Answers?

For most economists, it's necessary to work backward, starting with the data collection required to make comparisons among different treatments (i.e., cost–benefit analysis), considering how different systems for making medical care decisions can affect efficiency (e.g., indemnity insurance vs. managed care, network providers vs. solo providers), and then framing the questions. Tracing the flow of money over the first 13 chapters of this text reveals that while the data are important for understanding the system, the questions are fundamentally economic; they are about choices and thus have to do with values as well as numbers. Are some lives worth more than others? How much should a surgeon be paid for a one-hour operation if it saves a life? Which product of the health care system is more important—social justice or cancer mortality?

14.5.2 The Second Level of Economic Analysis: Who Makes the Decisions?

At a second level of analysis, economists are concerned with how to design a better health care system. At this level, the question isn't whether radiation is better than chemotherapy but whether capitation or fee-for-service payment leads to better decisions or whether group practice is more efficient than solo practice. The focus shifts from the particular decision being made to the issue of who is making the decision—physicians, patients, or payers.

14.5.3 The Third Level of Economic Analysis: What Are the Questions?

As economists trace how the flow of money follows the path of decision making, they begin to tease out the assumptions embedded in the current medical care system. Analysis at this third level becomes reflective: What does "better" mean? according to which value system? better for whom? Analysis transcends the current system as it is by asking What are the questions? Reaching beyond the veil of money and grasping the concept that every dollar spent on health care is a dollar earned by a health care provider makes it clear how the distribution of income and health are connected.

SELF-CHECK

- Briefly explain what it means to say that every decision involves a trade-off.
- Identify three levels of economic analysis.

14.6 Spending Money or Producing Health?

The distribution of health is unequal and has a profound impact on economic well-being. Some people work productively for years and die contentedly with wealth and happiness in old age, while others struggle for a few months or decades in agony as they are relentlessly drawn down into premature mortality. The question isn't whether the distribution of health is fair, or whether it determines or is determined by income, but whether it can be changed. More precisely, the questions are as follows:

▲ How can change be brought about by spending more on medical care? How much?
▲ What is that change worth?

The marginal productivity of medical care spending declines as more is spent. Increasing spending from $4,000 to $5,000 per person increases average life expectancy, but not by as much as increasing spending from $2,000 to

---

FOR EXAMPLE

Reaching a Consensus on Health Care Spending

Reaching a consensus on how much to spend becomes more complicated when there are two or more types of people who are to receive care. Suppose one group is relatively healthy and would maintain a high level of health, even if no money were spent on them, while another group begins at a disadvantage and, even with maximal effort, would still remain less healthy. If the same amount is spent per person on each group, the total and marginal impact of medical care will be very low in the healthy group, which seems wasteful, while the sicker group would still be forced to do without a lot of potentially beneficial care. To maximize the average healthiness of all people for a given health care budget, it would be necessary to equalize the marginal productivity of medical care (increase in health per additional dollar spent) across both groups, spending much more per person on the sicker people. Such an allocation of medical care resources might seem both fair and efficient, but it also might not. Suppose the healthy group consisted of employed people who paid insurance premiums while the sicker group were heroin and cocaine users. Most voters wouldn't be willing to cut funding for those who take care of themselves and go to work every day in order to provide more funding to people who stick needles in their arms. Further complications are posed by groups such as infants born with genetic defects who are likely to die young even with the best medical care. Should they be denied treatment on the grounds that it would not do them much good anyway?

$3,000, which, in turn, doesn't have as large an effect as going from $0 to $1,000. As more and more money is spent, fewer and fewer gains are achieved in life expectancy.

Although stating that the goal of medical care is to maximize health seems accurate and appropriate, a little reflection (or reading the first 13 chapters of this text) shows how inaccurate and irrelevant such a measure often is. If taken literally, maximizing health would mean that most hospitals in the United States would close so that more food, clothes, books, and medicine could be provided to China, India, Mozambique, and other less developed countries. It would also force most surgeons to give up their operating rooms in favor of sewage treatment plants, and force psychiatrists to give up the provision of therapy and the prescription of psychoactive drugs in favor of immunization campaigns and early childhood education. Stating that the goal of medical care is to maximize health for all is not only inaccurate but profoundly misleading. It confuses a measure of social welfare with the incentives of the groups that make up society to maximize their own welfare. Doctors, nurses, hospital supply company executives, National Basketball Association players, healthy industrial workers, college students, and other definable groups have multiple objectives, including the health of their families and their own incomes, many of which are more important to them than the advancement of global health.

It's relatively easy to understand why most Americans don't want all their hospitals to close and why most of the doctors who work in them are not eager to practice in Mozambique, even if they are certain that the number of additional life years produced would be higher. It's less obvious why Americans keep spending more and more on medical care if technological advances are making medicine more productive and efficient. Given that the baseline life expectancy at birth, even in the absence of medical care, is much higher now than it was a century ago, each year of life expectancy added becomes more difficult and more expensive to obtain; therefore, marginal productivity (i.e., gain in life expectancy per additional dollar spent) is much lower today than it was 50 or 100 years ago. If society optimized by choosing the point at which the value of health matched the price of health, and the value of health were the same, then less money would be spent as technology improved. Instead, we now spend more per person, implying that the incremental increase in health per additional dollar is even smaller. From the comparisons with Japan and England in Chapter 13, it appears that it would be possible to cut spending by one-third or more, with only a minor decrease in health, leaving average life expectancy in the United States almost unchanged.

It must be recognized that medical care has become largely a consumption good. Economists don't seek to explain increased spending on clothes in terms of warmth or durability or on gourmet takeout food in terms of calories and nutritional content, and they shouldn't try to explain all of the increase in medical expenditures in terms of health or life expectancy. Although it may seem inappropriate to compare arthroscopic surgery to the cut of a jacket, or organ transplants to organic vegetarian sushi, it is impossible to avoid the conclusion that medical care has a significant consumption component. Medicine is beginning to more and more resemble other service industries.

If surgery is sold like automobiles, and mental health like entertainment,[10] what role is there for the dismal science of economics? Perhaps economists relate to the public and politicians in a manner similar to the way personal trainers relate to their affluent and often overweight clients: as someone whose expertise is required in order to establish authority and make compliance with an unpleasant regime easier, even though all the exercises and advice are pretty simple and mostly well known in advance. It may be that economists, like politicians, are being paid to talk about the old-fashioned values of thrift and efficiency that everyone is eager to hear about, if not always to follow.

14.6.1 Allocation, Allocation, Allocation

When asked which three factors are most important in determining value, real estate appraisers reply, "location, location, and location." In a similar vein, health economists asked to determine the value of the money spent on health care must focus primarily on **allocation**: the distribution of resources, the distribution of health, the distribution of medical care, and the distribution of provider incomes. Although a high value is often placed on the quality of nursing care, the skill of the physician, or the use of new medical technology, none of these matters much if the care is provided to the wrong person or at the wrong time.

Health economists are asked to assess economic efficiency—how well the health care system has used the resources available to achieve its stated (and unstated) goals. The following list contains just a few of the questions that must be answered in this regard:

▲ Which diseases should be treated?
▲ Which people should be treated?
▲ How much care should be given?
▲ Who will pay?
▲ If the money is to come from taxes, who should be taxed most—those who benefit most or those who can most afford to pay?
▲ Should more money be spent on prevention or cure?
▲ How much should healers be paid?
▲ Should treatment be given by specialists or primary care providers?
▲ How should the power to make decisions be allocated?

Allocation is the subject of economics. Why, then, haven't economists been more successful in reforming health care? First, it must be recognized that the study of health economics has indeed improved efficiency to some degree. It has made the system better, although it is still far from perfect. Cost–benefit analysis has led to a reduction in the over-investment in hospitals, to the support and improvement of immunization programs, and to the more rapid and objective evaluation of new drugs. Assessment of incentives and risk bearing has led to the creation of new types of insurance and to the refinement of managed care contracting. The application of economics to decisions regarding individual allocation has only limited potential, however, because the most crucial issues in health are likely to involve the contentious questions of how the costs and benefits are to be distributed between different groups of producers and consumers.

It's quite possible to spend less on health care and simultaneously improve the average level of health by changing the allocation of resources. Yet just as U.S. citizens are unlikely to vote for a program that cuts Medicare in half and sends 80 percent of the remaining funds overseas to clinics in poor countries to raise average global life expectancy, almost any reallocation that improves efficiency makes some concerned group with decision-making power worse off and is, therefore, likely to be opposed, even if it clearly improves overall efficiency. The difficulty for health economists is that the question of how to improve efficiency is less relevant to reform of health care than the question of how to get the various interests to agree to make a change that, at the cost of harming some identifiable groups, yields an increase in average benefits.

14.6.2 Dynamic Efficiency

Changes are difficult to make, even when they are clearly beneficial overall, because groups that will be harmed find it difficult to be sure that their concerns are adequately weighed and that the harm done to them is somehow offset by benefits gained from other programs and policies. Assurances of fair treatment are more difficult to believe the more distant in time and more uncertain the compensating benefits are. Thus, while a group of elderly people may possibly be willing to accept less technologically advanced treatment for a reduction in their premiums and out-of-pocket costs, they might not be willing to make such a sacrifice in order to fund research that will only bring results 20 or 30 years in the future. Although this reluctance may be short-sighted, it's perfectly reasonable.

In medicine, the most important allocation may be that between current consumption and future productivity. The challenge is to structure a health care system for **dynamic efficiency,** or the use of inputs so as to maximize long-run value over time. In other words, dynamic efficiency involves creating technological and organizational change to improve health and productivity. Some current efficiency must be sacrificed for scientists to spend time tinkering to make new discoveries and to give managers the slack to come up with ideas for new products and service delivery systems.

SELF-CHECK

- Does the marginal productivity of medical care spending increase or decrease as more is spent?
- Briefly explain how changing the **allocation** of resources can improve the average level of health in the United States while at the same time resulting in lower spending.
- Briefly explain why even changes that are beneficial overall are difficult to make.
- Describe the value of **dynamic efficiency** to the future of health care.

14.7 Concluding Thoughts: The Future

What can be said about the future of health and medical care over the next 50 years? Here are some speculations on future trends:

- ▲ There will be greater longevity and better health.
- ▲ There will be more long-term and chronic care and less acute illness.
- ▲ Spending will increase overall, but a smaller fraction will be spent on the working population.
- ▲ There will be a decreased ability to shift costs by overcharging for treatment.
- ▲ A middle ground between public and private control will need to be established.
- ▲ Assessment of costs and outcomes will increase.
- ▲ There will be declining trust in medicine as an organized profession.
- ▲ Physicians will lead teams within organizations, with less autonomy and independence.
- ▲ Successful organizations will focus on information (e.g., biotechnology) and caring (e.g., hospice).
- ▲ Special characteristics previously found mostly in medical care will become more typical of many service organizations in a post-industrial economy.

It is relatively certain that there will be continued increases in longevity, greater technological capability to treat disease, and continuous increases in expenditure. While there will be more spending overall, the sources and uses of funding will change rather markedly, and it's probable that at some point, the annual rate of increase will moderate.

An older and healthier population implies more long term care, with greater emphasis on caring and rehabilitation. Thus, the fraction of medical spending accounted for by acute illnesses of the employed tax-paying population will fall. The tension between public and private financing is likely to remain unresolved, with payers operating under a mixture of market incentives and regulatory structures to provide a middle ground.

Physicians will become technical team leaders operating within a corporate organization rather than independent medical practitioners. Cost shifting in the form of marked-up prices and open-ended reimbursement will continue to wither and be replaced by new forms, such as mandated benefits pools. The use of economic information and cost accounting for comparative decision making will continue to increase. Greater knowledge about actual costs and the actual effectiveness of clinical practice will provide greater clarity in the questions raised about the trade-off between dollars and health. Some fields (e.g., dietary modification, parts of mental health and disability care) are being spun off and are less likely to be counted as integral parts of medicine. Others, such as information systems and genetic engineering, are becoming more integrated and will blur the traditional boundaries between what is medicine and what is information.

The special institutional features that set medicine and health apart from the rest of the economy may become less so over the coming years. In part, this is because medicine is becoming more organized and more corporate, more subject to a bottom-line assessment of cost and benefits. Yet the extent to which medicine is becoming like the rest of the economy is probably of far less importance than the extent to which the rest of the economy is becoming like medicine, where information, service, and public goods matter more than manufactured commodities. Previously, health economists have taken models from the study of industrial production and applied them to health and medical care. Ideas may increasingly flow in the other direction as the issues of special interest to health economists—uncertainty, agency, trust, service delivery, and quality—become central to the economy as a whole in a postindustrial era. Models developed for the study of medical care may in the future be applied to banking, entertainment, automation, fashion, and other industries.

SELF-CHECK

- How are changes in the characteristics of the population likely to influence future trends in health care economics?

- In the coming years, is health care more or less likely to become more like other sectors of the economy? Why?

SUMMARY

The major factors determining total health spending are national (macro) rather than individual (micro) in scope and include inflation, population, and GDP. Professional licensure, the prevalence of not-for-profit modes of operation, third-party reimbursement, and other institutional features make the health care sector slow in adjusting to changes in macroeconomic conditions. These delays in response create pressures for regulatory change. Yet many of the effects associated with the passage of health care cost-control regulations are actually delayed effects of inflation and recession. Real increases in health care spending are largely increases in labor. Much of the growth shows up in the form of new occupations, and some shows up as higher wages and professional incomes.

A primary role of health economists is to force the public and politicians to consider the trade-offs involved in every health and medical care decision. Who gets helped? Who gets hurt? Who makes money?

The increase in health and life expectancy that can be obtained from any given set of medical resources depends largely on the allocation of treatment to those most likely to benefit. Often, this isn't the group that is most able or willing to pay.

KEY TERMS

Allocation	The distribution of resources.
Capacity constraint	A lack of services to meet demand.
Dynamic efficiency	Use of inputs so as to maximize long-run value over time, taking account of the need for tinkering to bring about technological and organizational advances.
Dynamics	The process of change; the study of how change occurs over time, including the order, timing, and strength of interacting forces.

ASSESS YOUR UNDERSTANDING

Go to www.wiley.com/college/getzen to evaluate your knowledge of the dynamics of health spending.
Measure your learning by comparing pre-test and post-test results.

Summary Questions

1. The income elasticity of health care expenditures:
   (a) is significantly higher for nations than for individuals because national budget constraints are binding, while individuals can use insurance and cost shifting to avoid budget constraints.
   (b) is significantly higher for persons than for nations or large groups of people because the impact of health spending is a larger risk to an individual.
   (c) measures the amount of income it would take to purchase the same bundle of health care goods at different prices.
   (d) should be negative for individuals but positive for nations.

2. In times of unanticipated inflation:
   (a) health care generally adjusts more quickly than the rest of the economy because there are fewer collective bargaining agreements.
   (b) national health spending tends to adjust with a lag because of contractual provisions and budgeted government programs.
   (c) it appears that the health sector is claiming an increased share of GDP.
   (d) health care workers are temporarily made better off because their wages usually adjust faster than prices.

3. Attempts in the 1970s to slow the rate of increase in health expenditures were:
   (a) not very successful under President Nixon (1971–1974) because they did not employ actual limits on prices, only voluntary restraint.
   (b) successful primarily because of the tax increases required to pay for the Vietnam War, which reduced purchasing power.
   (c) largely unsuccessful because prices returned to rapid growth as soon as strict controls were lifted.
   (d) much more successful than the market impact of managed care in the 1990s in restraining expenditure growth.

4. Employment in the U.S. health care sector:
   (a) has grown more than twice as rapidly as total U.S. employment over the past 100 years.

(b) has remained a relatively constant proportion of total employment, but the proportion of national income earned in health care has risen steadily.

(c) grew extremely rapidly in 1965 and 1966 because of the enactment of Medicare and Medicaid, but then it tapered back off to the previous growth rate.

(d) contains a steadily rising proportion of physicians.

5. Economists leave questions regarding the allocation of resources to physicians and politicians, as the issue falls outside their area of expertise. True or False?

6. The marginal productivity of medical care spending declines as more is spent. True or False?

7. In the future of health care, which of the following is likely to be true?

(a) There will be greater ability to shift costs by overcharging for treatment.

(b) Less long-term and chronic care will be provided.

(c) There will be more spending overall, but a smaller fraction will be spent on the working population.

(d) Assessment of cost and outcomes will become less common.

Review Questions

1. Which adjusts more rapidly to changes in demand—the number of nurses or the number of physician? Briefly explain why.

2. What determines how much is spent on your health care—how sick you are or how much money you earn? What determines how much is spent, on average, in the United States—how sick people are or how much money they earn?

3. Are decisions regarding health care budgets and medical school enrollments based on the past or the future?

4. Why might it take longer to adjust health care expenditures downward than upward? Frame your answer in terms of the economic incentives facing those who make the decisions.

5. Did health care costs rise less rapidly after President Nixon introduced price controls in 1971? Why or why not?

6. What forces cause the public to want price controls?

7. What was the effect of Medicare PPS, which paid a fixed price per DRG after 1983, on the length of hospital stay? On outpatient surgery? On nursing home admissions? On total Medicare hospital expenditures? On total Medicare expenditures for all types of care?

8. Will health care be more efficient or less efficient in 2020 than it is today? Will people spend more money or less money on health care then than they do now?

9. Are health care funds spent to maximize health or to maximize the welfare of those who make the decisions?

10. Does the share of a person's income going to pay for health care rise or fall as income goes up? What about the share of a nation's income?

Applying This Chapter

1. Suppose that you read Sunday's newspaper and learn that price controls have been put in place to limit the cost of health insurance to $2,500 per employee, which is significantly below the current average. What effects would you predict to occur?

2. Although now well below the very high rates of the 1970s and 1980s, the continuing growth of health care expenditures has remained an important policy issue. Identify four realistic cost-containment strategies/proposals. Two of them must work primarily through the *demand* side of the market and two through the *supply* side of the market.

3. Suppose that you have been hired as the chief executive officer of a health maintenance organization (HMO). Explain how each of these concepts might be important in your task, either as a problem to be overcome or a tool to be used:

   (a) Price discrimination

   (b) Adverse selection

   If it arises as a problem, how would you overcome it? If it can be used as a tool, how would you make use of it? You must demonstrate both that you understand the basic concept and its relevance in this context.

4. Employees and employers are increasingly in conflict over the use of "cost-sharing" measures such as deductibles and coinsurance. These are ways of limiting employer health care benefit expenditures by affecting the demand (i.e., buyers') side of the market.

   (a) Compare and contrast deductibles and coinsurance as cost-containment strategies.

   (b) Suggest any alternative method of cost limitation that operates primarily on the *supply* (i.e., sellers') side of the market. Explain how it would contain costs and analyze its likely effectiveness.

YOU TRY IT

Societal and Individual Health Care Spending

In Chapter 13, comparisons were made regarding medical spending among different countries. The main reason Japan spends more on health care than Kenya (because Japan has more money) was so obvious, it hardly needed to be explained. Yet among the employees of General Motors, the janitors and clerks with low wages get the same kind of health care and spend just as much as the engineers and executives. Write a brief paper discussing why income matters so much in one case (comparisons between nations) and barely matters at all in another (comparisons between employees).

Evaluate Public Health Care Proposals

Suppose you have been appointed a consultant to the Centers for Medicare and Medicaid Services to give advice on the proper design of the public health care programs. You have been asked to consider three proposals for payment for inpatient hospital services, intended to promote appropriate access to hospital care at reasonable cost:

1. *Plan A: Pay the physician admitting the patient a fixed price, determined by diagnosis, for each patient.* Make the admitting physician responsible for paying for all costs of care (e.g., nursing, ancillary services, consultations from other physicians). There would be no coinsurance or deductible payment by the consumer, and the physician would be required to accept the fixed price as payment in full (i.e., no additional bill to the patient would be permitted). This would be similar to the way general contractors are paid for construction work, with the expectation that they will pay each of the subcontractors.

2. *Plan B: Pay the hospital a fixed price, determined by diagnosis.* Make the hospital responsible for paying all costs of care as for Plan A, including all physician services. There would be no coinsurance or deductible payment by the consumer, and the hospital would be required to accept the fixed price as payment in full (i.e., no additional bill to the patient would be permitted). This would be similar to the way most repair services are billed: Any professional work performed is simply included in the repair firm's price, and the firm compensates the workers.

3. *Plan C: Pay the hospital a per diem established in advance, regardless of diagnosis.* Pay physicians separately according to a negotiated fee schedule. This would be similar to the way that many managed care plans pay for hospital care, though they have many different ways of paying physicians.

Your task is to critically evaluate each of these proposals for its contribution to the general purposes of appropriate access and reasonable costs, and for its other effects, whether intended or not. Would you recommend any of these proposals? Would your analysis of these proposals change if this were an "all payer" system applying to all patients rather than just public patients?

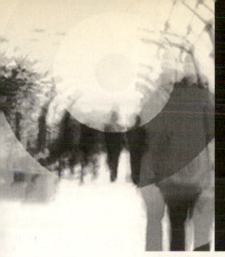

ENDNOTES

Chapter 1

1. Starr, Paul, *The Social Transformation of American Medicine* (New York: Basic Books, 1982).

2. U.S. Department of Health and Human Services, Centers for Medicare & Medicaid Services, National Health Accounts, *National Health Care Expenditures Projections: 2005–2015*. www.cms.gov/statistics/nhe. The CMS Office of the Actuary is the source for all expenditure estimates in this and subsequent chapters, unless noted otherwise.

3. Committee on the Costs of Medical Care, *Medical Care for the American People* (Chicago: University of Chicago Press, 1932); and Anderson, Odin W., *Health Services as a Growth Enterprise in the United States Since 1875* (Ann Arbor, MI: Health Administration Press, 1990).

4. Himmelstein, David U., Elizabeth Warren, Deborah Thorne, and Steffie Woolhandler, "MarketWatch: Illness and Injury as Contributors to Bankruptcy," *Health Affairs* Web Exclusive, February 2005.

5. The distribution of costs across individuals can be measured only for personal health care costs that are billed to individuals, not for overhead items such as public health, construction, and insurance administration. Such overhead items make up about 14 percent of national health expenditures. Hence, "personal health expenditures" account for only 86 percent of national health expenditures in Table 1-1 and elsewhere. In truth, even when charges are billed to an individual, many costs have overhead components and are difficult to unambiguously assign to a single person, although they are clearly concentrated on the most ill and are not evenly distributed. Many economists would argue that costs are more concentrated than statistics indicate because hospitals and physicians typically overcharge the least complex patients to subsidize the most difficult and complex cases.

6. Stiglitz, Joseph E., *The Economics of the Public Sector* (New York: W. W. Norton, 1986).

7. U.S. General Accounting Office, *Nursing Workforce: Emerging Nurse Shortages Due to Multiple Factors*, July 2001. www.gao.gov/archive/2001/d01944.pdf.

8. CBS News, *Foreign Nurses Sought to Fill Void*, June 29, 2004. www.cbsnews.com/stories/2004/06/29/health/main626643.shtml.

9. Source for all data in table: Howley, Kerry, "I Can't Afford to Get Sick," *Readers' Digest*, April 2006.

Chapter 3

1. Drummond, Michael, *Principles of Economic Appraisal in Health Care* (Cambridge, UK: Oxford University Press, 1981), p. 17. Good current examples of cost–benefit analyses and reviews of the literature can be found in journals such as *Health Economics, American Journal of Public Health, Medical Decision Making, New England Journal of Medicine,* and *Journal of the American Medical Association*.

2. Mark, Dan, "The Characteristics of Medical Innovation" in *Medical Innovation in the Changing Healthcare Marketplace: Conference Summary*, edited by Philip Aspden (Washington, DC: National Academy Press, 2002).

3. The "law of large numbers" says that the observed average will be close to the "true" mean if the number of observations is large enough.

4. Lee, Christopher, "Study Finds Health Care Good Value Despite Costs," *Washington Post*, August 31, 2006, p. A14.

5. Getzen, Thomas E., "Medical Care Price Indexes: Theory, Construction and Empirical Analysis of the U.S. Series 1927–1990," *Advances in Health Economics* 13:83–128, 1992.

6. Jones-Lee, Michael W., *The Economics of Safety and Physical Risk* (Oxford, UK: Blackwell, 1989), p. 67, based on data and extrapolations from Melinek, S. J., "A Method of Evaluating Life for Economic Purposes," *Accident Analysis and Prevention* 6:103–114, 1974.

7. Fanning, T. R., L. E. Cosler, P. Gallagher, J. Chiarella, and E. M. Howell, "The Epidemiology of AIDS in the New York and California Medicaid Programs," *Journal of Acquired Immune Deficiency Syndromes* 4:1025–1035, 1991.

8. Sanders, Gillian D., A. M. Bayoumi, V. Sundaram, S. P. Bilir, C. P. Neukermans, C. E. Rydzak, L. R. Douglass, L. C. Lazzeroni, M. Holodniy, and D. K. Owens, "Cost-Effectiveness of Screening for HIV in the Era of Highly Active Antiretroviral Therapy," *New England Journal of Medicine* 352 (6): 570–585, February 10, 2005.

Chapter 4

1. Frank, Robert H., *Passions Within Reason: The Strategic Role of the Emotions* (New York: Norton, 1988).

2. Stevens, Rosemary, *In Sickness and in Wealth: American Hospitals in the Twentieth Century* (New York: Basic Books, 1989); and Thompson,

John D., *The Hospital: A Social and Architectural History* (New Haven, CT: Yale University Press, 1975).

3. Glaser, William A., *Health Insurance in Practice: International Variations in Financing, Benefits, and Problems* (San Francisco: Jossey-Bass, 1991).

4. The distribution of costs across individuals can be measured only for personal health care costs that are billed to individuals, not overhead items, such as public health, construction, insurance administration, and so on. Such overhead items make up about 10 percent of national health expenditures; hence, the "all persons" average in Figure 4-1 is only 90 percent as large as the per capita average for all national health expenditures reported elsewhere. In truth, many costs have overhead components and are difficult to unambiguously assign to a single person, although they are clearly concentrated on the most ill and not evenly distributed. Many economists would argue that costs are even more concentrated than these statistics indicate because hospitals and physicians typically overcharge the least complex patients to subsidize the most difficult and complex cases.

5. Bureau of Labor Statistics, U.S. Dept. of Labor, *Employer Costs for Employee Compensation Summary*, September 22, 2006.

6. Workman, Lewis C., "Life Annuities," in *Mathematical Foundations of Life Insurance* (Atlanta: Life Office Management Association, 1982), pp. 155–195.

Chapter 5

1. Information on Kaiser Permanente is from the company's website, www.kaiserpermanente.org, accessed August 16, 2006.

2. Estimates of coverage are from Custer, William S., and Pat Ketsche, *The Changing Sources of Health Insurance*, Health Insurance Association of America, 2000 (www.hiaa.org); Employer Health Benefits, 2002 Annual Survey; Kaiser Family Foundation; and Health Research and Educational Trust, 2002.

3. The estimates, by type of coverage, are not mutually exclusive; people can be covered by more than one type of health insurance during the year. *Source:* U.S. Census Bureau, Current Population Survey, and Employee Benefit Research Institute.

4. Kaiser/Health Research and Educational Trust Survey of Employer Health Benefits, 2005.

5. "Higher-Income Medicare Beneficiaries to Pay Higher Part B Premiums Next Year," September 11, 2006, *Daily Health Policy Reports,* Kaisernetwork.org.

6. Laschober, M. A., M. Kitchman, P. Neuman, and A. A. Strabic, "Trends in Medicare Supplemental Insurance and Prescription Drug Coverage, 1996–1999," *Health Affairs* 21 (2): 11, April 2002.

7. Office of the Actuary, Centers for Medicare and Medicaid Services, *National Health Expenditure Accounts*. www.cms.gov/statistics/nhe.

8. The 19–24 age group is more than twice as likely to be uninsured as other age groups (35 percent versus 15 percent). Levy, Helen, and Thomas DeLeire, *What Do People Buy When They Don't Buy Health Insurance?* Harris Graduate School of Public Policy Studies working paper, University of Chicago, June 26, 2002.

9. State Health Access Data Assistance Center, University of Minnesota, "Covering Kids and Families: The State of Kids' Coverage," prepared for the Robert Wood Johnson Foundation, August 9, 2006. www.coveringkidsandfamilies.org/press/docs/2006StateofKidsCoverage.pdf.

10. Levy, Helen, and Thomas DeLeire, *What Do People Buy When They Don't Buy Health Insurance?* Harris Graduate School of Public Policy Studies working paper, University of Chicago, June 26, 2002.

11. Sources for this information are the Alan Guttmacher Institute and Planned Parenthood Federation of America.

Chapter 6

1. Freidson, Eliot, *Profession of Medicine* (New York: Dodd, Mead, 1970); and Fuchs, Victor R., *Who Shall Live? Health, Economics and Social Choice* (New York: Basic Books, 1983).

2. Most of the information here is from surveys done by the American Medical Association and reported in *Socioeconomic Characteristics of Medical Practice*, an annual/biennial monograph. A good sense of the entrepreneurial flavor of medical practice can be obtained by perusing several issues of *Medical Economics*, which is the *BusinessWeek* of physicians.

3. Office of the Actuary, Centers for Medicare and Medicaid Services, *National Health Expenditure Accounts*. www.cms.gov/statistics/nhe.

4. Hsiao, W. C., P. Braun, D. Dunn, and E. R. Becker, "Resource-Based Relative Values: An Overview," *Journal of the American Medical Association* 260 (16): 2347–2353, 1988; and Hsiao, William C., et al., "Results and Impacts of the Resource-Based Relative Value Scale," *Medical Care* 30 (11 Suppl.): NS61–NS79, 1992.

5. Medicaid Access Study Group, "Access of Medicaid Recipients to Outpatient Care," *New England Journal of Medicine* 330:1426–1430, May 19, 1994.

6. Hickson, G. B., W. A. Altmeier, and J. M. Perris, "Physician Reimbursement by Salary or Fee-For-Service: Effect on Physician Practice Behavior in a Randomized Prospective Study," *Pediatrics* 80:344–350, 1987.

7. Tu, Ha T., and Paul B. Ginsburg, "Losing Ground: Physician Income, 1995–2003," Tracking Report No. 15, June 2006. www.hschange.org/CONTENT/851.

8. *Ibid.*

9. American Medical Association, "Physician Characteristics and Distribution in the United States, 2006"; American Medical Association,

"Physician Socioeconomic Statistics, 2000–2002 and Earlier Years"; *Medical Economics,* compensation survey, 2006.

10. American Medical Association, *Physicians React to Projected Medicare Physician Payment Cuts.* www.ama-assn.org/ama/pub/category/16122.html.

11. American Medical Association, "Physician Socioeconomic Statistics, 2000–2002"; and *Medical Economics.*

12. Sloan, Frank A., "Physician Supply Behavior in the Short Run," *Industrial and Labor Relations Review,* 28:549–569, July 1975.

13. Glassman, Peter A., John E. Rolph, Laura P. Petersen, Melissa A. Bradley, and Richard L. Kravitz, "Physician's Personal Malpractice Experiences Are Not Related to Defensive Clinical Practices," *Journal of Health Politics, Policy and Law* 21 (2): 219–241, 1996.

14. Great-West Healthcare, *2006 Consumer Attitude Survey.* www.greatwest-healthcare.com/C5/StudiesSurveys.

15. Jensen, Michael C., and William H. Meckling, "Agency Costs in the Firm" and "Theory of the Firm: Managerial Behavior, Agency Costs and Ownership Structure," *Journal of Financial Economics* 3:305–360, 1976. The extensive economic analysis of agency has focused primarily on the manager of a firm who makes decisions on behalf of shareholders. Many of these models are applicable, but because medical outcomes are not as readily measured as the profits of a firm, and because death has even more moral overtones than bankruptcy, the doctor–patient bond has important aspects above and beyond those that characterize the owner–shareholder and supervisor–employee relationships.

16. Shryock, Richard, *Medical Licensing in America, 1650–1965* (Baltimore: Johns Hopkins University Press, 1967).

17. Rayack, Elton, *Professional Power and American Medicine: The Economics of the American Medical Association* (Cleveland: World Publishing, 1967).

18. American Board of Medical Specialties (www.abms.org).

19. Formal licensure actions against physicians are rather infrequent and are usually for misconduct (i.e., drug abuse, fraud, sexual advances) rather than poor quality of care, which has led some observers to conclude that the institution of licensure was never intended to improve quality. However, note that revoking of a driver's license is similarly rare. The quality of daily driving is measured by a 15-minute test when a person is first licensed, but not thereafter, and revocation of drivers' licenses reflects a similar pattern of egregious personal flaws rather than the traits associated with quality (vision, eye–hand coordination, etc.).

20. Freidson, Eliot, *Professional Dominance: The Social Structure of Medical Care* (New York: Atherton, 1970); and Freidson, Eliot, *Professional Powers: A Study in the Institutionalization of Formal Knowledge* (Chicago: University of Chicago Press, 1986).

21. Pennsylvania Health Care Cost Containment Council, *A Consumer Guide to Coronary Artery Bypass Graft Surgery*, Vol. IV, 1993 data. Harrisburg, PA: Pennsylvania Health Care Cost Containment Council, 1995.

Chapter 7

1. Enrollments and other data are taken from the September 6, 2006, "Medical Education" issue of the *Journal of the American Medical Association*.

2. Ganem, J., J. Krakower, and R. Beran, "Review of U.S. Medical School Finances, 1993–1994," *Journal of the American Medical Association* 274 (9): 723–730, September 6, 1995.

3. American Association of Medical Colleges, *AAMC Medical Student Education: Cost, Debt, and Resident Stipend Facts,* October 2005. It is worth noting that while the average doctor under age 35 was at least $200,000 in debt, just 10 percent of that debt was for student loans, while 90 percent was for home mortgage, indicating that tuition was not financially burdensome relative to current and expected income; see Farber, Lawrence, "How Financially Secure Are Young Doctors?" *Medical Economics* August 24, 1998, pp. 34–43.

4. Fein, Rashi, *The Doctor Shortage: An Economic Diagnosis* (Washington, DC: Brookings Institute, 1967).

5. U.S. Department of Health and Human Services, *Fifth Report to the President and Congress on the Status of Health Personnel in the United States* (Washington, DC: U.S. Government Printing Office, 1984).

6. U.S. Department of Health and Human Services (DHHS), Office of Graduate Medical Education, *Report of the Graduate Medical Education National Advisory Committee to the Secretary,* DHHS Pub No. 81–651 (Washington, DC: U.S. Government Printing Office, 1981). This became widely known as the GMENAC Report.

7. Barzansky, Barbara, and Sylvia I. Etzel, "Educational Programs in U.S. Medical Schools, 2004–2005," *Journal of the American Medical Association* 294 (9): 1068–1074, September 7, 2005.

8. Rayack, Elton, "The Physicians Service Industry," Chapter 6 in Walter Adams, ed., *The Structure of American Industry,* 5th edition (New York: Macmillan, 1982), pp. 407–408.

9. American Medical Association, *Physician Characteristics and Distribution in the United States, 2006.*

10. Wolinsky, Frederick, and William Marder, *The Organization of Medical Practice and the Practice of Medicine* (Ann Arbor, MI: Health Administration Press, 1985).

11. Reinhardt, Uwe, *Physician Productivity and the Demand for Health Manpower* (Cambridge, MA: Ballinger, 1974).

12. Getzen, Thomas, "A 'Brand Name' Firm Theory of Medical Group Practice," *Journal of Industrial Economics* 33 (2): 199–215, 1984.

13. Clapesattle, Helen, *The Doctors Mayo* (Minneapolis: University of Minnesota Press, 1941).

14. Lutz, Sandy, "Troubled Times for Psych Hospitals," *Modern Healthcare* 21 (50): 26–27, 30–33, December 16, 1991; and "NME Totals Costs of Psych Woes," *Modern Healthcare* 23 (43): 20, October 25, 1993.

15. Mitchell, Jean M., and Jonathan H. Sunshine, "Consequences of Physician's Ownership of Health Care Facilities—Joint Ventures in Radiology," *New England Journal of Medicine* 327:1497–1501, 1992.

16. Physicians are allowed to buy stocks and make other forms of investments in laboratories, hospitals, and medical businesses, but they cannot be partners or get special treatment different from nonphysicians who are not in a position to refer patients.

17. Kessel, Reuben, "Price Discrimination in Medicine," *Journal of Law and Economics* 1 (2): 20–53, October 1958.

18. Care for Ohio, *Twice the Price: \What Uninsured and Underinsured Patients Pay for Hospital Care,* March 2005. www.careforohio.org.

Chapter 8

1. Fein, Rashi, *The Doctor Shortage: An Economic Diagnosis* (Washington, DC: Brookings Institute, 1967).

2. American Hospital Association, *Hospital Statistics 2006*, Table 3.

3. The prices that patients pay for services are even less important than Table 8-1 suggests because much of the 3 percent is actually deductibles, copayments, and other charges that are, in effect, insurance premiums or taxes and not directly related to the prices of the services chosen.

4. State Medicaid plans used the DRG system but generally paid fewer dollars for each patient. In time, this underpayment led to complaints and a series of lawsuits. Temple University Hospital sued the state of Pennsylvania under the Boren Amendment to the Social Security Act, which obligated states to make payments sufficient to cover the cost of efficiently provided services. The hospital eventually won—creating a precedent that hospitals around the country quickly followed (and that forced state budgets into deficits). Hence, although, in concept, a charge system gives all the power to the seller and an administered price system (e.g., DRGs) gives all the power to the buyer, in reality, both sides are at least to some extent constrained by the political process and public opinion.

5. Aaron, Henry J., and Robert D. Reischauer, "The Medicare Reform Debate: What Is the Next Step?" *Health Affairs* 14 (4): 8–30, Winter 1995.

6. National Coalition on Health Care, www.nchc.org.

7. Cooper, R. A., et al., "Current and Projected Workforce of Nonphysician Clinicians," *Journal of the American Medical Association* 280 (9): 788–794, 1988; and Druss, B. G., et al., "Trends in Care by Nonphysician Clinicians in the United States," *New England Journal of Medicine* 348 (2): 130–137, January 9, 2003.

8. This sidebar was researched and prepared by Patrick M. Bernet, Ph.D. candidate at Temple University.

9. Wolinsky, Frederick, and William Marder, *The Organization of Medical Practice and the Practice of Medicine* (Ann Arbor, MI: Health Administration Press, 1985).

10. Getzen, Thomas, "A 'Brand Name' Firm Theory of Medical Group Practice," *Journal of Industrial Economics* 33 (2): 199–215, 1984.

11. Lutz, Sandy, "Troubled Times for Psych Hospitals," *Modern Healthcare* 21 (50): 26–27, 30–33, December 16, 1991; and "NME Totals Costs of Psych Woes," *Modern Healthcare* 23 (43): 20, October 25, 1993.

12. Asch, Steven M., et al., "Comparison of Quality of Care for Patients in the Veterans Health Administration and Patients in a National Sample," *Annals of Internal Medicine* 141 (12): 938–945, December 21, 2004; and Arnst, Catherine, "The Best Medical Care in the U.S.: How Veterans Affairs Transformed Itself—And What It Means for the Rest of Us," *BusinessWeek* July 17, 2006.

Chapter 9

1. Becker, E. R., and B. Steinwald, "The Determinants of Hospital Case-Mix Complexity," *Health Services Research* 16 (1): 439–458, 1981.

2. Sloan, Frank, Roger Feldman, and Bruce Steinwald, "The Effects of Teaching on Hospital Costs," *Journal of Health Economics* 2 (1): 1–28, 1983; and Berman, Howard, and Louis Weeks, *The Financial Management of Hospitals,* 5th ed. (Ann Arbor, MI: Health Administration Press, 1990).

3. Care for Ohio, *Twice the Price: What Uninsured and Underinsured Patients Pay for Hospital Care,* March 2005. www.careforohio.org.

4. The adjustment calculation used here is arbitrary and intended for illustrative purposes only; it is not an estimation of actual cost penalties. The important point is that being over or under the optimal level of planned output causes a disproportionate increase in per-unit costs.

5. Strunk, Bradley, Paul B. Ginsburg, and Michelle I. Banker, "The Effect of Population Aging on Future Hospital Demand," *Health Affairs* 25:141–149, 2006.

6. Granneman, T. W., R. S. Brown, and M. V. Pauly, "Estimating Hospital Costs: A Multiple-Output Analysis," *Journal of Health Economics* 5 (2): 107–127, 1986; Cowing, T. G., A. G. Holtman, and S. Powers, "Hospital Cost Analysis: A Survey and Evaluation of Recent Studies," *Advances in Health Economics and Health Services Research* 4:257–303, 1983.

7. Cutler, David M., Allison B. Rosen, and Sandeep Vijan, "The Value of Medical Spending in the United States, 1960–2000," *New England Journal of Medicine* 355:920–927, August 31, 2006.

8. Pauly, Mark, and Michael Redisch, "The Not-for-Profit Hospital as a Physicians Cooperative," *American Economic Review* 63:87–99, 1973.

9. A current research project of the Bing Center for Health Economics, RAND Health. www.rand.org/health/centers/bing/research.html.

10. Pauly, Mark V., *The Doctor's Workshop* (Philadelphia: University of Pennsylvania Press, 1980).

11. Luft, H., J. Robinson, D. Garnick, S. Maerki, and S. McPhee, "The Role of Specialized Clinical Services in the Competition Among Hospitals," *Inquiry* 23 (1): 83–94, 1986.

12. Bays, Carson W., "The Determinants of Hospital Size: A Survivor Analysis," *Applied Economics* 18:359–377, 1986.

13. American Hospital Association (AHA), *Hospital Statistics* (Chicago: AHA, various years).

14. *Ibid.*

15. CON, UR, PSROs, DRGs, and other regulations have all taken many different forms in different state or national programs over time. The brief discussion here refers to general conclusions about that type of regulation rather than any particular specific program. The interested reader should consult one of the many comprehensive reviews that have been written, such as those in Joskow, Paul, *Controlling Hospital Costs: The Role of Government Regulation* (Cambridge, MA: MIT Press, 1981); Abernathy, D., and D. A. Pearson, *Regulating Hospital Costs: The Development of Public Policy* (Ann Arbor, MI: Health Administration Press, 1979); the relevant chapters of Rosko, Michael, and Robert W. Broyles, *The Economics of Health Care: A Reference Handbook* (New York: Greenwood Press, 1988); or Folland, Sherman, Allen Goodman, and Miron Stano, *The Economics of Health and Health Care* (Upper Saddle River, NJ: Prentice Hall, 2001).

16. Salkever, David, and Thomas Bice, *Hospital Certificate-of-Need Controls: Impact on Investment, Costs and Use* (Washington, DC: American Enterprise Institute, 1979).

Chapter 10

1. *2005 eHMO-PPO/Medicare-Medicaid Digest,* www.managedcaredigest.com. This is a standard compilation of HMO statistics that has been published for a number of years under various titles and corporate sponsors.

2. The U.S. Bureau of Labor Statistics employee compensation measures have varied over the years, and the various issues of the *BLS Handbook of Methods* should be examined to understand the vagaries of comparison (www.bls.gov). Braden, Bradley R., and Stephanie L. Hyland, "Cost of Employee Compensation in Public and Private Sectors," *Monthly Labor Review* 116 (5): 14–21, 1993.

3. The United States ranked 26th in male life expectancy among 191 nations in 2000 (28th for females), a bit behind most other developed countries. The risk of dying between ages 15 and 59, a perhaps more significant measure, was even worse (36th for males, 38th for females). Overall, the World Health Organization ranked the performance of the

U.S. health system 37th in the world (*World Health Report 2000,* www.who.int/whr). See also Fuchs, Victor, "The Best Health Care System in the World?" *Journal of the American Medical Association* 268 (7): 916–917, 1992; Hadley, Jack, *More Medical Care, Better Health?* (Washington, DC: The Urban Institute Press, 1982); and Organization for Economic Cooperation and Development (OECD), *OECD Health Data: Comparative Analysis of Health Systems* (Paris: OECD, 2002).

4. Sekhri, Neelam K., "Managed Care: The U.S. Experience," *Bulletin of the World Health Organization* 78 (6): 830–844, 2000. www.who.int.

5. Cutler, David M., Mark McClellan, and Joseph P. Newhouse. "How Does Managed Care Do It?," *RAND Journal of Economics* 31 (3): 526–548, Autumn 2000; Alman, Daniel, Richard Zeckhauser, and David M. Cutler, *Enrollee Mix, Treatment Intensity and Cost in Competing Indemnity and HMO Plans,* National Bureau of Economic Research working paper No. 7832, August 2000, www.nber.org; and Flood, Ann Barry, et al., "How Do HMOs Achieve Savings?," *Health Services Research* 33 (1): 79–99, April 1998.

6. *Managed Care Digest 2001,* www.managedcaredigest.com; Miller, Robert H., and Harold Luft, "Managed Care Plans: Characteristics, Growth and Premium Performance," *Annual Review of Public Health* 15:437–459, 1994.

7. *Managed Care Digest: HMO-PPO Digest 1995* (Kansas City, MO: Hoechst Marion Roussel, 1995). In an integrated CPGP HMO, administrative and medical expenses all occur within the same organization and cannot meaningfully be separated. In reports, Kaiser or Group Health often say their administrative expenses are very low, 2 percent or so, but this low figure is a result of counting only the central office staff, and not all the clerks, secretaries, medical directors, information specialists, and so on who are at work in the clinics.

8. *Managed Care Digest: HMO-PPO Digest 1995* (Kansas City, MO: Hoechst Marion Roussel, 1995).

9. Hsu, John, et al., "Unintended Consequences of Caps on Medicare Drug Benefits," *New England Journal of Medicine* 354:22, June 1, 2006.

10. In principle, an integrated closed HMO could be run as a for-profit corporation benefiting stockholders, a division of a voluntary hospital chain, or a consumer co-op with all profits used to increase community benefits. In practice, the residual ownership interest has de facto resided primarily with the senior physician group, even when they are technically employees of the HMO.

11. The term *PPO* is commonly used to refer to two things: an insurance plan and a corporate entity. The two are distinct. Your PPO insurance may actually have contracts with a dozen PPO organizations. Conversely, a single PPO organization with 50 physicians may have contracts with more than one insurance company (and at different prices).

12. Gold, Marsha, et al., "A National Survey of the Arrangements Managed-Care Plans Make with Physicians," *New England Journal of Medicine*

333:1678–1683, 1995; Anderson, Gerard, et al., "Setting Payment Rates for Capitated Systems: A Comparison of Various Alternatives" *Inquiry* 27 (3): 225–233, 1990.

13. Starr, Paul, *The Social Transformation of American Medicine* (New York: Basic Books, 1982).

14. Luft, Harold, *Health Maintenance Organizations: Dimensions of Performance* (New York: Wiley, 1981); Miller, Robert H., and Harold Luft, "Managed Care Plan Performance Since 1980: A Literature Analysis," *Journal of the American Medical Association* 271 (19): 1512–1519, 1994; Hill, J., et al., *The Impact of the Medicare Risk Program on the Use of Services and Costs to Medicare* (Princeton, N.J.: Mathematica Policy Research, 1992); and Freeborn, D. K., and C. R. Pope, *Promise and Performance in Managed Care: The Prepaid Group Practice Model* (Baltimore: Johns Hopkins University Press, 1994).

15. Wilensky, Gail, and Louis Rossiter, "Patient Self-Selection in HMOs," *Health Affairs* 5 (4): 66–80, 1986; Berki, S. E., and M. L. Ashcraft, "HMO Enrollment: Who Joins and Why: A Review of the Literature," *Milbank Memorial Fund Quarterly* 58:588–632, 1980; and Grazier, Kyle, et al., "Factors Affecting Choice of Health Care Plans," *Health Services Research* 20 (6): 659–682, 1986.

16. Retchin, S. M., and B. Brown, "The Quality of Ambulatory Care in Medicare Health Maintenance Organizations," *American Journal of Public Health* 80:411–415, 1990; Udvarhely, I. S., et al., "Comparison of the Quality of Ambulatory Care for Fee-for-Service and Prepaid Patients," *Annals of Internal Medicine* 327:424–429, 1991; Ware, J. E., et al., "Comparison of Health Outcomes at a Health Maintenance Organization With Those of Fee-for-Service Care," *Lancet* 1986, pp. 130–136; Mahar, Maggie, "Time for a Checkup: HMOs Must Now Prove That They Are Providing Quality Care," *Barron's*, March 4, 1996, pp. 29–35; and Robinson, Ray, "Managed Care in the United States: A Dilemma for Evidence-Based Policy?" *Health Economics* 9 (1): 1–7, January 2000.

17. Davis, Karen, Karen Scott Collins, Cathy Schoen, and Cynthia Morris, "Choice Matters: Enrollees' Views of Their Health Plans," *Health Affairs* 14 (2): 99–112, 1995; and Rubin, H. R., et al., "Patients Ratings of Outpatient Visits in Different Practice Settings: Results from the Medical Outcomes Study," *Journal of the American Medical Association* 262:57–63, 1989.

18. Hurley, Robert, Deborah Freund, and John Paul, *Managed Care in Medicaid: Lessons for Policy and Program Design* (Ann Arbor, MI: Health Administration Press, 1993).

19. Miller, Robert H., and Harold Luft, "Managed Care Plans: Characteristics, Growth and Premium Performance," *Annual Review of Public Health* 15:437–459, 1994; and Baker, Laurence C., "Managed Care Technology Adoption in Health Care: Evidence from Magnetic

Resonance Imaging," *Journal of Health Economics* 20 (3): 395–421, 2001.

20. Miller, Robert H., and Harold Luft, "Managed Care Plan Performance Since 1980: A Literature Analysis," *Journal of the American Medical Association* 271 (19): 1512–1519, 1994.

21. Council on Ethical and Judicial Affairs, American Medical Association, "Ethical Issues in Managed Care," *Journal of the American Medical Association* 273 (4): 330–335, 1995; Emanuel, Ezekiel, and Nancy Dubler, "Preserving the Physician–Patient Relationship in the Era of Managed Care," *Journal of the American Medical Association* 273 (4): 323–329, 1995; and Rodwin, Marc, "Conflicts in Managed Care," *New England Journal of Medicine* 332 (9): 605–607, 1995.

22. See Rovner, Julie, "The Safety Net: What's Happening to Health Care of Last Resort?" *Advances* No. 1, 1996; and Larkin, Howard, "Employed but Uninsured: Why Business Is Cutting Back on Health Insurance," *Advances* No. 1, 1996. (*Advances* is the quarterly newsletter of the Robert Wood Johnson Foundation, Princeton, NJ.)

23. Enthoven, Alain, "Consumer Choice Health Plan," *New England Journal of Medicine* 298:650–658, 709–720, 1978; and Enthoven, Alain, *Theory and Practice of Managed Competition in Health Care Finance* (Amsterdam: North-Holland, 1988).

24. Enthoven, Alain, "Management of Competition in the FEHPB," *Health Affairs* 8 (3): 33–50, 1989.

Chapter 11

1. Arno, Peter S., Carol Levine, and Margaret M. Memmott, "The Economic Value of Informal Caregiving," *Health Affairs* 18 (2): 182–188, March 1999.

2. Benjamin, A. E., "An Historical Perspective on Home Care," *Milbank Quarterly* 71 (1): 129–166, 1993.

3. Centers for Disease Control and Prevention, National Center for Health Statistics, *Health United States, 2002.*

4. MetLife, "Key Long-Term Care Costs Increase More Than 5% from 2004," 2005 MetLife Mature Market Institute Survey Reports, www.metlife.com.

5. Kane, Robert L., Joseph G. Ouslander, and Itamar B. Abrass, *Essentials of Clinical Geriatrics* (New York: McGraw-Hill, 1989), pp. 30–44.

6. Hughes, Susan, "Home Health Care," in Connie Evashwick, ed., *The Continuum of Long-Term Care* (Albany, NY: Delmar Publishers, 1996), pp. 61–81.

7. "Yearly Long Term Care Costs Move Above $70,000 in 2006, According to Annual Benchmark Study by Genworth Financial, USA," *Medical News Today,* March 28, 2006, www.medicalnewstoday.com.

8. HCFA detailed breakdown of nursing home input price index weightings, Bureau of Labor Statistics Employment Statistics Survey.

9. Burwell, Brian, William H. Crown, Carol O'Shaunessy, and Richard Price, "Financing Long-Term Care," in Connie Evashwick, ed., *The Continuum of Long-Term Care* (Albany, NY: Delmar Publishers, 1996), p. 199.

10. Aaronson, William, "Financing the Continuum of Care: A Disintegrating Past and an Integrating Future," in Connie Evashwick, ed., *The Continuum of Long-Term Care* (Albany, NY: Delmar Publishers, 1996), p. 225.

11. Note that any brief description of Medicaid must be qualified because there are more than 50 state Medicaid payment systems, with numerous clauses, exceptions, and special programs.

12. Liu, Korbin, Pamela Doty, and Kenneth Manton, "Medicaid Spend-Down in Nursing Homes," *The Gerontologist* 30 (10): 7, 1990; and Temkin-Greener, H., M. Meiner, E. Petty, and J. Szydlowski, "Spending Down to Medicaid in the Nursing Home and in the Community," *Medical Care* 31 (8): 663–679, 1993.

13. Burwell, Brian, *Middle-Class Welfare: Medicaid Estate Planning for Long-Term Care Coverage* (Lexington, MA: Systemetrics, 1991).

14. Moses, S., "The Fallacy of Impoverishment," *The Gerontologist* 30 (1): 21–25, 1990.

15. Nyman, John, "The Private Demand for Nursing Home Care," *Journal of Health Economics* 8 (2): 209–231, 1989; John Nyman, "Excess Demand, the Percentage of Nursing Home Patients, and the Quality of Nursing Home Care," *Journal of Human Resources* 23 (1): 76–92, 1988; and Katz, S., A. B. Ford, R. W. Moskowitz, B. A. Jackson, and M. W. Jaffee, "Studies of Illness in the Aged. The Index of ADL: A Standardized Measure of Biological and Psychosocial Function," *Journal of the American Medical Association* 185:94ff, 1963.

16. U.S. General Accounting Office (GAO), *Nursing Homes: Admission Problems for Medicaid Recipients and Attempts to Solve Them*, GAO Reports #GAO/HRD-90-135, September 1990.

17. Alzheimer's Association, *Statistics About Alzheimer's Disease*, www.alz.org/AboutAD/statistics.asp.

18. Kaiser Commission on Medicaid and the Uninsured, *Private Long-Term Care Insurance: A Viable Option for Low and Middle-Income Seniors?*, February 2006, www.kff.org/uninsured/7459.cfm.

19. Lubitz, James, et al., "Three Decades of Health Care Use by the Elderly, 1965–1998," *Health Affairs* 20 (2): 19–21, March 2001.

20. Getzen, Thomas E., "Population Aging and the Growth of Health Expenditures," *Journal of Gerontology: Social Sciences* 47 (3): S98–S104, 1992.

21. Spillman, Brenda C., and James Lubitz, "The Effect of Longevity on Spending for Acute and Long-Term Care," *New England Journal of Medicine* 342:1409–1415, May 11, 2000.

22. Lakdawalla, Darius, and Tomas Philipson, "The Rise in Old-Age Longevity and the Market for Long-Term Care," *American Economic Review* 92 (1): 295–306, March 2002.

Chapter 12

1. The first edition version of this chapter was prepared with the assistance of Thomas Abbott, Ph.D. senior economist, Outcomes Research Management, Merck & Co. Major revisions have been made for this edition, and the responsibility for all representations, opinions, and statistics rests with the primary textbook author, T. E. Getzen.

2. Kaufman, David W., et al., "Recent Patterns of Medication Use in the Ambulatory Adult Population of the United States," *Journal of the American Medical Association* 287 (3): 337–344, January 16, 2002.

3. Kaiser Family Foundation, *Prescription Drug Trends*, June 2006, www.kff.org/rxdrugs/3057.cfm.

4. Centers for Medicare and Medicaid Services, *National Health Care Expenditures Projections: 2005–2015,* www.cms.hhs.gov/NationalHealthExpendData.

5. Kaiser Family Foundation, *Prescription Drug Trends*, Exhibit 3.2, June 2006, www.kff.org/rxdrugs/3057.cfm.

6. Kaiser Family Foundation and Health Research and Educational Trust, *Annual Surveys of Employer-Sponsored Health Benefits, 2000–2005,* www.kff.org/insurance/7315/index.cfm.

7. Standard & Poor's, *Standard & Poor's Industry Surveys—Health*: *Pharmaceuticals*, June 27, 2002, p. 3, www.standardandpoors.com; and Centers for Medicare and Medicaid Services, *Health Care Industry Update: Pharmaceuticals*, 2003.

8. Kaiser Family Foundation, *Prescription Drug Trends*, June 2006, www.kff.org/rxdrugs/3057.cfm.

9. Centers for Medicare and Medicaid Services, *National Health Care Expenditures Projections: 2005–2015,* www.cms.hhs.gov/NationalHealthExpendData.

10. *Ibid.*

11. Families USA, *Big Dollars, Little Sense: Rising Medicare Prescription Drug Prices*, June 20, 2006, www.familiesusa.org.

12. Kaiser Family Foundation, *Prescription Drug Trends*, Exhibit 3.2, June 2006, www.kff.org/rxdrugs/3057.cfm.

13. *Ibid.*, Exhibit 1.4, Iglehart, John K., "Medicare and Prescription Drugs," *New England Journal of Medicine* 344 (13): 1010–1015, March 29, 2001.

14. Kaiser Family Foundation, *Prescription Drug Trends*, Exhibit 4.13, Exhibit 4.15, June 2006, www.kff.org/rxdrugs/3057.cfm.

15. Standard & Poor's, *Standard & Poor's Industry Surveys—Health; Pharmaceuticals*, June 27, 2002, www.standardandpoors.com. Standard & Poor's Corporation generously made available access to a number of its proprietary industry reports.

16. Langreth, Robert, and Matthew Herper, "Pill Pushers: How the Drug Industry Abandoned Science for Salesmanship," *Forbes*, May 8, 2006, pp. 94–102.

17. "Fortune 500 Top Companies," *Fortune*, April 17, 2006.

18. Langreth, Robert and Matthew Herper, "Pill Pushers: How the Drug Industry Abandoned Science for Salesmanship," *Forbes*, May 8, 2006, pp. 94–102.

19. "Luxury Goods," *The Economist*, March 23, 2002, p. 65.

20. Standard & Poor's, *Standard & Poor's Industry Surveys—Health: Pharmaceuticals*, June 27, 2002, www.standardandpoors.com.

21. Cockburn, Iain M., and Rebecca M. Henderson, "Scale and Scope in Drug Development: Unpack the Advantages of Size in Pharmaceutical Research," *Journal of Health Economics* 20 (6): 1033–1057, November 2001.

22. Malaria R&D Alliance, *Malaria Research and Development: An Assessment of Global Investment*, November 2005, www.malariaalliance.org.

23. Sorenson, Alan T., "An Empirical Model of Heterogenous Consumer Search for Retail Prescription Drugs," NBER working paper 8548, www.nber.org (Cambridge, MA: National Bureau of Economic Research).

24. Becker, Cinda, "Drugmakers Fight for Good Name," *Modern Healthcare* August 27, 2001, pp. 28–33; Standard & Poor's, *Standard & Poor's Industry Surveys—Health: Pharmaceuticals*, June 27, 2002, p. 3, www.standardandpoors.com.

25. Lu, Z. John, and William S. Comanor, "Strategic Pricing of New Pharmaceuticals," *The Review of Economics and Statistics 1998*, pp. 108–118.

26. Hensley, Scott, "AMA, Prescription Drug Makers Agree Ethics Policy Needs Better Implementation." *The Wall Street Journal*, January 21, 2002.

27. Stephen S. Hall, "The Claritin Effect: Prescription for Profit," *New York Times*, Magazine Section, March 11, 2001, pp. 40ff; and Benko, Laura, "Ugly Wait at the Counter: Insurer Pushes to Make Allergy Drugs Nonprescription," *Modern Healthcare*, August 6, 2001, pp. 22–23.

28. Kaiser Family Foundation, *Impact of Direct-to-Consumer Advertising on Prescription Drug Spending*, June 10, 2003, www.kff.org/rxdrugs/6084-index.cfm.

29. Standard & Poor's, *Standard & Poor's Industry Surveys—Health: Pharmaceuticals*, June 27, 2002, pp. 3, 5, www.standardandpoors.com.

Chapter 13

1. World Health Organization, *World Health Report 2002*, www.who.int/whr/2002/en.

2. In converting local expenditures and income into U.S. dollars, two methods are used. The value in local currency can be converted using the foreign exchange rate (i.e., the rate at which dollars are traded for local currency in the market), or it can be converted in terms of purchasing power parity (PPP), the amount required to purchase an equivalent amount of goods and services. In India, gross national GDP per capita was $450 measured in terms of foreign exchange, but $2,149 in terms of the value of goods. This is largely because the cost of food, transportation, and so on is much lower there than the price of such goods in the United States, converted at the currency market exchange rate (e.g., whereas 100 rupees = US$2.08, that amount cannot buy a good meal in the United States but would be sufficient to purchase more than three good meals in India).

3. World Health Organization, *World Health Report 2002*, www.who.int/whr/2002/en; and the World Bank, *World Bank Development Report 2000*.

4. The World Bank, *World Development Report 1993: Investing in Health* (New York: Oxford University Press for the World Bank, 1993). This report provides comparative data on a number of health issues not available elsewhere and thus is used here despite the age of the data (mostly 1990). Making comparisons requires not only that the data exist but also that the data be made comparable in terms of definitions, time periods, and so on, which is a tremendous task for 191 countries.

5. Fuchs, Victor, "The Health Sector's Share of the Gross National Product," *Science*, February 2, 1990, pp. 534–38.

6. Getzen, Thomas, "Population Aging and the Growth of Health Expenditures," *Journal of Gerontology* 47 (3): S98–S104, 1992.

7. Getzen, Thomas E., "An Income-Weighted International Average for Comparative Analysis of Health Expenditures," *International Journal of Health Planning and Management* 6:3–22, 1991.

8. Preston, Samuel H., *Fatal Years: Child Mortality in Late Nineteenth-Century America* (Princeton, NJ: Princeton University Press, 1991).

9. The World Bank, *World Development Report 1993: Investing in Health* (New York: Oxford University Press for the World Bank, 1993).

10. Data taken from the World Bank's HNPStats, at www.worldbank.org/hnpstats, and the World Health Organization's website, at www.who.int/countries.

11. Roemer, Milton I., *National Health Systems of the World* (New York: Oxford University Press, 1991), which includes information reproduced from Bloom, G. M., M. Segal, and C. Thube, *Expenditure and*

Financing of the Health Sector in Kenya (Nairobi: Ministry of Health, 1986). The World Bank Statistics, used for most of the tables in this chapter, estimate national health spending in Kenya at $375 million for 1990, of which 63 percent came from the public sector. Roemer argues that private-sector spending is much less visible and usually underreported because no regular statistics are kept. Bloom et al., through extensive surveys and several alternate methods, estimate that private-sector spending actually slightly exceeded public-sector spending, 51 percent to 49 percent, in 1986. Table 13.2 takes the World Bank estimate of public spending of $237 million, derived from government budget reports, as correct. Private-sector spending is then estimated to be 51 percent of the total, or $247 million, following Bloom et al. The percentages of total spending within each category in Bloom et al. for the year 1986 are then applied to the $484 million total to create breakdowns by category. The net effect of the adjustment for underreported private expenditures is to raise the estimate of per capita health expenditures in Kenya from $16 per person to $20 per person.

12. The World Bank, *World Development Report 1993: Investing in Health* (New York: Oxford University Press for the World Bank, 1993); and Bloom, G. M., M. Segal, and C. Thube, *Expenditure and Financing of the Health Sector in Kenya* (Nairobi: Ministry of Health, 1986).

13. UNAIDS: The Joint United Nations Programme on HIV/AIDS, *Fact Sheet: Sub-Saharan Africa*, 2006.

14. Republic of Kenya Ministry of Health website, *HIV/AIDS in Kenya*, www.health.go.ke/aids.htm.

15. This section was revised by Julio Frenk, MD, PhD, Minister of Health, and Octavio Gomez, MD.

16. Roemer, Milton, *National Health Systems of the World* (New York: Oxford University Press, 1991), pp. 345–351.

17. *Ibid.*

18. WHO Regional Office, *European Health Report 2002*, www.euro.who.int/document/e76907.pdf.

19. Organisation for Economic Co-operation and Development (OECD), *OECD Health Systems: Facts and Trends 1960–1991* (Paris: OECD, 1993).

20. Abel-Smith, Brian, *The Reform of Health Care Systems: A Review of Seventeen OECD Countries* (Paris: Organisation for Economic Co-operation and Development, 1994), p. 49.

21. Rublee, Dale A., "Medical Technology in Canada, Germany and the United States: An Update," *Health Affairs* 13 (4): 113–117, 1994.

22. Hurst, Jeremy, *The Reform of Health Care: A Comparative Analysis of Seven OECD Countries* (Paris: Organisation for Economic Co-operation and Development, 1992), pp. 140–151. See also Maynard, Alan, and Karen Bloor, "Introducing a Market to the United Kingdom's National Health Service," *New England Journal of Medicine* 334:604–608, 1996.

23. The fact that so many health policy experts in so many countries all agree on the essential elements of what the future of health care organizations and financing will and should be is probably reassuring, although such a consensus has not always guaranteed either insight or good results in the past.

24. This section was contributed by Ato Z. Okamoto, MD, MPH, National Institute of Public Health, Saitama, Japan.

25. Some of the information presented here came from conversations with Naoki Ikegami, MD, Professor of Health Administration at Keio University, and is well presented in Ikegami, Naoki, and John Campbell, "Medical Care in Japan," *New England Journal of Medicine* 333 (19): 1295–1299, 1995. See also Powell, Margaret, and Masahira Anesaki, *Health Care in Japan* (New York: Routledge, 1990); and Sonoda, Kyoichi, *Health and Illness in Changing Japanese Society* (Tokyo: University of Tokyo Press, 1988).

26. The World Bank, *World Development Report 1993: Investing in Health* (New York: Oxford University Press for the World Bank, 1993), p. 145; Organisation for Economic Co-operation and Development (OECD), *OECD Health Data 2002* (Paris: OECD, 2002).

27. Pollack, Andrew, "Who's Reading Your X-Ray?" *The New York Times*, November 16, 2003.

Chapter 14

1. Getzen, Thomas E., "Health Care Is an Individual Necessity and a National Luxury: Applying Multilevel Decision Models to the Analysis of Health Care Expenditures," *Journal of Health Economics* 19:259–270, 2000.

2. Getzen, Thomas E., "Macro Forecasting of National Health Expenditures," *Advances in Health Economics and Health Services Research* 11:27–48, 1990.

3. Goodman, William C., "Employment in Services Industries Affected by Recessions and Expansions," *Monthly Labor Review*, October 2002, pp. 1–15.

4. Ginsburg, Paul, "Impact of the Hospital Stabilization Program on Hospitals," in M. Zubkoff, I. E. Raskin, and R. S. Hanft, eds., *Hospital Cost Containment: Selected Notes for Future Policy* (New York: PRODIST for Milbank Memorial Fund, 1978), pp. 293–323.

5. Congressional Budget Office, *Rising Health Care Costs: Causes, Implications and Strategies* (Washington, DC: U.S. Government Printing Office, 1991).

6. Davis, Karen, Gerard Anderson, Diane Rowland, and Earl Steinberg, *Health Care Cost Containment* (Baltimore: Johns Hopkins University Press, 1990).

7. All data in this section are from various publications of the U.S. Census Bureau and Bureau of Labor Statistics.

8. All data in this section are from various publications of the U.S. Bureau of Labor Statistics.

9. Samuelson, Paul, and William Nordhaus, *Economics*, 14th ed. (New York: McGraw-Hill, 1992), p. 19.

10. In the words of Dr. John R. Ball, "Health care used to be something perceived as mystical. Now it's something closer to marketing a product or a service," as quoted in Eric Hollreiser, "Nation's Oldest Hospital Coping With New Age," *Philadelphia Business Journal*, March 22, 1996, p. 25.

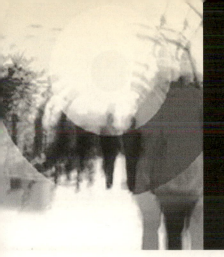

GLOSSARY

Actuarially fair premium   The predicted cost divided by the number of people in the group.

Adverse selection   A situation in which those at high risk for medical problems are more likely to buy insurance than those at low risk.

Agency   An exchange relationship in which one party (the agent) makes decisions on behalf of another.

Allocation   The distribution of resources.

Assignment   An agreement by a physician to take payment directly from Medicare and to accept the amount as payment in full.

Balance bill   The practice of billing a patient for the amount over and above what Medicare pays for a particular service.

Benefit–cost principle   The principle that people tend to make choices that make them better off in a way they value.

Capacity constraint   A lack of services to meet demand.

Capitation   Payment of a fixed amount per enrolled insurance plan member per month, regardless of the number of services each member uses.

Case-mix reimbursement   Adjustment of reimbursement provided by a state to a nursing home to account for differences in patient diagnoses and sometimes for the severity of illness as well.

Certificate-of-need (CON) legislation   Legislation that required approval of any increase in the number of hospital beds.

Circular flow of funds   A system in which every dollar that a consumer spends ultimately ends up in the hands of someone else who wants to spend it.

Closed-panel HMO   A managed care plan that provides all care in-house, using its own doctors and hospitals.

Coinsurance   The amount of a medical bill not paid for by insurance but by the patient.

Contract   An agreement to trade.

Copayment   A specified amount a patient must pay for each service received.

Cost–benefit analysis (CBA)   A set of techniques for assisting in the making of decisions that translates all relevant concerns into market (dollar) terms.

Cost-effectiveness analysis (CEA)   A form of CBA that analyzes the cost side of a decision but doesn't translate the benefits (e.g., lives saved, illnesses prevented, a patient's additional days of activity, the extent to which a patient's sight is restored) into dollars. CEA is used in decision making to determine which alternatives are less expensive yet effective.

Cost reimbursement   Payment for services based upon a hospital's actual costs.

Cost shifting   The process of using excess revenues from one set of services or patients to subsidize other services or patient groups.

Cream skimming   The process of providing only the services that are overpriced, not the ones that are more costly and subsidized.

Deductible   An amount that must be paid by the patient out of his or her own pocket before the insurance company begins to pay.

Demand   The relationship between price and quantity.

Demand curve   A graph that shows the total quantity of a good that buyers wish to buy at each price.

Demand side   The consumer.

Derived demand   Demand for a good due to its use rather than for itself (e.g., the demand for x-ray film is derived from the demand for medical diagnoses, which in turn is derived from a consumer's demand for health).

Diagnosis related group (DRG)   A system of reimbursement that compensates by the case (rather than per day or per charged item) based on the diagnosis of the treatment.

Diseconomies of scale   The principle that the average cost per unit rises as the quantity produced increases.

Dynamic efficiency   Use of inputs so as to maximize long-run value over time, taking account of the need for tinkering to bring about technological and organizational advances.

Dynamics   The process of change; the study of how change occurs over time, including the order, timing, and strength of interacting forces.

Economies of scale   A situation in which the average cost per unit decreases as output increases.

Expected value   An estimate of what is likely to happen.

Fee-for-service payment   Payment of a specified amount for each health care visit or procedure.

Fee schedule   A list that specifies how much an insurance company will pay physicians for particular services.

Firm demand   The demand for each firm in a particular market.

Fixed budget   A budget that doesn't change with volume.

Flexible budget   A budget that changes with volume.

Food and Drug Administration (FDA)   The U.S. federal agency that has jurisdiction over the labeling, manufacture, and sale of food and drugs for human consumption.

Fundamental theorem of exchange   A theorem stating that any voluntary exchange between persons must make both of them better off because they willingly agreed to trade.

Gatekeeper system   A system in which a primary physician manages and approves all services for a patient who enrolls in his or her practice.

Generic drug   A drug that is identical in chemical composition to a brand-name pharmaceutical preparation but is produced by competitors after the firm's patent expires and is usually sold for much less than the brand-name drug.

Global budget   A fixed grant amount intended to cover all of a hospital's costs.

Grant   Donated funds that are intended for a specific purpose.

Health maintenance organization (HMO)   An organization that contracts to provide comprehensive medical services (not reimbursement) for a specified fee each month.

Health savings account (HSA)   A tax status given to a variety of savings and investment vehicles that allows tax deferred deposits up to stated yearly limits, tax-deferred interest, and tax-free withdrawals for qualified medical expenses.

Independent practice association (IPA) HMO   An HMO formed by non-exclusive contracts with many providers who operate independently.

Individual demand   The demand by each individual in a particular market.

Individual reimbursement   A reimbursement system in which the patient pays all the charges, sends copies of the bills to the insurer, and is reimbursed for the medical expenses that are covered.

Kickback   A surreptitious payment in order to obtain business.

Law of demand   A concept stating that the quantity demanded will always fall as prices rise (assuming that all other conditions remain constant).

Licensure   The establishment of legal restrictions specifying which individuals or firms have the rights to provide services or goods.

Loading factor   The difference between the actual premium and the actuarially fair premium.

Malpractice   Physician failure to meet professional standards.

Managed care organization (MCO)   An HMO, a PPO, or another organization that accepts financial risk for and manages medical care.

Managed care plan   A type of insurance plan in which a manager controls the number and type of services covered in return for more affordable premiums.

Margin   The change in xxxx. A one-unit increase.

Marginal benefit   The value to consumers of one more unit of service.

Marginal cost   The increase in total cost caused by the production of one more unit.

Marginal revenue   The change in a firm's total revenue that results from a one-unit change in sales.

Market   The point at which buyers and sellers exchange dollars for goods and services.

Market demand   The sum of all individuals in a market.

Medicaid   A combined state/federal program that insures people whose incomes are insufficient to pay for health care, primarily those individuals on welfare and elderly people in nursing homes.

Medicare   A federal government insurance program that provides hospital (Part A), medical (Part B), and prescription drug (Part D) benefits to persons over age 65 and some qualified people with disabilities.

Medicare resource-based relative value scale (RBRVS)   A Medicare-established point value system for services, based on physician time, intensity of effort, practice costs, and costs of advanced specialty training.

Need   A professional determination of the quantity that should be supplied.

Operating budget   A budget that projects all anticipated expenses for the next year.

Opportunity cost   What must be given up in order to do or obtain something; the highest-valued alternative that must be forgone.

Optimum   The point at which the net gain (Benefits − Costs) is largest.

Per diem   Per-day payment for services.

Pharmacoeconomics   Cost–benefit analysis of drugs; assessment of the market for a drug.

Pharmacy benefits managers (PBMs)   Subcontractors chosen by insurance companies to develop prescription drug benefit plans, administer claims, and manage relationships with pharmaceutical companies (i.e., manufacturers) and retail pharmacies.

Preferred provider organization (PPO)/point of service plan (POS)   A managed care plan that offers enrollees a discount for using hospitals and physicians within an approved network of contracted providers.

Price discrimination   The practice of charging different people different prices for the same good or service.

Price elastic   Demand in which the quantity demanded changes a lot for any small change in price.

Price inelastic   Demand in which the quantity demanded barely budges when the price rises.

Private goods   Goods that are consumed or financed individually.

Private health insurance   Insurance that is based on a contract between an individual and an insurance company.

***Pro forma* financial statements**   Projections of incomes, assets, and fund balances for a set period of years in summary format.

Public goods   Goods that are consumed or financed collectively (e.g., clean air, national defense, discovery of penicillin) either because it's impossible to include/exclude any consumer who doesn't pay or because once the goods are produced, there's no additional cost for additional consumers.

Relative value scale   A fee schedule that gives medical services unique point values.

Risk aversion   The willingness to incur a relatively small but certain expense (the premium) to avoid the risk of a catastrophic loss.

Risk pooling   Forming a group so that individual risk can be shared among many people.

Social insurance   Insurance that extends and formalizes the informal obligations of citizens to society expressed in charitable giving.

Spending down   The process of spending or giving away assets by elderly persons so as to qualify for Medicaid reimbursement of LTC expenses.

Staff HMO   An HMO in which physicians work exclusively for the HMO and are often on salary.

Strategic budget   A budget that focuses on long-run changes and plans.

Supply curve   A graph showing the total quantity of a good that sellers which to sell at each price.

Supply side   The seller.

Terms of trade   Terms that specify what the buyer is to give the seller and what the seller is to give the buyer in return.

Two-party transaction   An exchange between a buyer and seller, usually trading money for goods or services.

Unit elastic   Demand in which the percentage change in price is equal to the percentage change in quantity.

Withhold   A pool of money for providers that is held back and distributed by an HMO only if total expenses for the year end up at or below acceptable levels.

INDEX

Cost reimbursement